Philadelphia MAGAZINE'S
1997 Guide to Good Health

The advice and recommendations in this guide are provided by *Philadelphia Magazine* for your general information only. For any medical problem you should consult your physician.

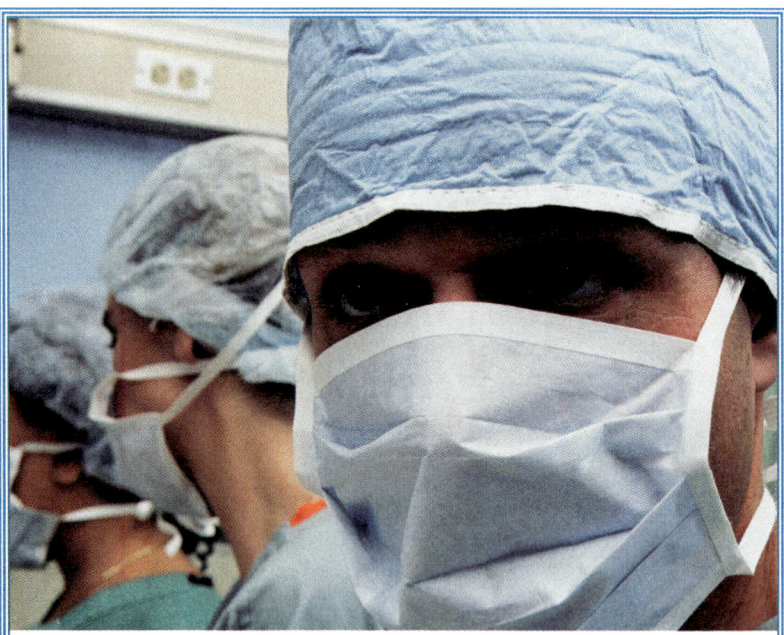

Independence Blue Cross And Pennsylvania Blue Shield Salute Our Own "Top Docs"

Every day, thousands of the finest primary care physicians and specialists in the region take good care of our members. And for an organization that provides coverage for more than 2.4 million people, that's a vitally important job.

We're dedicated to quality care and professional service. And that's why we have our own "Top Docs" on our staff; fifteen Medical Directors, including primary care physicians and specialists in such fields as Pediatrics, Internal Medicine, Family Practice and General Surgery.

Ably assisted by over 200 professional nurses, our medical team evaluates and monitors the quality and appropriateness of care given by our vast network of hospitals and physicians.

Our Medical Management Team is deeply involved in preventive care programs such as adult and infant immunization rates, incentives for breast cancer screening, award winning perinatal care, smoking cessation and fitness programs.

It's a process that is helping to set a new standard for the finest in health care.

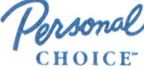
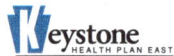
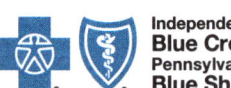

Independence Blue Cross, Pennsylvania Blue Shield and Keystone Health Plan East are independent licensees of the Blue Cross and Blue Shield Association.
® Registered marks of the Blue Cross and Blue Shield Association, an Association of Independent Blue Cross and Blue Shield Plans.

Table of Contents

SECTION ONE
Prevention Is the Best Medicine

9	CHAPTER 1	**Testing, Testing ...** *What medical tests do you really need?*
17	CHAPTER 2	**Storm Warnings** *Common cancer signs, and where to find help*
23	CHAPTER 3	**Behind Closed Doors** *What every medicine cabinet should have*

SECTION TWO
Choosing a Doctor

41	CHAPTER 4	**Finding Dr. Right** *A shopper's guide to selecting a personal physician*
47	CHAPTER 5	**Top Docs** *A review of the area's outstanding doctors*
61	CHAPTER 6	**Centers of Excellence** *The best local facilities for specialty care*

SECTION THREE
Choosing a Hospital

83	CHAPTER 7	**Inside Story** *The lowdown on diagnostic techniques*
93	CHAPTER 8	**Check It Out Before You Check In** *Mini-profiles of area hospitals*
142	CHAPTER 9	**Emergency!** *What to do when time is critical*

SECTION FOUR
You Are What You Eat

150	CHAPTER 10	**A Carrot a Day** *Area nutritionists answer 16 questions about eating right*
156	CHAPTER 11	**Dining for Life** *How to eat healthy when you're eating out*

SECTION FIVE
The Healthy Woman

165	CHAPTER 12	**In Sickness and in Health** *Straight talk about female problems*
177	CHAPTER 13	**A Change of Thought on Change of Life** *The pros and cons of hormone replacement therapy*

187	CHAPTER 14	**Women's Services**	
		A rundown of area centers, hotlines and support groups	

SECTION SIX
The Healthy Child

199	CHAPTER 15	**Accidents Will Happen ...**
		Tips for handling emergencies with children
203	CHAPTER 16	**Your Attention, Please**
		Advice and support for the child with ADHD

SECTION SEVEN
Mind Over Matter

214	CHAPTER 17	**The Drug Zone**
		Feeling sad? Hyper? Paranoid? Take a pill
224	CHAPTER 18	**Where to Go for Help**
		Psychiatric treatment centers

SECTION EIGHT
Making Sense for Seniors

234	CHAPTER 19	**The Dosage Dilemma**
		How to keep your medications straight
241	CHAPTER 20	**The Lowdown on Life-Care**
		A guide to the latest trend in continuing care

SECTION NINE
For Your Information

253	CHAPTER 21	**Home Sweet Home**
		Help that makes house calls, including home health care
259	CHAPTER 22	**The Road Back**
		Resources for rehabilitation services
263	CHAPTER 23	**We've Got Your Number**
		Special programs, support groups and health services
314		**Index**

ADVERTISER RESOURCE

161	**List of Advertisers**
284	**Professional Profile Section**
	Special advertising directory

Contributors

Award-winning journalist, broadcaster and best-selling author **Carol Saline** created *Philadelphia Magazine's Guide to Good Health* in 1992. "After ten years of writing about medical issues," says Saline, "I knew there was a need in the Philadelphia area for a comprehensive, accessible directory to health services." Saline is currently working on the book *Mothers and Daughters*, the follow-up to *Sisters*, which was on the *New York Times* best-seller list for more than a year. All articles in the *Guide*, unless otherwise noted, were written by Saline.

Steven Benowitz has written about science and medicine for a wide range of publications, including *Science News*, the *University of Chicago Magazine*, the *World Book Health and Medical Annual* and *The Scientist*, where he currently serves as senior editor.

Joyce Brazino specializes in health-care program development and medical copywriting. Her background includes clinical patient care, public health education and extensive hospital-based public relations and marketing experience.

Joan Capuzzi, who has an academic background in medicine, writes and edits for several scientific publications. She has also written for such publications as the *Philadelphia Inquirer*, *Business Philadelphia* and the *Philadelphia Business Journal*.

Lynn Selhat is a marketing/public relations writer specializing in health-care issues. Her work includes developing patient education information for pharmaceutical companies and other health-care clients.

Elisabeth Torg, a health and medical writer with 12 years' experience, specializes in women's health. She is the co-author of *Total Health for Women* and a contributing author to *The Female Body* and *Age Erasers for Women*, all published by Rodale Press. Torg has also been published in *Glamour*, *Prevention's Guide for New Moms* and *New Business Opportunities*.

1997 Guide to Good Health, produced by *Philadelphia Magazine*

EDITOR, *Jodie Green;* ASSOCIATE EDITORS, *Barbara Brynko, Nancy Houtz;* ART DIRECTORS, *Ken Newbaker, Rosemary Tottoroto;* ILLUSTRATOR, *Dan Yaccarino;* COPY EDITOR, *Lillian C. Haas;* TYPESETTER, *Timothy Haas*

ASSOCIATE PUBLISHER, *Carmen N. Hist;* ASSISTANT TO THE ASSOCIATE PUBLISHER, *Michele Murati;* SENIOR ACCOUNT EXECUTIVES, *Michele S. Freiberg, Deborah S. Hoxter, Deborah K. Long, Amy Huskey Marrone, Eileen Turner;* ACCOUNT EXECUTIVES, *Jodi L. Kaiser, Deborah A. McGraw, Joseph T. Sosnowski;* PROFESSIONAL LISTINGS, *Christina Martin;* PRODUCTION DIRECTOR, *Deborah Cassell;* PRODUCTION COORDINATOR, *Jill Maharam;* TRAFFIC COORDINATOR, *Peter O'Steen;* ADVERTISING DESIGNER, *Carla Coutts-Miners;* ASSISTANT ADVERTISING DESIGNER, *Hedy Sirico*

PHILADELPHIA MAGAZINE: CHAIRMAN, *D. Herbert Lipson;* PRESIDENT AND PUBLISHER, *David H. Lipson Jr.;* EDITOR, *Eliot Kaplan;* VP/TREASURER, *Frederick B. Waechter Jr.;* ASSOCIATE PUBLISHER/DIRECTOR OF ADVERTISING, *Marian Hettel*

DIRECTOR OF MARKETING, *Stephanie Lafair Smith;* PROMOTION DIRECTOR, *Sherry L. Litwer;* PROMOTION AND MARKETING COORDINATOR, *Cara I. Meyers;* CIRCULATION MANAGER, *A. Carmen Conrad;* CONTROLLER, *Mary F. Gruszka;* MANAGER OF INFORMATION SYSTEMS, *Daniel J. Shimberg;* CREDIT MANAGER, *Pat John Romanelli*

Philadelphia Magazine's Guide to Good Health (ISBN 0-9635666-3-6) is published annually at 1818 Market Street, Philadelphia, PA 19103-3682; 215-564-7700. All contents of this guide © 1996 by *Philadelphia Magazine*, a division of METROCORP™. Printed in U.S.A.

Section

Prevention Is the Best Medicine

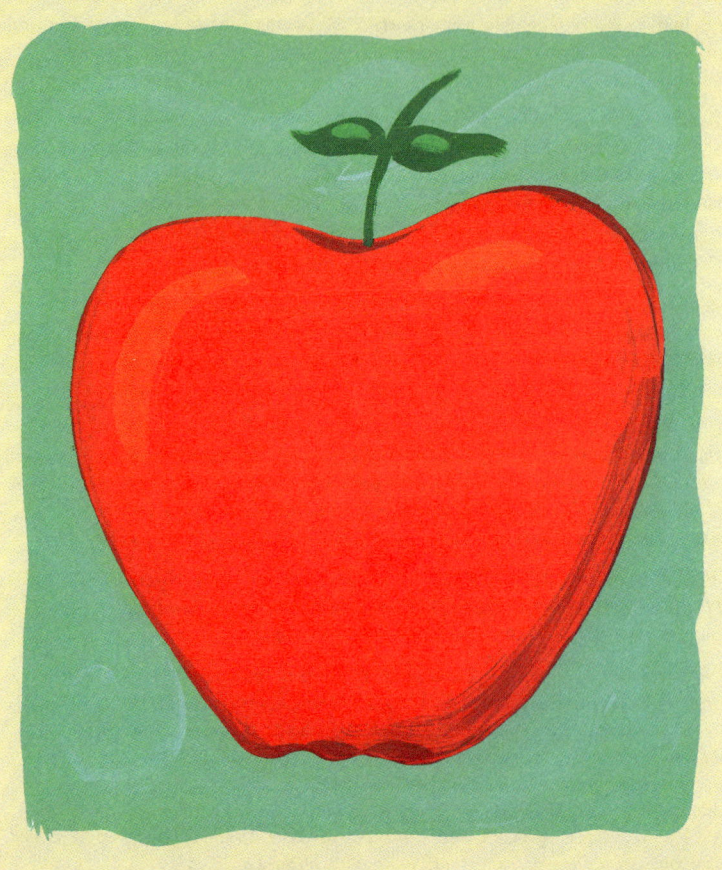

One

Chapter 1
Testing, Testing ...
What medical tests do you really need?

Chapter 2
Storm Warnings
Common cancer signs, and where to find help

Chapter 3
Behind Closed Doors
What every medicine cabinet should have

GRADUATE HOSPITAL
GASTROENTEROLOGY ASSOCIATES, P.C.

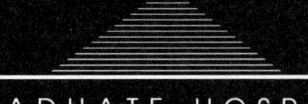

We enjoy a reputation as caring, hardworking physicians who give the best care that academic medicine can offer. All members of the section practice general gastroenterology. We also offer areas of subspecialization (within the field of gastroenterology) so that patients with atypical or complicated gastrointestinal problems may also receive expert care from clinicians experienced in that area.

Pepper Pavilion
1800 Lombard Street, Suite 100
Philadelphia, PA
(215) 893-2532

2300 S. Broad Street
Suite 202
Philadelphia, PA
(215) 336-9420

47 Copley Road
Upper Darby, PA
(610) 352-4426

George Ahtaridis, M.D.
Motility abnormalities of the esophagus, stomach, small and large bowel, fecal incontinence.

Steven Greenfield, M.D.
Chronic liver disease, gallstones, gastrointestinal manifestations of AIDS.

S. Philip Bralow, M.D.
Gastrointestinal malignancies.

Jeffrey N. Retig, M.D.
Pancreatic and biliary disorders, inflammatory bowel disease, therapeutic endoscopy

Anthony Infantolino, M.D.
Gastrointestinal malignancies, inflammatory bowel disease, special expertise in endoscopic ultrasound/laser and therapeutic endoscopy.

David Katzka, M.D.
Diseases of the esophagus, and gastrointestinal motility disorders, inflammatory bowel disease.
"Top Doctor - Gastroenterology PHILADELPHIA Magazine 1996

Donald Castell, M.D.
Diseases of the esophagus.
"Top Doctor - Gastroenterology PHILADELPHIA Magazine 1996

CHAPTER 1

Testing, Testing . . .

. . . and more testing. Billions of dollars' worth of medical tests may be unnecessary. And that includes the all-purpose annual physical

Just try to remember the last time you visited a doctor and didn't wind up having some kind of medical test. Feeling tired? Let's do a complete blood workup for $300. Complaining of headaches? Go get a CAT scan for $846. Just a routine checkup? At the least you'll have a urinalysis and a chest X-ray—$60 for the basic front view, $157 for a four-sided picture. And heaven forbid you've got some tightness in your chest, because you'll probably need an EKG for $121, a stress test for $400 and maybe even a heart catheterization for a whopping $3,900.

Okay, I'm exaggerating—but only slightly. The point is, patients have come to expect, even request, excessive testing, in part because their insurance foots the bill. Granted, the doctor's arsenal of 1,500 available medical tests has removed a lot of the guesswork from health care. But it seems the overreliance on testing has burgeoned into too much of a good thing, in part because tests are sometimes used to produce income or avoid lawsuits rather than to obtain information.

"No one would suggest that there is anything wrong with a diagnostic test when symptoms indicate a need, but otherwise these tests are just money-makers," says Dr. Edward Pinckney, a California internist and author of *A Patient's Guide to Medical Tests*. Pinckney believes too many tests are fishing expeditions used by doctors in lieu of careful examinations of patients. That's akin to the view of Dr. John Eisenberg, chairman of the department of medicine at Georgetown Medical Center: "More important than an EKG in your pocket," he says, "is developing a relationship with a doctor who knows you, your lifestyle and your family history, and counsels you according to your risks."

Dr. Katalin Roth, vice chairwoman for general medicine at Pennsylvania Hospital, points out: "Third-party payers [insurance companies] do not reimburse doctors for ten minutes of health counseling. But you get paid $100 for doing an EKG and as much as $250 for a flexible sigmoidoscopy. The way health care is financed, there's little incentive for doctors to spend time talking about important areas like prevention." And as for whether Americans need all the tests they get, according to former Secretary of Health and Human Services Louis Sullivan, "Increasingly we're finding that a substantial portion of the care that's being ... billed for is of unproven medical necessity and effectiveness."

What drives excess testing?

We asked Dr. Arnold Relman, former editor of the *New England Journal of Medicine*, why American doctors do so much testing. One of his explanations was exactly what we'd expected: the profit motive. But the whole answer goes much deeper. An enormous amount of unnecessary testing is motivated by a fear of malpractice litigation. Just in case something goes wrong with a patient, doctors can't afford to be held liable for insufficient diagnostic studies. They engage in exhaustive testing to avoid being accused of negligence.

In addition, the inclination to overtest is fueled by our obsession with expert opinions. "Americans with health insurance love to see specialists," Relman says. "In this country, 75 percent of physicians are specialists who, by their very nature, are trained to do special tests. An awful lot of headaches and chest pains could be handled for far less money by general practitioners."

False negatives, false positives

Indeed, many medical tests are highly inaccurate. Some of the most common screenings are riddled with false-positive or false-negative results. "What does it mean psychologically to be called hypercholesterolemic [suffering from abnormally high cholesterol] when you're perfectly healthy, or to suffer through the false-positive of a mammography?" asks Harvard Medical School's Dr. Robert Lawrence. Lawrence chaired the government's Preventive Services Task Force, which questioned the validity of a plethora of routine tests. "This kind of thing does real damage to people. We in modern medicine find great comfort in doing lab tests and concluding things that may not be valid. The measurable tends to drive out the important, and the behavioral issues threatening health [things like smoking, drinking and diet] get ignored because they aren't quantifiable."

Improper readings are frequently the fault of the laboratory, although that has improved now that government regulations mandate inspections at some 300,000 laboratories. Just as problematic is how to interpret what's normal. It's quite common for someone to fall outside the so-called normal range and yet be perfectly healthy. "We do so much blood testing," explains Dr. Marie Savard, a local internist, "because it's an inexpensive screening that occasionally picks up kidney disease or diabetes, or liver problems that indicate alcoholism. What's being asked in this era of cost containment is whether those few that are helped by an unexpected finding offset the expense and worry for the far greater numbers who are wrongly diagnosed."

Is this test necessary?

What can you do to break the overused-test pattern? The People's Medical Society advises asking your doctor why a test has been requested. Is it because you're a high-risk patient? If not, why bother? What is the test supposed to reveal? How reliable is the lab where the test will be processed, and what's the margin of error for the results? Are there risks? If so, are there safer alternatives that will yield comparable information? Finally, if something wrong *is* discovered, can it be treated?

If there is one trend in testing you want to seriously reconsider, it's the idea of an unnecessary annual physical. Many, many people see a doctor every year even though they're perfectly healthy. Major studies and reams of research indicate that this staple of American health care may have outlived its usefulness as a general rule. The head-to-toe yearly physical, first introduced in 1914 by the Metropolitan Life Insurance Company for its employees and policyholders, may, like the appendix, have become an anachronism.

The truth about routine exams

That doesn't mean people should see a doctor only if they're sick. But the all-inclusive, expensive ($400 to $500) routine exam no longer makes either medical or economic sense. "The word *routine* checkup implies nonthinking," says Georgetown Medical Center's Eisenberg. "It's a tragedy that people so often get the tests they don't need, but they don't get the tests they do need. The traditional knee-jerk evaluation without regard to risk factors is bad medicine."

Instead, what doctors and their patients ought to be practicing is an individualized approach to health care based on something called risk assessment.

Using a variety of criteria, doctors today can place patients in high- or low-risk categories; those labels in turn will dictate who needs to be examined for what problems. As Savard explains, "Today we evaluate patients by looking at their family history, their lifestyle—do they smoke or drink?—various genetic and environmental factors, even their emotional makeup. Then we decide how often to see them and what tests they need. For somebody who has no risks and no symptoms, there are just a few basic areas that need occasional checking. Beyond that, risk factors should be used to determine precisely what needs periodic monitoring." One category of high-risk patient is the person with a family history of a particular disease. If that applies to you, you'll want to discuss with your doctor the following tests: for colon cancer, fecal occult blood, sigmoidoscopy or colonoscopy; for diabetes, a fasting plasma glucose; for heart disease, an electrocardiogram; for osteoporosis, a bone mineral content.

Test cases: Mammography and prostate screenings

The question of when to begin mammographies and how often to get them is currently under hot debate. Using the high-risk/low-risk model, a woman whose mother or sister had breast cancer would fall into a high-risk category, requiring annual mammograms as early as age 35. Yet a woman with no family history of breast cancer would fall in a low-risk group and could postpone her first mammography until she's well over 40. Currently the American Cancer Society and the National Cancer Institute recommend mammograms every one or two years for women between 40 and 49. But new studies have challenged whether this frequency is actually useful, and the guidelines are under scrutiny. Simultaneously, other experts claim that women between 40 and 49 should have yearly mammograms because cancers grow faster in younger women. Let your risk factors be your guide, and when you do have a mammogram, choose a facility accredited by the American College of Radiology.

The PSA blood test for prostate cancer is similarly confusing. It's recommended for men over 50 by the American Cancer Society, because it ferrets out prostate cancer among high-risk men better than the old digital rectal exam. But the test isn't cheap—$30 to $70—and it's difficult to interpret because it gives misleading signals. So aggressive use among low-risk men is not only wasteful but may lead to rounds of more tests and uncalled-for treatment. *The Philadelphia Inquirer* reported that some doctors think the number of patients who actually live longer as a result of early cancer treatment may be smaller than those unnecessarily harmed.

The value of seeing a family doctor once a year for a preset battery of tests first came into question more than a decade ago with a landmark report issued for the Canadian National Health Service. Another study in London compared 3,292 patients who'd had regular health checkups with 3,132 who hadn't; the results showed no appreciable difference in the health of one group compared to the other. But the strongest argument against routine physicals rose from an exhaustive research project undertaken from 1984 to 1989 by the United States Preventive Services Task Force. After collating and reviewing some 2,400 worldwide studies of the screening and monitoring tests commonly used by doctors—things like X-rays, blood work and EKGs—it concluded that a vast majority are a waste of time and money.

By contrast, there was a rather short list of mandatory age- and gender-related evaluations suggested for healthy adults in the average or low-risk categories. In general, upon reaching the ripe old age of 20 everybody should visit the dentist annually and get a one-time full-body examination for moles that might develop into melanoma, the deadliest of skin cancers. Anyone found at risk should thereafter be checked annually.

The bare essentials

The government's most recent task force revamped previous guidelines for testing and preventive medical services. The task force advised physicians to perform fewer tests and put more energy into counseling as a diagnostic tool. The following list, which is in no way definitive or representative of all health plans, provides guidelines for "well" patient testing. Your physician may modify this schedule depending on your family medical history or illnesses.

AGE 19-39	*Every 1-3 years* **Discuss with doctor:** weight, height, blood pressure and cholesterol screening, diet, physical activity, tobacco/alcohol/drug use, sexual practices *Every 5 years* Glaucoma screening (after age 35) *Every 10 years* Tetanus shot **For women:** Annual pelvic exam/Pap smear, baseline mammography screening (at 35 to 40 years)
AGE 40-64	*Every 1-3 years* **Discuss with doctor:** weight, height, blood pressure and cholesterol screening, diet, physical activity, tobacco/alcohol/drug use, sexual practices *Every 5 years* Glaucoma screening, flexible sigmoidoscopy (every 3 to 5 years after age 45 to examine lower bowel and rectum) *Every 10 years* Tetanus shot **For women:** pelvic exam/Pap smear, mammogram/breast exam (every 1 to 2 years) **For men over 50:** annual prostate screening
AGE 65 AND OVER	*Every year* **Discuss with doctor:** weight, height, blood pressure and cholesterol screening, diet, physical activity, tobacco/alcohol/drug use, sexual practices, urinalysis, thyroid screening, rectal exam, influenza and pneumonia immunization (once during lifetime) *Every 3 years* Flexible sigmoidoscopy *Every 5 years* Glaucoma screening *Every 10 years* Tetanus shot **For women:** annual pelvic exam/Pap smear, mammogram **For men:** prostate screening

Be wise and immunize

Dr. Katalin Roth includes certain inoculations as part of her recommendations for routine health care: a tetanus booster every ten years after age 20, a flu and pneumonia vaccine after 65 and a revaccination for rubella (German measles) for anyone who received the vaccine between 1957, when it was first introduced, and 1965; the original formulation doesn't give complete protection. Roth, an advocate of preventive medicine, sums up the attitude among enlightened doctors toward the old-fashioned routine checkup: "I think if an individual has had a blood pressure reading, a cholesterol check and a good family history to assess risks and everything is normal, that person does not need a complete physical with lab tests every year. Those executive physicals are unnecessary. It is useful for everybody to check in occasionally with a doctor who knows them, and a woman should see a gynecologist annually who can manage the rest of her general health care."

The American Academy of Pediatrics makes the following recommendations for immunization:

Birth	Hepatitis B
1–2 months	Hepatitis B
2 months	Diphtheria/tetanus/pertussis (DTP), polio, hemophilus influenza B (bacterial meningitis)
4 months	Diphtheria/tetanus/pertussis (DTP), polio, hemophilus influenza B (bacterial meningitis)
6 months	Diphtheria/tetanus/pertussis (DTP)
6–18 months	Hemophilus influenza B (bacterial meningitis), polio, hepatitis B
12–15 months	Hemophilus influenza B (bacterial meningitis), measles/mumps/rubella
1–12 years	Varivax (chicken pox)
15–18 months	Diphtheria/tetanus/pertussis (DTP)
4–6 years	Diphtheria/tetanus/pertussis (DTP), polio
11–12 years	Measles/mumps/rubella
13+ years	Varivax (chicken pox)
14–16 years	Diphtheria/tetanus

Can we talk?

When patients do visit the doctor, it would be valuable if, in addition to poking and prodding, physicians increased their talking and listening. The task force strongly urged family doctors to spend less of their average 12-minute visits with patients on tests and pulse-taking and more on counseling, particularly in those areas where behavioral changes can really modify risks. These include discussions about diet, aerobic exercise, tobacco and drugs, using seat belts, practicing safe sex and buying smoke detectors.

Critics of the task force's strong pro-counseling position complained that the government spent money in studying preventive health measures only to conclude that doctors ought to spend more time advising patients about diet and seat belts. Lawrence's retort: "If we did more of that we'd have a healthier nation and wouldn't need to do all this screening in the first place."

FOX CHASE CANCER CENTER AND ITS NETWORK OF COMMUNITY CANCER CENTERS

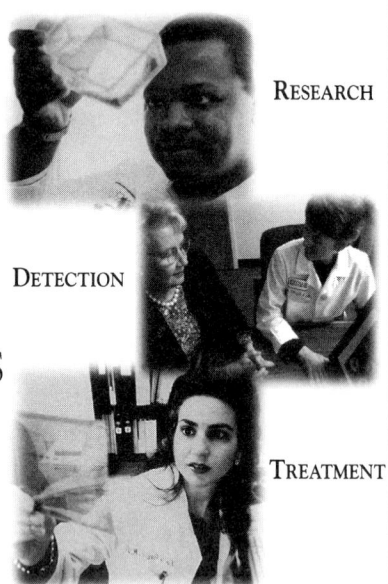

RESEARCH

DETECTION

TREATMENT

PENNSYLVANIA
- Delaware County Memorial Hospital, Drexel Hill
- Montgomery Hospital Medical Center, Norristown
- North Penn Hospital, Lansdale
- Paoli Memorial Hospital, Paoli
- Pinnacle Health System, Harrisburg
- Reading Hospital and Medical Center, Reading
- Shadyside Hospital, Pittsburgh
- St. Luke's Health Network
  Bethlehem • Palmerton • Quakertown
- St. Mary Medical Center, Langhorne

NEW JERSEY
- Community-Kimball Health Care System
  Toms River • Lakewood
- Hunterdon Medical Center, Flemington
- Memorial Hospital of Burlington County, Mt. Holly
- Riverview Medical Center, Red Bank
- St. Francis Medical Center, Trenton
- South Jersey Health System
  Millville • Bridgeton • Elmer

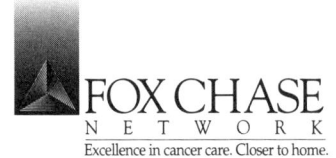

Excellence in cancer care. Closer to home.

For Network information call 1-800-639-0600

Visit our web site at http://www.protonet.fccc.edu

FOX CHASE NETWORK, providing cancer care in partnership with nineteen community cancer centers, is the area's leader in cancer outreach. Network cancer centers, through their affiliation with Fox Chase Cancer Center, bring the latest in cancer research, detection and treatment to the communities they serve. Fox Chase Cancer Center is designated a Comprehensive Cancer Center by the National Cancer Institute.

Discoveries Through Research
FOX CHASE NETWORK cancer centers have access to important new research through their affiliation with Fox Chase Cancer Center. Everyday, scientists at Fox Chase are coming closer to discovering new ways to prevent, detect and treat cancer.

Increasing Survival by Early Detection
Many cancers can be treated successfully if detected early. FOX CHASE NETWORK cancer centers offer programs to educate people about cancer risk and to help them reduce risk.

Developing New Treatments
FOX CHASE NETWORK cancer centers offer access to clinical trials available only at Fox Chase or approved research centers. Using new cancer drugs and therapies, clinical trials enable Network physicians to apply new knowledge and advances to patient treatment.

CHAPTER 2

Storm Warnings

Catching cancer early could save your life

The American Cancer Society estimates that more than 550,000 people in the United States will die of cancer this year. Cancers caused by cigarette smoking and alcohol abuse are the most preventable. Stop smoking and drinking! Equally important to prevention are certain routine screenings—mammographies, mole checks, fecal occult blood tests, etc. Along with self-examinations, they detect cancers at an early stage, when treatment is more likely to be effective.

A wide spectrum of cancer treatments is available at many area hospitals (see Chapter 8). For complicated or advanced cases requiring cutting-edge, high-tech care, you may want to contact a National Cancer Institute-designated comprehensive cancer center. These hospitals are heavily engaged in research as well as clinical trials of experimental protocols for which you may be eligible. There are 27 in the United States, two of which are in Philadelphia:

Fox Chase Cancer Center
7701 Burholme Avenue, Philadelphia, PA 19111; 215-728-6900

University of Pennsylvania Cancer Center
6 Penn Tower, 3400 Spruce Street, Philadelphia, PA 19104; 1-800-383-UPCC (8722)

Danger zones

While it takes a physician to diagnose cancer, your own watchfulness is the best early-warning system. See your doctor if you have:

A change in bowel or bladder habits.

A sore that doesn't heal.

Unusual bleeding or discharge.

A thickening or lump in the breast or any other body part.

An obvious change in a wart or mole.

A nagging cough or hoarseness.

Indigestion or difficulty swallowing.

The skinny on skin cancer

If you are a sun worshiper, don't skip this section. In fact, anybody who spends time in the sun—sailing, playing tennis, working outdoors—has to face the fact that he's exposing himself to potential skin cancer. The reason is quite simple: Skin cancer is caused by exposure to ultraviolet (UV) rays, whether from the sun in your backyard or the tanning bed at your salon. And it looks like we're all overdoing it in one way or another: According to the National Cancer Institute, close to 50 percent of all Americans who live to age 65 will get skin cancer at least once. The only way to reduce your odds, says Dr. Paul Engstrom of Fox Chase Cancer Center, is to reduce the amount of time you spend unprotected from UV rays. "Skin cancers are becoming more and more common," he says, "with about 800,000 new cases occurring each year. But it is also one of the most preventable forms of cancer there is, because we know exactly what causes it."

Most at risk are Caucasians with light-color eyes and hair and fair complexions that don't tan easily. Least at risk are those with naturally dark skin, whose rich pigmentation protects them from UV radiation. For all people, though, sun damage is cumulative: It can take 20 years or more for a cancerous lesion to evolve from that bad sunburn you received as a child. While the most commonly occurring forms of skin cancer are rarely fatal, if ignored they can extend below the skin to the bone and cartilage, causing considerable damage and disfigurement.

Three varieties of skin cancer

The most common type, basal cell carcinoma (*carcinoma* is cancer that starts in the tissue of an organ lining) arises from basal cells in the epidermis. It's slow-growing and rarely spreads—unlike squamous cell carcinoma, the second-most-common form of skin cancer, which begins in the squamous cells of the epidermis and can, if neglected, spread to other parts of the body. Together, these cancers are referred to as "nonmelanoma skin cancers" to distinguish them from melanoma, which develops in the skin's melanocytes (the cells that produce the pigment). Melanoma is the most serious form of skin cancer because it can spread to other parts of the body through the lymph systems; left untreated, it is usually fatal.

The warning signs

With basal cell and squamous cell cancers, the first sign is a change in the skin, especially a new growth or a sore that won't heal. These types of skin cancers may start as firm red lumps or as small, smooth, shiny, pale or waxy bumps; either type may crust or bleed. They may also begin as flat red spots that are rough, dry or scaly.

The first warning sign of a melanoma is most often a change in the size, shape or color of a mole, or the appearance of a new mole. A normal mole is a brown, black or tan spot on the skin that can be flat or raised, round or oval. Any change in a mole should be brought to the attention of your doctor immediately, according to the following "ABCD" characteristics outlined by the National Cancer Institute.

Asymmetry: The shape of one half of the mole does not match the other half.

Border: The edges are ragged, notched or blurred.

Color: The color is uneven. For example, shades of black, brown or tan are present, or areas of white, red or blue can be seen.

Diameter: There is a change in size.

Other signs of melanoma can include scaling, oozing or bleeding of a mole or a change in the way the mole feels; it may become hard, lumpy, itchy, swollen or tender. In men, melanoma occurs most often on the trunk of the body; in women, on the arms and lower legs.

Diagnosis and treatment

Skin cancers are usually diagnosed via biopsy, the surgical removal of all or part of the growth. The tissue is examined microscopically and a diagnosis is made. The stage of the disease is based on the thickness of the tumor, the depth of skin penetration and whether the cancer has spread to nearby lymph nodes or other parts of the body.

More than 95 percent of nonmelanoma skin cancers are completely curable; the choice of treatment depends on the size and type of growth, its location and whether it has the potential to spread. The most common methods of removal include surgery, which may involve skin grafting if the area affected is large; curettage, a common "scooping out" method used to treat very small growths; and cryosurgery, in which liquid nitrogen is sprayed on the growth to freeze and kill abnormal cells. Radiation therapy, chemotherapy and laser treatment are also used, depending on the type of cancer and its stage of advancement. All may result in scarring.

People who have had nonmelanoma skin cancer are at risk for recurrence of the original cancer and development of new ones, so they should be examined regularly by their physicians and also examine their own skin on a monthly basis for new growths or changes.

What's done may be undone

Sun damage is cumulative, and the best you can do is start taking care of your skin today to reduce your lifetime risk of getting the disease. However, for some precancerous conditions (those in which cells show the kind of abnormal growth that is a precursor to skin cancer), there is hope. Retinoic acid (known commercially as Retin-A, the "miracle" antiwrinkle cream) has been shown to reverse some squamous cell cancers. And current research evaluating the effectiveness of massive doses of vitamin A and its precursor, beta-carotene, in patients with rare skin diseases is showing promise as well.

The best way to avoid getting skin cancer is to reduce your exposure to UV rays. Avoid the sun during the hours of the day when it's strongest—those hours when your shadow is shorter than you are. The remainder of the day, wear a sunscreen with a sun protection factor (SPF) of at least 15. Wear a wide-brim hat and cover your arms and legs with clothing whose weave is tight enough to seal out the sun's rays. And remember that snow, ice, sand and concrete reflect from 10 to 50 percent of the sun's damaging rays. It should go without saying, says Fox Chase's Engstrom, that children should never go into the sun without protection. "We've got to reschool society from day one that a suntan is *not* a sign of physical beauty," he says. "Any tan at all is a sign that the skin has marshaled a defense against UV rays." So teach your kids that using a sun block is as routine and necessary as brushing their teeth. In 30 years, they'll thank you for it.

Warning signs of other cancers

Each type of cancer has its own particular configuration of symptoms. Don't panic if you suddenly begin to experience one of them; many cancer signs are also common to benign illnesses. However, do take note of the following warnings, and if they persist, the American Cancer Society recommends checking in with your doctor.

Lung cancer: Persistent cough, sputum streaked with blood, chest pain, recurring pneumonia or bronchitis.

Colon and rectal cancer: Rectal bleeding, blood in the stool, change in bowel habits.

Breast cancer: Persistent breast changes, such as a lump, thickening, swelling, dimpling, skin irritation, distortion, scaliness, pain or tenderness of the nipple.

Prostate cancer: Weak or interrupted urine flow; frequent urination, especially at night; blood in the urine; pain or burning on urination; continuing pain in lower back, pelvis or upper thighs.

Uterine and cervical cancer: Bleeding outside of the normal menstrual period or after menopause, unusual vaginal discharge.

Leukemia: Early signs may include fatigue, paleness, weight loss, repeated infections, bruising, nose bleeds or other hemorrhages.

Hodgkin's disease: Swollen glands, itching, night sweats, weight loss and fever.

Non-Hodgkin's lymphoma: Swollen glands, anemia, weight loss and fever.

Bladder cancer: Blood in the urine. Usually associated with increased frequency of urination.

Oral cancer: A sore or red or white patch that bleeds easily and/or doesn't heal, a lump or thickening.

FYI: Cancer Information Services

The American Cancer Society's information service number is 1-800-ACS-2345. Call for free booklets about cancer and information about services and activities in your area.

The National Cancer Institute maintains a vast information network available to the public, and since your tax dollars pay for it, you ought to take advantage:

Cancer Information Service (CIS)
1-800-4-CANCER

A free service available Monday through Friday, 9 to 4:30; the Delaware Valley office is managed by the Fox Chase Cancer Center. Callers speak to an NCI-trained and -certified professional, who can provide up-to-date information on prevention, detection and diagnosis; referrals to hospitals and specialists; and free publications.

Physicians Data Query (PDQ)
301-496-7403

This comprehensive database contains a wealth of current information about cancer prognosis, staging and treatment, clinical trials, standard therapy protocols and physicians and organizations active in cancer research and treatment. The database is accessible 24 hours a day from your personal computer, if you have a modem, through the online MEDLARS system. Prices vary according to distributor and search time. If you don't have a PC, call 1-800-338-7657 for a library in your area that subscribes to the NCI's databases.

CancerFax
301-402-5874

This is another way to use PDQ. Call from your fax machine telephone for a list of code numbers. The only charge is the cost of a telephone call from your fax machine to the CancerFax computer in Bethesda, Maryland.

The Center for Advancement in Cancer Education
610-642-4810

This nonprofit agency operates out of a cluttered office in Wynnewood and disseminates information about what's happening worldwide in alternative cancer therapies. Its director, Susan Silberstein, watched her young husband die of cancer and decided she wasn't going to bury with him all that she'd learned in researching nontraditional ways to treat the disease. "There are lots of ways you can make a tumor disappear, at least temporarily," she says, "but if you don't repair the body chemistry, you aren't cured." Most cancer patients die of malnutrition, toxemia and opportunistic infections, not of a tumor. The center endorses approaches that are host-oriented rather than tumor-oriented. That means they don't deal with the disease per se but with ways to fight it by balancing body chemistry and boosting the immune system. Silberstein can tell you about programs that fit into one of three categories: clinical nutrition, botanical medicine and psychoneuroimmunology. For cancer patients who've exhausted the conventional medical menu of chemo and radiation therapy or who are seeking a holistic treatment that offers a better quality of life, Silberstein has much to offer.

Wellness Community
610-664-6663

The California-based operation now has a branch in Philadelphia. Gilda Radner was among the 15,000 cancer patients who have found solace in this free program, which offers support groups, seminars on nutritional cooking, new cancer therapies and even classes in guided imagery. No medical services are provided, because the sole purpose of the Wellness Community is to help sick people fight their disease through mental strength and freedom from stress.

The Common Thread
1-800-959-5555

Sometimes navigating the crowded waters of cancer services can be nearly as daunting as the disease. The Common Thread, a regional program of the Crozer-Keystone Health System, helps cancer patients and their families reach all aspects of the fragmented cancer marketplace—including rehab therapies, support groups, genetic education, social services, educational programs, home care, bereavement counseling and pain management—and get the care they need. It has offices in Springfield, Upland and Drexel Hill.

ELM Lifelines
609-654-4044

This Medford, New Jersey-based private, nonprofit outpatient group provides cancer counseling and a support program. They offer weekly two-hour sessions; emotional support; relaxation and visualization; nutrition and exercise; stress management; coping strategies; and health, healing and wellness materials.

CHAPTER 3

Behind Closed Doors

What every medicine cabinet should have

You've probably got a well-stocked liquor cabinet and a bulging pantry, but is your medicine cabinet ready for an emergency? For that matter, do you have something on hand for the cold you just caught? Every medicine cabinet needs certain staples. But before stocking up, you ought to clean out.

Dispose of all prescription medicines, over-the-counter medicines and birth-control products that have passed their expiration. Get rid of any leftover antibiotics—you really shouldn't have any, because you were supposed to finish the prescription. Throw away eye drops that are not crystal clear or have floating clumps. Get rid of any discolored creams. Trash aspirin that smells of vinegar; this is a sign that moisture in the bottle has caused the pills to decompose. To be safe, don't just toss this stuff into your garbage can. Instead empty all bottles of pills and liquids and all tubes of cream into the toilet—out of your reach, and your children's.

Store your medicines—the new ones—in a cool, dry, dark place, preferably one that can be locked if small children are in the house. Here's a basic list, with some brand-name examples, of what you should keep on hand:

Aspirin: The world's oldest painkiller, it's ubiquitous but also dangerous. Aspirin can cause bleeding and stomach distress, so be careful how much you take. Children younger than 15 should never take aspirin because of its link to Reye's syndrome.

Acetaminophen: Tylenol. Its advantage over aspirin is that it does not contain salicylic acid, the ingredient responsible for stomach problems. However, it does not reduce inflammation anywhere near as well as aspirin does. And acetaminophen is not nearly as harmless as believed. Massive overdoses may cause liver poisoning in some patients.

Ibuprofen: Motrin, Advil. These drugs are designed to reduce inflammation from arthritis, muscular aches and sprains, and menstrual cramps. They're less likely to cause upset stomachs than aspirin.

Antibiotic ointments: Neosporin. Preventing or treating infection.

Antihistamine: Benadryl, Chlor-Trimeton. For mild allergic symptoms or reactions to bee stings and other insect bites. May cause drowsiness.

Cold medication: Actifed, Drixoral. Most of these combine an antihistamine and a decongestant. Note that if you have a condition like high blood pressure, glaucoma or asthma, you should consult your doctor before taking a decongestant.

Cough medicine: Lots of hospitals use Robitussin.

Antacid: Maalox Plus, Mylanta, Zantac 75. For mild cases of upset stomach, indigestion and/or gas. Liquid antacids are more effective and work more quickly.

Antidiarrheal medicine: Pepto Bismol, Kaopectate, Imodium A-D. Some doctors recommend leaving diarrhea untreated for a day or so to just let it run its course. Be sure you drink lots of water because dehydration, a common side effect, can be more dangerous than the diarrhea itself.

Syrup of ipecac: To induce vomiting in cases of accidental poisoning. Vomiting is not recommended for all types of poisoning, so always call the Poison Control Center (215-386-2100) before giving ipecac.

Antiseptic: Hydrogen peroxide, for cleaning cuts and scrapes.

Skin creams and/or antiseptic creams: Americaine. For minor skin rashes and irritation.

Itch remedies: Calamine, the yucky pink lotion you grew up with, is still the best sting remover around for bites and poison ivy.

Sunscreen: Choose one with an SPF of 30 or higher; most doctors are recommending an SPF of 45. Then use it!

Ace bandages: Get the 3- to 4-inch size. That's best for wrapping a strain or sprain or holding a splint in place on the way to the hospital.

Eyewash: Bausch and Lomb makes a good one for cleansing the eye to relieve irritation, burning or itching.

Other supplies: Assorted Band-Aids and gauze pads; cotton balls or swabs for applying antiseptics.

Thermometer

The
University of Pennsylvania
Health System is pleased
to bring you

PENN**Health** *Aware*

your 24-hour, free,
confidential source
for health information.

It's as easy as 1-800-789-PENN.

PENN**Health** and PENN**Health** *Aware* are a community service for the Greater Philadelphia Region, from the University of Pennsylvania Health System.

A special advertising section.

PENNHealth *Aware*

When you dial 1-800-789-PENN...

You will be offered two choices. One of the nice features of PennHealth is that you can speak to one of our staff almost immediately, without listening to one of those lengthy phone "menus."

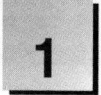

When you press "1," you will speak to one of our PennHealth Referral nurses or counselors.

When you press "2," you may select a topic on PennHealth *Aware*, our health information library with hundreds of useful, practical and confidential health topics.

Here's how easy it is:
- Dial 1-800-789-PENN.
- Press 2.
- Enter the four-digit code for your health topic. (Listed in this Directory.)
- You may speak to a counselor at any time by pressing the * star key.
- You may listen to up to 4 health topics.

1-800-789-PENN

For a world of health information, follow these simple steps:

[ABC 2] Backup
When you'd like to hear a message repeated, press "B" for "Backup" (or the "2" key). You may do this at any time while you're listening to a message.

[GHI 4] Go
If you decide not to listen to a topic you have entered, press "G" for "Go" (or the "4" key) followed by the number of the message you want to hear.

[JKL 5] Jump
If you want to skip to the end of the message in the category you're listening to, press "J" for "Jump" (or the "5" key) to jump forward.

[JKL 5] Cancel
If you make a mistake entering a code, simply press the # key to cancel your entry, then enter the correct code. To end a call, press the # key.

[PRS 7] Repeat
If you missed the first part of a message and you'd like to hear it repeated, press "R" for "Repeat" (or the "7" key).

[JKL 5] To Speak to a PennHealth Referral Counselor
If you'd like to speak with one of our PennHealth Referral Counselors at any time during a message, just press the * star key. Counselors will speak with you 8:30 am - 5:00 pm, Monday through Friday. During non-office hours you may leave a message and your call will be returned.

Don't have a touch-tone phone?

If you would like to listen to PennHealth Aware but you don't have a touch-tone phone…just stay on the line and one of our referral counselors will connect you with the topics of your choice, from 8:30 am to 5 pm, Monday through Friday.

PENNHealth *Aware*

PENNHealth *Aware*
Health Topic Directory

Aging

4111	Alzheimer's Disease
7808	Blood Pressure Medication and Depression
4112	Depression
1568	Diuretics
7822	Drug Interactions
7826	Extended Care Facilities
7827	Family Care Givers
4123	Getting Enough Water
7829	Health Confidence - Taking Charge of Your Health
7837	Hip Fracture
4122	Home Healthcare
7840	Home Safety Tips
7841	Hospice Care
2152	How Can I Help My Aging Parent?
4124	Immunizations
4113	Incontinence
4114	Living Independently
7855	Medicare - Part A
7856	Medicare - Part B
7857	Medication Safety
1571	Nitroglycerin for Angina
7859	Nursing Homes
4125	Nutrition
4116	Parkinson's Disease
4120	Physical Changes
7865	Planning for Retirement
4117	Preventing Falls
1572	Prostate Problems
7877	Skin Problems
4126	Sleep Problems
7879	Snoring/Sleep Apnea
7880	Social Security & SSI
4127	Stress
7883	Stroke Risk
4118	Taking Medication
4119	Talking to Your Doctor

Alcohol Problems

4131	Alcoholism - Causes
4132	Alcoholism - Information and Resources
4133	Alcoholism - The Disease of Denial
4134	How Much is Too Much?
4136	Recovery - The Twelve Step Approach
4137	Symptoms of Alcoholism
4138	Teenage Drinking

Allergies

1875	Allergic Shock
1876	Allergy Testing
1877	Egg and Milk Testing
1878	Food Allergies
1879	Hay Fever
1880	Insect Bites and Stings
1881	Poison Ivy and Poison Oak
1882	Skin Allergies
1883	What is an Allergy?

Back and Neck Problems

4191	Back Exercises
4192	Back Pain - Causes
4193	Exercises for the Desk Bound
4194	Lift It Right
4195	Neck Exercises
4196	Preventing Back Pain
4197	Self-Care for Back Pain
4198	Whiplash

Bones, Joints and Muscles

4231	Arthroscopic Surgery
4232	Bursitis
4233	Carpal Tunnel Syndrome
4239	Gout
4234	Hip Replacement
4235	Knee Replacement
4240	Lupus
4236	Muscle Cramps and Spasms
4237	Overuse Injuries
4176	Rheumatoid Arthritis
4238	Sprains and Strains

Brain and Nervous System

1436	Bell's Palsy
1437	Brain Tumor
1438	Brain Aneurysms
1439	Carotid Artery Disease
1496	Cerebral Angiography
1440	Diseases of the Spine
1441	Epilepsy
1442	Lou Gehrig's Disease
1400	Memory Disorders
4253	Meningitis
1443	Neurological Institute
1444	Narcolepsy
1445	Paralysis After an Injury
4256	Parkinson's Disease - Symptoms
1446	Pinched Nerves
4258	Stroke
6164	Stroke - Are You At Risk?
6165	Stroke - What is It?

ABC 2 BACKUP   **JKL 5 JUMP**   **WXY 9 REPEAT**

1-800-789-PENN

6166	Stroke Quiz	1513	Penn's Cancer Network
6167	Stroke and Apoplexy	1258	Premalignant Skin Lesions
6168	Stroke-Induced Mental Impairments	1559	Prostate Problems
1447	Stroke-Induced Physical Impairments	1259	Prostate Specific Antigen (PSA)
1448	"Think First"	6450	Protecting Yourself from Cancer
1449	Vascular Malformations	1560	Radiation Therapy

Cancer

		1417	Regaining Sense of Control
1501	About Penn's Cancer Center	6452	Risk Factors for Cancer
1539	Bladder Cancer	4280	Seven Warning Signs
1250	Bone Marrow Transplant	1511	Skin Cancer
1541	Bone Scan	4282	Smoking and Cancer
1542	Brain Tumor	6459	Stomach Cancer
1500	Breast Cancer	1512	Support Services
1502	Cancer Evaluation Centers	6465	Throat Cancer
1503	Cancer Risk Evaluation - Breast and Ovarian Cancer	1260	Thyroid Cancer
1504	Cancer Screenings	1565	Uterine Cancer
1544	Cervical Cancer	1514	What is a Clinical Trial?
1545	Cervical Polyps and Cysts	1515	What Is Cancer?
1505	Chemotherapy	1261	What is an Oncologist?

Cosmetic/Reconstructive Surgery

1546	Colon Cancer	4351	Abdominoplasty (Tummy Tucks)
6418	Colonoscopy	4358	Body Contouring
6419	Colposcopy	1900	Blepharoplasty (Eyelids)
6421	Diet and Cancer Risk	4352	Breast Enlargement or Reduction
1413	Digestive Changes During Treatments	4353	Breast Reconstruction
1507	Educational Programs	1901	Facelifts
1588	Endometrial Cancer	1903	Hand Surgery
1547	Endometrial Polyps	1904	Head & Neck Surgery
6424	Esophageal Cancer	1905	Laser Surgery
1548	Fluoroscopy	1906	Cosmetic/Lasers
1415	Handling Stress	4355	Liposuction
6426	Hodgkin's Disease	1902	Rhinoplasty

Diabetes

1251	Immunotherapy	1519	Diabetes - Type I
1252	Kidney Cancer	1520	Diabetes - Type II
6428	Leukemia - Acute	1521	Diabetes and Exercise
6429	Leukemia - Chronic	6960	Carbohydrates
6430	Liver Cancer	6962	Eating Tips for Traveling
1550	Lumps - Breast	6963	Guide to Foods & Labels
1551	Lumps - Skin	1522	Hyperglycemia
1552	Lung Cancer	1523	Hypoglycemia (Insulin Shock)
1553	Lymph Nodes - Enlarged	6964	Proteins for Meals & Snacks
1554	Lymphomas	6965	Use of Alcohol
1253	Malignant Melanoma	1524	What Is Diabetes?

Digestive System

1556	Mammography		
1254	Multiple Myeloma	4411	Colitis
1414	Myths About Cancer Pain	4412	Constipation
1255	Nutrition and Cancer		
6443	Ovarian Cancer		
1256	Pancreatic Cancer		
1557	Pap Smear		
1558	Pelvic Examination		

  GO   CANCEL   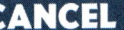 COUNSELOR

PENNHealth *Aware*

4413 Diarrhea
4422 Diverticulosis and Diverticulitis
4414 Gastritis (Stomach Upset)
4415 Heartburn
4416 Hemorrhoids
4417 Hiatal Hernia
4418 Indigestion
1516 Irritable Bowel Syndrome
4420 Rectal Itching
4421 Ulcers - Overview

Ear, Nose and Throat

4451 Dizziness From Inner Ear Disorders
4452 Ear Infection in Children
1525 Ear Wax
1526 Laryngitis
4455 Nosebleed-Causes
4456 Ringing in the Ear-Causes
4457 Sinus Problems
4458 Strep Throat
1527 Tonsillitis/Sore Throat

Eating Disorders

4472 Anorexia-How it is Harmful
4473 Bulimia-How it is Harmful
4471 Compulsive Overeating
4474 Recognizing Anorexia
4475 Recognizing Bulimia
4476 Treating Anorexia
4477 Treating Bulimia

Exercise & Fitness

4491 Athletic Shoes
7409 Back Exercises
7410 Back Pain
7411 Balanced Diet
7417 Cardiovascular Conditioning
4494 Dynamic vs. Static Exercise
4495 Exercise Essentials
4497 Exercise and Your Heart
4496 Exercise and Weight Control
4498 Fitness Values of Common Activities
7437 Foot Advice for the Jogger
7438 Foot Care Basics
4499 How to Check Your Pulse
7448 Neck Exercises
7450 Preventing Sports Injuries
7452 Rowing
7453 Runner's Knee
7454 Running or Jogging
7455 Stair Climbing

7456 Step Training
7457 Strength Training
4500 Tips for Safe Exercising
7467 Torn Ankle Ligaments
4493 Your Personal Fitness Plan
7475 Weight Training

Eyes & Vision

1528 Cataracts
1529 Double Vision
1531 Glaucoma
4515 Radial Keratotomy
4516 Something in Your Eye
4517 Spots and Floaters
4518 Sunglasses - More than Fashion
1530 Symptoms Demanding Immediate Attention

Family Planning

4536 Adoption Options
1352 Birth Control Pills
4532 Child Spacing
4534 Condoms
4533 Contraception
4535 Natural Family Planning
4537 Tubal Ligation
4538 Vasectomy

Foot Care

4551 Athlete's Foot
4552 Bunions
4553 Calluses and Corns
4554 Fitting Shoes Properly
4555 Foot Care Basics
4556 Hammertoes
4557 Ingrown Toenails
4558 Plantar Warts

HIV/AIDS

4612 HIV Infection and AIDS - What Are They?
4616 HIV - Myths and Misconceptions
4615 HIV Information and Referral
1750 Testing for HIV
4617 Minorities and HIV
4618 Safe Sex and HIV
4620 Women and HIV

Headaches

1272 Cluster Headaches
4632 Migraine Headaches
4633 Sinus Headaches
4634 Tension Headaches

ABC 2 BACKUP   **JKL 5** JUMP   **WXY 9** REPEAT

PENNHealth *Aware*

Health Quizzes

- 4651 Alcohol Awareness
- 7406 Arthritis
- 6711 Caffeine
- 7809 Cataracts
- 4653 Diabetes Awareness
- 4654 Fitness Awareness
- 4658 HIV/AIDS Awareness
- 4655 Healthy Diet
- 4656 Healthy Heart
- 4657 Healthy Pregnancy
- 6768 Sleep Disorders
- 4660 Stress Management
- 4661 Weight Control

Hearing

- 4681 Assistive Listening Devices
- 4682 Detecting a Hearing Problem
- 4683 Hearing Aids
- 4687 Hearing Loss Sensorineural
- 1259 Hearing Loss from Otosclerosis
- 4686 Hearing Loss in Children
- 4688 Noise and Hearing
- 4689 Protect Your Hearing

Heart

- 1811 Abdominal Aortic Aneurysm
- 4291 Abnormal Heartbeat
- 1812 Arterial Occlusive Disease
- 1813 Bacterial Endocarditis
- 6107 Breathlessness
- 6109 Cardiac Arrest
- 6110 Cardiac Catheterization & Angiogram
- 1815 Cardiomyopathy
- 1422 Cardiovascular Risk Assessment
- 4293 Chest Pain (Angina)
- 4294 Chest Pain (Other Than Angina)
- 6116 Cholesterol, "Good" & "Bad"
- 6117 Cholesterol Testing
- 6118 Cigarettes - Enemies of a Healthy Heart
- 1816 Congenital Heart Disease
- 4295 Coronary Artery Disease
- 1817 Coronary Intensive Care
- 4296 Decrease Your Risk
- 4297 Early Warning
- 6130 Eating for a Healthy Heart
- 6128 Electrocardiogram (EKG)
- 6132 Exercise Makes Your Heart Stronger
- 4298 Heart Attack - Are You at Risk?
- 6138 Heart Attack - Know What To Do
- 6139 Heart Murmur
- 4299 High Cholesterol
- 1578 High Blood Pressure Medicines
- 4300 High Blood Pressure Treatments
- 4301 High Blood Pressure and Heart Disease
- 6145 Holter Monitoring
- 6146 Low Blood Pressure
- 6147 Low Cholesterol Diet
- 6148 Low Sodium Diet
- 6149 Mitral Valve Prolapse
- 1818 Myocarditis
- 1579 Nitroglycerin for Angina
- 6153 Pacemakers
- 6154 Palpitations
- 1800 "Penn HeartBeat"
- 6155 Pericarditis (Heart Inflammation)
- 6157 Peripheral Vascular Disease
- 6158 Phlebitis & Thrombosis
- 4302 Preventing Heart Disease
- 6160 Reversing Heart Disease
- 1801 What A Hypertension Program Can Do For You

Infectious Diseases

- 4735 Fifth Disease
- 4721 Hepatitis
- 4722 Herpes - Lips, Mouth, and Eyes
- 4732 Herpes Encephalitis
- 4733 Legionnaires' Disease
- 4723 Lice
- 4724 Lyme Disease
- 1200 Lyme Disease Test
- 4725 Pericarditis (Heart Inflammation)
- 4734 Pinworms
- 4726 Rheumatic Fever
- 4727 Ringworm
- 4728 Rubella
- 4729 Salmonella Infections
- 4736 Scabies
- 4336 Shingles
- 4730 Tetanus
- 1210 Tuberculosis

Legal

- 1152 Advance Directives
- 1154 Living Will
- 1153 Power of Attorney

Managed Care

- 1107 How Does My Health Plan Work at the University of Pennsylvania Health System?
- 1108 Managed Care Plans Participating with the University of Pennsylvania Health System

GHI 4 **GO**   # **CANCEL**   ✱ **COUNSELOR**

PENNHealth *Aware*

1109 Questions Regarding Your University of Pennsylvania Medical Center Bill	**6720** Exhibitionism
1110 What is Managed Care?	**6721** Explosive Behavior
	5133 Facing Financial Troubles

Medications

- **1649** Antacids
- **1650** Antibiotics
- **1651** Aspirin
- **1652** Steroids
- **1653** Diuretics
- **4746** Drug Interactions
- **1654** Generic or Brand Names - Which to Buy?
- **1655** High Blood Pressure Medicines
- **4749** Laxatives
- **4750** Over-the-Counter Medications
- **1656** Questions to Ask Your Doctor About Any Medicine
- **1657** Sleep Inducers
- **1658** Tranquilizers
- **1659** You and Your Pharmacist

Men's Health

- **4761** Balding or Hair Loss
- **1460** Impotence
- **4763** Incontinence
- **4765** Penile Inflammation
- **4766** Premature Ejaculation
- **1461** Prostate Problems
- **4768** Sexual Response, Male
- **1462** Sterilization, Male
- **1260** Testicular Self-Exam

Mental Health

- **6701** Aggressive Behavior
- **6702** Agoraphobia
- **6703** Amnesia
- **6704** Anorexia - How it is Harmful
- **1495** Anti-Depressant Medications
- **6706** Antisocial Behavior
- **6707** Anxiety
- **6708** Bulimia - How it is Harmful
- **6709** Burnout
- **6711** Caffeine Quiz
- **6713** Children's Insecurities
- **6714** Compulsive Gambling
- **6715** Counseling Can Help
- **6716** Delirium
- **6717** Depression and Its Symptoms
- **6718** Disappointment
- **6719** EEG (Electroencephalogram)

- **6722** Family Communication
- **6723** Fetishism
- **6724** Gender Identity Disorder
- **6725** Grief and Loss
- **6726** Hallucinations
- **6727** Headache Prevention Quiz
- **5134** How Friends Buffer Stress
- **6728** Hypnosis
- **6729** Hypochondria
- **6730** Hysteria
- **6731** Insomnia
- **6732** Irritability
- **6733** Kleptomania
- **6734** Lethargy
- **6735** Letting Go of Resentment
- **6736** Lying - Pathologic
- **6737** Manic or Bipolar Depression
- **6738** Masochism
- **6739** Memory Loss
- **6740** Mental Exercises for Stress
- **6741** Mental Health Professionals
- **6743** Multiple Personality Disorder
- **6744** Narcissism
- **6745** Nervous Breakdown
- **6746** Nervousness
- **6747** Nightmares and Terrors
- **6748** Obsession and Compulsion
- **6749** Panic Attacks
- **6750** Paranoia
- **6751** Pedophilia
- **6752** Personality Change
- **6753** Phobias - Causes and Symptoms
- **6754** Phobias - Treatment
- **6755** Post-traumatic Stress Disorder
- **6756** Power of a Positive Attitude
- **6757** Psychogenic Pain
- **6758** Psychosis
- **6759** Psychosomatic Illness
- **6760** Pyromania
- **6761** Relaxation Techniques
- **6762** Sadism
- **6742** Seasonal Affective Disorder
- **6763** Schizophrenia
- **6764** Self-Esteem
- **6765** Senility - Causes and Symptoms
- **6766** Senility Prevention
- **6767** Separation Anxiety
- **6768** Sleep Disorders Quiz
- **6769** Sleepwalking

ABC 2 **BACKUP**	JKL 5 **JUMP**	WXY 9 **REPEAT**

PENNHealth *Aware*

6770	Spouse Abuse	6969	Food Poisoning Prevention
6771	Stress - What is It?	6940	Food Pyramid
6772	Stress Management Quiz	6941	Great Grains
6773	Suicide	4825	Healthy Snack Foods
6774	Suicide Warning Signs	4836	How You Think is How You Eat
5131	10 Stress Busters	4826	Kicking the Junk Food Habit
6775	Transvestism	1466	Know Your Nutrients
1497	Valium (Diazepam)	6951	Low Cholesterol Diet
6777	Voyeurism	6952	Low Sodium Diet
5138	What is Stress?	4820	Low Fiber Diet
6778	When You Feel Like Hitting	6956	Nutrition Fads & Foibles

Newborn Care

		4837	Nutrition at the Supermarket
		6967	Overcoming Backsliding
4801	Breast-Feeding	6969	Overweight Child
1744	Care of Your Newborn at Home	4828	Reading Food Labels
4802	Crying	6975	Recognizing Anorexia
1463	Diaper Rash	6976	Recognizing Bulimia
4804	Fathering an Infant	4829	Safe Weight Loss
4805	Formula Feeding	6977	Snacking for Weight Control
4806	Jaundice	4838	Sugar Substitutes
4807	Mothering an Infant	6981	Teaching Your Body to Burn More Calories
1464	Rashes	4839	Vegetarianism
4809	Sleep Patterns in Newborns	4830	Are Vitamin and Mineral Supplements Really Necessary?
4810	Spitting Up	4831	Water - Essential for Good Health

Nutrition

		6989	Weight Control During the Holidays
4821	A Guide to Eating Well	6994	What is Obesity?
4822	Basics of a Balanced Diet	6995	When Others Pressure You to Eat
4832	Caffeine	6996	When You Choose Beef
1582	Calories	5297	Why Fad Diets Don't Work

Oral / Maxillofacial Surgery

4823	Checking Out "Health" Foods
6912	Compulsive Overeating
6913	Cooking with Less Fat & Oil
6914	Cooking with Less Salt
1465	Curbing Your Sweet Tooth
6916	Cutting Out the Fat
6918	Diet & Cancer Risk
6919	Diet & Coronary Disease
4885	Eating Right During Pregnancy
6922	Dining Out Tips
4834	Eating Well for Less
6929	Fake Fats
6930	Fasting/Liquid Diets
4835	Fat Facts
6932	Fat Makes You Fat
6933	Fat-Free Foods
6934	Feeding Your Child
6936	Fiber & Weight Loss
4154	Food Allergies
6938	Food Poisoning

1201	Aesthetic Dentistry
1202	Implants
1203	Maxillofacial Prosthesis
1205	Oral Lesions
1206	Orthognathic Surgery
1208	Sleep Apnea
1209	TMJ and/or Facial Pain
1210	Cosmetic/Laser
1211	Wisdom Teeth

Parenting and Family Life

4841	Building Your Child's Self-Esteem
4842	Communicating With Your Teen
4843	Discipline and Punishment
4844	Helping Siblings Get Along
4845	Separation Anxiety
4846	Suicide Warning Signs
4848	Talking to Your Kids About Drinking and Drugs
4849	Talking to Your Kids About HIV

GHI 4	GO	# CANCEL	* COUNSELOR

PENNHealth *Aware*

4850	Talking to Your Kids About Sex	7767	Tics - Outlet for Anxiety
4851	When You Feel Like Hitting	7770	Viral Infections
4852	Your Teenage Daughter is Pregnant	7771	Whooping Cough

Pediatrics

Pregnancy and Childbirth

7712	Alcohol Affected or Drug Addicted Babies	1740	Breastfeeding Tips
7713	Autism	1741	Breastfeeding and Sore Nipples
7714	Baby Teeth	1742	Care for Mom After Delivery
1353	Bedwetting	1744	Care of Your Newborn Baby
1354	Chickenpox	1745	Childbirth and Parent Education Classes
7706	Child at 7 Months	4881	Choosing an Obstetrician
7707	Child at 8 Months	1742	Common Myths About Breastfeeding
7708	Child at 9 Months	4882	Danger Signs
7709	Child at 10 Months	4883	Drinking During Pregnancy
7710	Child at 11 Months	4884	Drugs During Pregnancy
7711	Child at 12 Months	4885	Eating Right During Pregnancy
1355	Childproofing Your Home	4886	Exercise During Pregnancy
7774	Choking - Older Than One Year	4887	Fetal Development
7775	Choking - Younger Than One Year	1746	Labor - Warning Signs
1356	Choosing Childcare	4888	Membrane Leakage
1357	Croup	4889	Morning Sickness
7722	Dental Care for Infants	4890	Overcoming Fear of Childbirth
7723	Dental Care for Kids	1491	Physical Therapy Tips
7724	Diabetes in Children	4891	Postpartum Blues
7726	Drowning Alert	4896	Pregnancy and Traveling
7727	Dyslexia	4897	Pregnancy: Blood Tests
1498	Diaper Rash	4898	Pregnancy: Early Stages
1358	Earache in Children	4899	Pregnancy: Urine Tests
7729	Exercise - Are Your Kids Getting Enough?	1747	Premature Labor
7731	Fat - What's Normal?	4892	Prenatal Care
7730	Feeding Your Child	4893	Prenatal Tests and Exams
1359	Fever/Treatment	4894	Sex During Pregnancy
1360	Head Lice	4895	Smoking During Pregnancy
1361	Hearing Loss		

Preparing for Emergencies

1362	Hyperactivity	4901	Animal Bites
7753	Reye's Syndrome	4902	Bee Stings
7754	Rheumatic Fever	4903	CPR
7755	Safety Seats for Children	4904	Chemical Burns
7756	Scald Injuries from Tap Water	4905	Chemicals in Eyes
7757	Sleep Patterns	4923	Children Who Stop Breathing
7758	Sleeplessness	4906	Choking - Over One Year Old
7760	Speech Development, 2 Years and Under	4925	Choking - Under One Year Old
7759	Speech Development, Ages 2 - 5	4907	Cuts and Scrapes - Shallow
7761	Speech Problems	4916	Electrical Shock
7772	Stop Breathing - Children	4917	Eye Injuries
7773	Stop Breathing - Infants	4908	Fever
7762	Sudden Infant Death Syndrome	4918	Food Poisoning
7763	Teething	4909	Heart Attack
7764	Temper Tantrums	4910	Heat Stress
7765	Terrible Twos	4911	Home First Aid Supplies
7766	Thumb Sucking	4924	Infants Who Stop Breathing

ABC 2 BACKUP **JKL 5** JUMP **WXY 9** REPEAT

PENN Health *Aware*

4912	Minor Burns and Scalds	5117	Body Fat Tests
4913	Nosebleed	7512	Cardiovascular Conditioning
4914	Poisoning	7513	Circuit Strength Training
4915	Rape	7515	Cross Training
4922	RICE	7516	Cycling Injuries
4919	Sore Throat	5118	Eating Before Exercise
4920	Splinters	5119	Electrical Nerve Stimulation
7772	Stop Breathing - Children	5120	Exercise Testing
7773	Stop Breathing - Infants	7519	Elbow Injuries
4921	Sunburn	5121	Fluid Replacement
		5112	Foot Advice for Joggers

Respiratory Problems

		7530	Foot Care Basics
1906	Asthma	7531	Foot Injuries
1916	Broncoscopy	5122	Growth Hormone
1917	Quit Smoking Program	7534	Hamstring Injuries
1918	Sarcoidosis	7535	Hand Injuries
1389	Surgical Treatment for Emphysema	7536	Head Injuries
1919	Tuberculosis	7537	Heel Spur
		7538	Hip Injuries

Sexually Transmitted Diseases

		7540	Knee Injuries
		7543	Lower Back Injuries
1468	Chlamydia	7544	Lower Leg Injuries
4952	Gonorrhea	7546	Neck Exercises
4953	Herpes	7547	Neck Injuries
4954	Prevention	7548	Orthopaedic Examination Before Exercise
1469	Syphilis	7553	Plantar Fasciitis
1470	Vaginitis	5113	Preventing Injuries
4957	Venereal Disease	7555	Pronated Foot
		7557	Running Injuries

Skin Health

		5125	Temperature and Humidity
1710	Acne	5114	Tendinitis
1711	Canker Sores and Fever Blisters	5115	Treatment with RICE
1712	Dandruff	7558	Shin Splints
1713	Impetigo	7559	Shoulder Injuries
1714	Itching Skin	5124	Sports Drinks
4974	Moles	7570	Warm-Up/Cool Down
4975	Psoriasis	7571	Weight Training
1715	Retin-A		

Travel Medicine

4977	Seborrhea		
1716	Sunburn	1303	Altitude Sickness
1717	Warts	1305	Food and Water Precautions
		1309	Health Care Abroad/ Insurance

Sports Medicine

		1311	Hepatitis A Vaccine
7501	Aerobic Dance Injuries	1301	Immunizations
5116	Altitude & Exercise	1306	Insect Repellants
7504	Ankle Injuries	1302	Malaria
7505	Arthritis or Rheumatism?	1304	Pneumovax
5111	Athlete's Foot	1307	Tips for Travel Abroad
7506	Athletic Amenorrhea	1300	Travel Medicine at Penn
1585	Dysmenorrhea	1308	Travelers Diarrhea
7508	Back Exercises	1310	Yellow Fever Vaccine

GHI 4 GO   **# CANCEL**   **✱ COUNSELOR**

PENNHealth *Aware*

Urinary & Genital Systems

- **5261** Bladder Stones
- **5262** Blood in Urine
- **5270** Cystitis
- **2213** Cystogram
- **5271** Genital Warts
- **5268** Hernia - Inguinal
- **5272** Human Papillomavirus
- **1476** Kidney Stones
- **1477** Kidney/ Urinary Tract Infections
- **1478** Lithotripsy
- **1410** Prostate Specific Antigen Levels (PSA)
- **5266** Urinary Catheterization
- **5269** Urinary Obstruction
- **1479** Women and Urinary Infections

Women's Health

- **7102** Absence of Periods
- **7103** Anorexia - How it is Harmful
- **7104** Battered Women
- **1611** Bleeding Abnormalities - Postmenopausal
- **1612** Bleeding Abnormalities Between Periods
- **1613** Breast Discharge
- **1614** Breast Disease - Fibrocystic
- **7110** Breast Self - Examination
- **7111** Bulimia - How it is Harmful
- **1615** Cervical Cancer
- **1616** Cervical Dysplasia
- **1617** Cervical Polyps and Cysts
- **7116** Cervicitis
- **7117** Cesarean Section
- **1483** Contraception Methods
- **1619** D&C/Hysteroscopy
- **1588** Endometrial Cancer
- **1620** Endometrial Polyps
- **1621** Estrogen Replacement Therapy
- **1622** Feminine Hygiene
- **7128** Fertility Drugs
- **1623** General Physical for Women
- **7130** Genetic Counseling
- **1624** Hot Flashes
- **1619** Hysteroscopy/D&C
- **1625** Mammography
- **7142** Mastitis
- **1626** Menopause
- **1627** Menopause Problems
- **7146** Miscarriage
- **7147** Mothering an Infant
- **1628** Osteoporosis
- **1629** Pap Smear
- **1630** Pelvic Examination
- **7161** Pregnancy Planning
- **7162** Pregnancy Recovery Quiz
- **7163** Pregnancy Tests
- **7164** Pregnancy and Work
- **7165** Premenstrual Tension
- **1635** Urinary Infections
- **1631** Uterine Cancer
- **1632** Uterine Fibroids
- **7182** Vaginal Infections
- **1633** Vaginitis
- **1634** Vaginitis - Postmenopausal
- **7188** Women Living Alone
- **7189** Women and HIV
- **7191** Yeast Infections

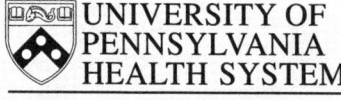

The future of medicine.℠

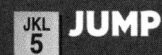

PENNHealth *Aware*

Your 24-hour, free, confidential source for health information.

It's as easy as 1-800-789-PENN.

| GHI 4 GO | # CANCEL | * COUNSELOR |

Section

Choosing a Doctor

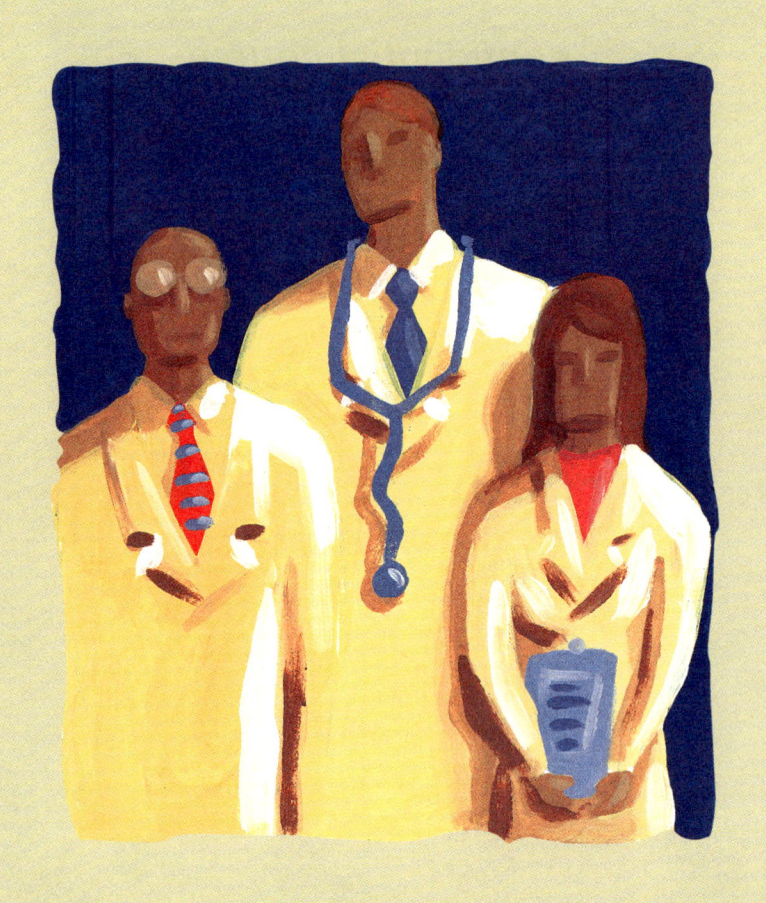

Two

Chapter 4
Finding Dr. Right
A shopper's guide to selecting a physician

Chapter 5
Top Docs
A review of the area's outstanding doctors

Chapter 6
Centers of Excellence
The best local facilities for specialty care

America's #1 Adult Heart Transplant Center... Again.

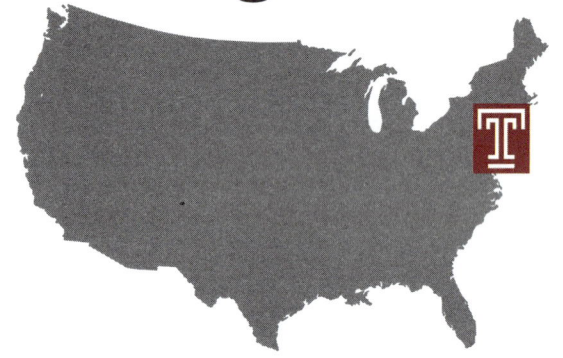

During 1995, Temple University Hospital physicians again performed more adult heart transplants than any other hospital in the United States.* More than all of the other Delaware Valley hospitals combined.

With more than a decade of heart transplantation experience, Temple is a leader in transplant techniques, unique cardiac surgery procedures and cardiac research.

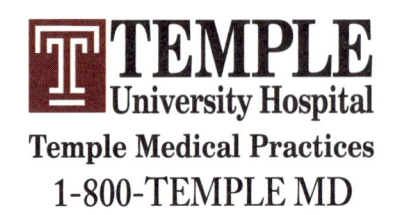

TEMPLE University Hospital
Temple Medical Practices
1-800-TEMPLE MD

*Source: Intersearch Corporation-Health Sciences Group, Horsham, PA

CHAPTER 4

Finding Dr. Right

A shopper's guide to selecting a personal physician

On the short list of life's important decisions, choosing Dr. Right may well rank up there with choosing a spouse. Like the latter, a doctor can be a confidant, adviser and caretaker. While love is just about the only radar for finding a life partner, you can use a more rational method for your medical needs.

More people are now finding themselves in managed care plans, in which insurers pay set fees to doctors to oversee the basic health needs of their patients. Fee-for-service as we have always known it is vanishing, except among those who can afford it. In this new era of health care, your most important doctor is an updated version of the old-fashioned family doc. In the past, if you broke your leg you called an orthopedist to set it. Under managed care the first person to contact becomes your primary-care physician, who will assess your needs and make an appropriate referral to an orthopedist who participates in your plan.

Managed care plans allow you to choose your own primary-care doctor, and because practitioners usually participate in more than one plan, you should have a good list of choices. Proponents of managed care claim that as a larger percentage of people enroll in these plans, costs should drop and, at the least, basic care should improve, because everyone will develop a long-term relationship with a doctor who knows his or her medical and personal history. Does diabetes run in your family? Are you prone to bouts of depression? What medicines are you taking routinely, and do you have any allergies? The doctor you rush to see only when you're ill has very little context for diagnosis and little time or interest in the all-important area of prevention.

I've never understood why so many people put a greater effort into selecting a car or a stereo system than into selecting a doctor. Begin your doctor shopping by considering some of the following:

Office location: Is the office near your home or workplace? Convenient to public transportation? If not, does it have ample parking?

Solo or group practice: If you don't like the busy atmosphere and the chance you will not always see the same doctor, a group practice may not be for you. On the other hand, solo practitioners may not be available weekends or in emergencies.

Hours: Are the office hours compatible with your work schedule? Can you be seen at night?

Hospital privileges: Where does the doctor admit patients and is it a place you'd want to be? If he's in more than one hospital, how does he choose who goes where?

Fees and insurance: What does the doctor charge for initial visits and for follow-ups? Does she accept your insurance plan, and what portion of the fee might you have to absorb? Who does the paperwork and submits the bills?

Once you've narrowed the prospects, schedule a get-acquainted visit. You wouldn't buy a car over the phone, and you shouldn't "buy" a doctor that way either. If the doctor won't agree to meet with you, view it as a warning sign. Once you arrive, check out the office. Are the personnel friendly and the place clean and attractive? How long do patients sit in the waiting room before being seen?

When you meet the doctor, have your questions ready. You'll want to know who covers for him or her on nights and weekends. Would he make an emergency house call? Does she have telephone hours to answer questions? Will you have access to your medical records? State laws regarding release of medical records vary. Pennsylvania law grants hospital patients direct access to their medical records, but private physicians are not required to give you this information, although they may send it to another doctor who requests it. What may not be yours legally certainly belongs to you rightfully, so be sure to establish your physician's policy up front. It will become especially important if you ever fire the doctor and discover your records can't leave with you.

Don't be embarrassed to ask the doctor about his or her qualifications. Where did he go to school? Is she board-certified? This term means that the doctor has received extensive training in a particular area and has passed oral and written examinations administered by the American Board of Medical Specialties. While board certification is not a guarantee of quality medicine, it's certainly a valuable indicator in terms of training and knowledge. Some physicians claim to be board-certified when in fact they're simply affiliated with professional organizations or belong to one of the 100 or so alternative, less-stringent boards. This misrepresentation is particularly rampant in the field of plastic surgery. A study published by the *New England Journal of Medicine* found that 12 percent of the doctors advertising in the Yellow Pages were not certified by the ABMS, and nearly half the plastic surgeons lacked ABMS certification. (You can check if a doctor is legitimately boarded by calling 1-800-776-CERT.)

If your concern is the doctor's legal track record, you can research his malpractice claims in a book called *10,289 Questionable Doctors*, published by Public Citizen Health Research Group. It's available in the reference section of the business, science and industry department at the Free Library on Logan Square. On the other hand, be warned that doctors can also check up on your litigation record. A legal service based in Philadelphia researches the number of malpractice suits a patient has filed, thus allowing the doctor to decide if you're worth the risk of treating.

Finally, perhaps the most critical question of all: Do you and the doctor have the right chemistry? Remember, you're beginning what you hope will be a cordial, long-term relationship, so examine the doctor's human qualities. You want a good listener, someone who talks *to you* rather than *at you*—or down to you—someone articulate, considerate, pleasant. Is this the kind of person who might come into the waiting room and apologize for running late? Nowhere is it written that doctors are immunized against courtesy.

After all this work, you still might find you've made a mistake. In that case, vote with your feet and move on.

Firing a doctor

Patients have an awful time grappling with the idea of changing doctors. They feel embarrassed; they don't quite know what to say; they don't know where else to go. None of these is a sufficient reason to remain with a doctor who isn't meeting your needs or providing the care you're paying for. The doctor is probably much more important to your life than you are to his. I can think of few services people continue to accept with displeasure to the degree they'll keep seeing a doctor they don't like or no longer trust.

If you're uncomfortable confronting the doctor or hurting her feelings, announce your intentions by phone or by letter or to the office manager so that you can request a copy of your medical records. They are full of valuable information your new doctor should have. While you're at it, you'd do the doctor a service by explaining why you're unhappy: The nurses overbook patients and you're sick of waiting an hour every time you schedule a visit. The doctor is never available when you call and in a hurry when you're there. Your appointments seem to last about 30 seconds. She's raised her fees once too often. You aren't getting the care or attention you deserve. While you're flattered being spoken to as if you had a medical degree from Harvard, you can't understand the doctor's explanations. Your son just graduated from medical school and opened an office around the corner. Bye.

Second opinions

Sometimes you can allay doubts about the level of care your doctor is providing by getting a second opinion. And second opinions are absolutely in order when you're considering elective surgery, you've been advised you need major surgery or you're uncertain about a proposed treatment plan. Research by the Rand Corporation, a

California think tank, indicates that as many as one in three medical and surgical procedures is inappropriate, suggesting that it's worth the trouble to get another view.

I'd advise against taking a name for a second opinion from the doctor who's given you the first one. (That's where *Philadelphia Magazine*'s top doctors list comes in handy; see Chapter 5.) Too often the referral goes to a pal in the old boys' network. In the worst circumstances, the referring doctor kicks back a piece of the fee, and in the best, there's an unspoken promise to support the original diagnosis—especially when surgery is involved. You wash my back and I'll wash yours.

Also think about taking your bones to someone in a different hospital from the one your specialist is affiliated with. Because philosophies within a given department are frequently similar, you should check out another perspective. And consider reaching beyond your original specialist's discipline. Every specialist has a bias. Internists are more disposed to medical approaches, while surgeons tend to solve problems by cutting them out. Even among surgeons, an orthopedist might take a different tack from a sports medicine specialist.

When a disfiguring or difficult treatment plan is suggested, don't hesitate to consult elsewhere for alternative strategies. Many problems can be treated medically as well as surgically, so explore your options. If you decide the side effects aren't worth the gains, speak up and say no. A friend of mine was told by a leading cardiologist that he had several clogged arteries and ought to schedule bypass surgery immediately. He took his angiogram results to someone else who recommended trying chelation therapy first. Six months later he swears his cholesterol is down and his arteries are open.

Your second opinion may confirm the first or it may not. Keep looking until a consensus relieves your confusion. And don't panic if you're part of a manage care plan and want to get a second opinion. Consult your primary-care physician about your concerns; he or she may be able to arrange referrals for a second opinion, if necessary. Or you may choose to find another physician, if you have a flexible plan that allows freedom of choice. Best bet: Call your managed care plan to find out how second opinions are handled.

Patient's responsibilities

Certainly the responsibility for delivering quality medicine belongs to doctors, but there's plenty of evidence that people who assertively engage as partners in their treatments have better outcomes. In fact, doctors have told me they actually prefer active to passive patients. Clearly you can improve your chances of having a better doctor by becoming a good patient. That means it's your job to:

_____
Be on time for appointments.
_____
Expedite the efficiency of your visit by preparing your complaints and questions before you get to the office—writing them out, if necessary, to jog your memory.

Take your medication as prescribed, and know the names of the drugs you take. Don't expect doctors to educate you about the medicines they prescribe. It's up to you to ask what the side effects are, how long before the drug works, whether it interacts with other medications and whether it's best taken on an empty or full stomach. Pharmacists can also be very helpful with drug information.

When talking to the doctor, discuss your symptoms in descending order of concern. A study showed that doctors start to formulate their diagnosis within the first minute of an examination.

Should you require surgery, there are several things you'll want to inquire about. How many of these particular operations has the surgeon done? This is especially important with some of the newer laparoscopic surgeries, where there is a definite learning curve and you don't want to be at the front end. How often does he or she do this procedure? At least two or three times a week is an acceptable base. What's the success rate and rate of complications? Pray he tells the truth.

In general, treat your medical care like any product in the marketplace and exercise the dictum "caveat emptor." You should question why a particular test has been ordered, what it will reveal and how the results will change your treatment plan. Why put yourself through discomfort simply to satisfy a doctor's curiosity? And when it's suggested that you try some state-of-the-art procedure, play the skeptic. Not all newfangled techniques—lasers, implants, laparoscopes—are an improvement over the standard ways. They may be more exciting and challenging for the doctor but of no real advantage to you.

As in everything else, knowledge is power. If you've been diagnosed with a disease or condition, go to the library and read about it. Information on a wide range of medical research can be obtained from CRISP (Computer Retrieval of Information on Scientific Projects), a service of the National Institutes of Health, at 301-594-7267. Some organizations charge a fee and do the research for you, such as the Health Resource (501-329-5272) and Planetree Health Resource Center (415-923-3680).

Years ago there was a standing joke that many physicians held the notion that the initials M.D. stood for *medical deity*. There's a lot less of that attitude around these days, partly because patients have gotten smarter and become health consumers. How fortunate that Philadelphians live in the midst of an outstanding medical center where the shopping opportunities couldn't be better.

Thomas Jefferson University

DEPARTMENT OF SURGERY

1025 Walnut Street, Philadelphia, PA 19107

Francis E. Rosato, MD, Chairman

For more than a century and a half, Jefferson surgeons have been setting standards for surgical care in this country through landmark advances in research, diagnosis and treatment.

➤ **Division of Cardiothoractic Surgery** 955-6996
*Richard N. Edie, MD
Thomas L. Carter, MD
James T. Diehl, MD
John D. Mannion, MD

➤ **Division of Colorectal Surgery** 955-5869
*Robert D. Fry, MD
Jan Rakinic, MD

➤ **Division of General Surgery** 955-6925
*Francis E. Rosato, MD
Donna J. Barbot, MD
James E. Colberg, MD
Murray J. Cohen, MD
Herbert E. Cohn, MD
Diane R. Gillum, MD
John C. Kairys, MD
Pauline K. Park, MD
Reuven Rabinovici, MD
Ernest L. Rosato, MD
Jerome J. Vernick, MD

➤ **Department of Pediatric Surgery** 955-7635
*Philip J. Wolfson, MD
E. Stanton Adkins, III, MD
Aviva Katz, MD
Stephen G. Murphy, MD
John Noseworthy, MD

➤ **Division of Transplant Surgery** 955-4888
*Michael J. Moritz, MD
Vincent T. Armenti, MD, PhD
John S. Radomski, MD
Gary A. Wilson, MD

➤ **Division of Trauma** 955-2600
*Jerome J. Vernick, MD
Murray J. Cohen, MD
Paul G. Curcillo, III, MD
Reuven Rabinovici, MD

➤ **Division of Vascular Surgery** 955-4912
*R. Anthony Carabasi, MD
Paul J. DiMuzio, MD
Mark B. Kahn, MD
Stanton N. Smullens, MD

Board Certified Surgeons.
*Division Directors.

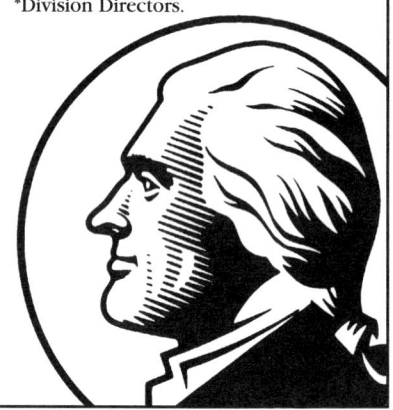

CHAPTER 5

Top Docs

Here are the specialists area doctors themselves would choose

Say one thing about Philadelphia, it's a great place to get sick. The health industry accounts for almost 15 percent of all private-sector jobs in the region and a payroll of more than $6 billion. The five-county area has roughly 80 hospitals, some 70 manufacturers of medical instruments, 60 or so biomedical research firms, more than 40 pharmaceutical companies and more than 10,000 physicians. If you have to pick one of them, why not the best?

Finding the best doctor has never been easy. You can ask a friend, ask a doctor or hazard a surf through the classifieds—or you can use *Philadelphia Magazine*'s list of doctors other doctors have recommended. Since we started publishing our choices back in the mid-'80s, this list has become one of the area's most trusted consumer resources. Doctors admit that even they use it for referrals.

Our methodology is fairly simple. This year we mailed 5,000 surveys to randomly selected area physicians—and nearly 1,000 sent them back. We asked doctors to tell us whom they'd send a family member to for everything from arthritis to a urinary tract infection. Their answers created a working list we honed through more than 100 personal interviews with outstanding specialists we'd cited in previous years.

Is it perfect? No. Are there excellent docs quietly working in the smaller suburban hospitals who aren't on it? Without a doubt. The list always has a preponderance of doctors in academic centers, because such places attract more cutting-edge practitioners. Should you change doctors if yours isn't listed? Only if you aren't satisfied. Most medical problems don't need the attention of a top doc. In fact, often you may be better off with a skilled and caring general practitioner than a superb and overworked specialist.

This year you'll notice the absence of some old names and the addition of some new ones. Some great doctors who've reduced their patient care hours or moved into administrative positions—for example, psychiatrists Aaron Beck, Peter Whybrow and Charles O'Brien—have been deleted. We wanted people whose primary focus is seeing patients in a clinical setting, which automatically removed many outstanding researchers like Karl Rickels.

Don't be surprised if a doctor has moved to another hospital by the time you read this. Seismic shifts are occurring in the medical field—to keep abreast we'd have to list the doctors' hospital affiliations on Velcro. Please use the following as a resource, not a bible. If there's a physician here who nearly killed your mother, we're sorry. That's what malpractice suits are for. And if your beloved doctor's name is missing, consider yourself lucky. It will be easier to book your next appointment.

The following abbreviations are used for area hospitals:

Abington—ABINGTON MEMORIAL HOSPITAL; *Allegheny*—ALLEGHENY UNIVERSITY HOSPITALS (FORMERLY MEDICAL COLLEGE OF PENNSYLVANIA/HAHNEMANN UNIVERSITY HOSPITAL SYSTEM); *Belmont*—BELMONT CENTER FOR COMPREHENSIVE TREATMENT; *Brandywine*—BRANDYWINE HOSPITAL; *Bryn Mawr*—THE BRYN MAWR HOSPITAL; *Charter Fairmount*—CHARTER FAIRMOUNT INSTITUTE; *Chester County*—THE CHESTER COUNTY HOSPITAL; *Chestnut Hill*—CHESTNUT HILL HOSPITAL; *CHOP*—CHILDREN'S HOSPITAL OF PHILADELPHIA; *CMC*—COOPER HOSPITAL/UNIVERSITY MEDICAL CENTER; *Crozer-Chester*—CROZER-CHESTER MEDICAL CENTER; *Delco Memorial*—DELAWARE COUNTY MEMORIAL HOSPITAL; *Doylestown*—DOYLESTOWN HOSPITAL; *Einstein*—ALBERT EINSTEIN MEDICAL CENTER; *Episcopal*—EPISCOPAL HOSPITAL; *Fox Chase*—HOSPITAL OF FOX CHASE CANCER CENTER; *Frankford*—FRANKFORD HOSPITAL; *Friends*—FRIENDS HOSPITAL; *Germantown*—THE GERMANTOWN HOSPITAL AND MEDICAL CENTER; *Graduate*—THE GRADUATE HOSPITAL; *Holy Redeemer*—HOLY REDEEMER HOSPITAL AND MEDICAL CENTER; *Institute*—THE INSTITUTE OF PENNSYLVANIA HOSPITAL; *Jeanes*—JEANES HOSPITAL; *Jeff*—THOMAS JEFFERSON UNIVERSITY HOSPITAL; *Lankenau*—THE LANKENAU HOSPITAL; *Magee*—MAGEE REHABILITATION HOSPITAL; *Mercy Catholic*—MERCY CATHOLIC MEDICAL CENTER; *Montgomery*—MONTGOMERY HOSPITAL; *Moss*—MOSSREHAB; *Nazareth*—NAZARETH HOSPITAL; *Paoli*—PAOLI MEMORIAL HOSPITAL; *Penna*—PENNSYLVANIA HOSPITAL; *Phoenixville*—PHOENIXVILLE HOSPITAL; *Presby*—PRESBYTERIAN MEDICAL CENTER OF THE UNIVERSITY OF PENNSYLVANIA HEALTH SYSTEM; *Renfrew*—THE RENFREW CENTER; *Scheie*—SCHEIE EYE INSTITUTE; *St. Chris*—ST. CHRISTOPHER'S HOSPITAL FOR CHILDREN; *Taylor*—TAYLOR HOSPITAL; *Temple*—TEMPLE UNIVERSITY HOSPITAL; *UPMC*—UNIVERSITY OF PENNSYLVANIA MEDICAL CENTER; *VA*—VETERANS AFFAIRS MEDICAL CENTER; *Wills*—WILLS EYE HOSPITAL; *West Jersey*—WEST JERSEY HEALTH SYSTEM

Medical Specialists

Allergy and Immunology
PAUL ATKINS, *UPMC*; FREDERICK COGEN, *Holy Redeemer*; ELIOT H. DUNSKY, *Allegheny* (SP: ASTHMA); MARC F. GOLDSTEIN, *Allegheny* (SP: INTERNAL MEDICINE); GEORGE R. GREEN, *Abington*; DAVID M. LANG, *Allegheny*; ARNOLD LEVINSON, *UPMC* (SP: IMMUNOLOGY); STEPHEN MCGEADY, *Jeff* (SP: IMMUNOLOGY); JOSEPH E. PAPPANO, *Bryn Mawr*; ALBERT ROHR, *Bryn Mawr*; SHERYL F. TALBOT, *Penna*; BURTON ZWEIMAN, *UPMC*

TOP DOCTORS
The Very Best in 70 Specialties ▪ PLUS: Rising Stars

Philadelphia
MAY 1996 $2.95

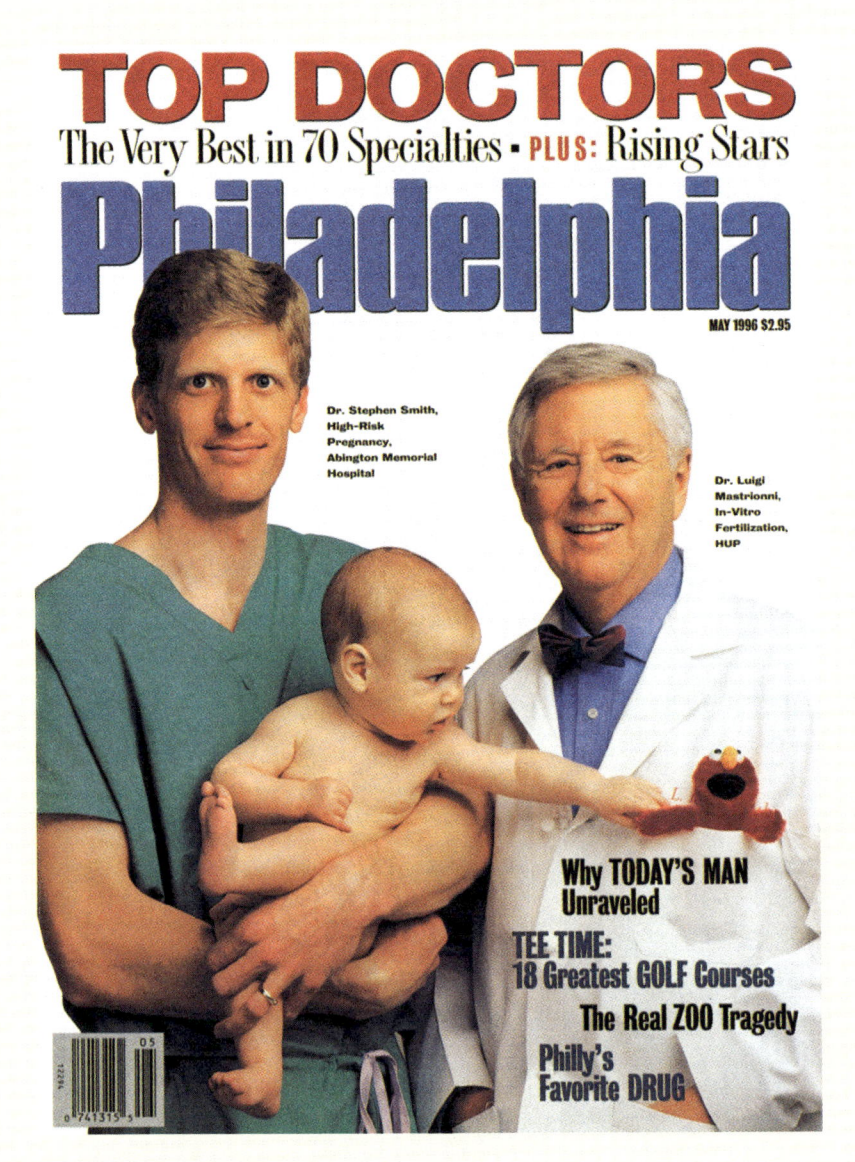

Dr. Stephen Smith, High-Risk Pregnancy, Abington Memorial Hospital

Dr. Luigi Mastrionni, In-Vitro Fertilization, HUP

Why TODAY'S MAN Unraveled
TEE TIME: 18 Greatest GOLF Courses
The Real ZOO Tragedy
Philly's Favorite DRUG

The magazine Philadelphians live by.

For subscription information call Carmen Conrad at (215) 564-7700 ext. 2067.

Anesthesiology

STAN AUKBURG, *UPMC* (SP: VASCULAR TRANSPLANTS, THORACIC); JAMES BAUMGARDNER, *UPMC* (SP: NEURO-ANESTHESIOLOGY); EUGENE BETTS, *CHOP*; JAMES E. DUCKETT, *Presby*; NORIG ELLISON, *UPMC* (SP: CARDIOTHORACIC); F. MICHAEL FERRANTE, *UPMC* (SP: PAIN MANAGEMENT); DAVID FISH, *Fox Chase* (SP: CRITICAL CARE); EVAN FRANK, *Jeff* (SP: PAIN MANAGEMENT); BRETT GUTSCHE, *UPMC* (SP: OBSTETRICS); DAVID MAGUIRE, *Jeff* (SP: CARDIOVASCULAR); LEE MALIT, *Lankenau* (SP: CARDIOVASCULAR); THOMAS D. MULL, *Bryn Mawr*; STANLEY MURAVCHICK, *UPMC* (SP: PLASTIC SURGERY); J. STEPHEN NAULTY, *UPMC* (SP: OBSTETRICS, PAIN MANAGEMENT); SUSAN NICOLSON, *CHOP* (SP: CARDIAC); DEBORAH E. RITTER, *Jeff* (SP: CARDIO-VASCULAR); HENRY ROSENBERG, *Allegheny*; JOSEPH SAVINO, *UPMC* (SP: CARDIOTHORACIC, INTENSIVE CARE); ALAN JAY SCHWARTZ, *Allegheny* (SP: CARDIAC); JOSEPH SELTZER, *Jeff*; DAVID S. SMITH, *UPMC* (SP: NEUROSURGICAL); LINDA SUNDT, *Jeff* (SP: CARDIAC); DOUGLAS A. SWIFT, *Penna* (SP: CARDIOTHORACIC)

Cardiology

ALFRED A. BOVE, *Temple* (SP: HEART FAILURE); SUSAN C. BROZENA, *Allegheny* (SP: TRANSPLANT); ALFRED BUXTON, *Temple* (SP: ELECTROPHYSIOLOGY); HOWARD EISEN, *Temple* (SP: TRANSPLANT); WILLIAM S. FRANKL, *Allegheny*; IRVING HERLING, *UPMC*; MARIELL JESSUP, *Allegheny* (SP: HEART FAILURE); JAMES KITCHEN, *Lankenau*; MORRIS KOTLER, *Einstein*; WILLIAM K. LEVY, *Abington*; EVAN LOH, *UPMC* (SP: HEART FAILURE); FRANCIS MARCHLINSKI, *Allegheny* (SP: ELECTROPHYSIOLOGY); MARK ROSENTHAL, *Abington* (SP: ELECTROPHYSIOLOGY); ZEL ROTHSTEIN, *Phoenixville*; BERNARD SEGAL, *Allegheny*; HARVEY L. WAXMAN, *CMC*

Cardiac Catheterization

JAMES A. BURKE, *Temple* (SP: INTERVENTIONAL); MARC COHEN, *Allegheny*; SHELDON GOLDBERG, *Jeff* (SP: INTERVENTIONAL); RONALD S. GOTTLIEB, *Graduate* (SP: INTERVENTIONAL); HOWARD HERRMANN, *UPMC* (SP: INTERVENTIONAL CARDIOLOGY); JOHN W. HIRSHFELD, *UPMC*; ANCIL JONES, *Crozer-Chester*; PETER KURNIK, *CMC*; WILLIAM G. KUSSMAUL, *Allegheny* (SP: INTERVENTIONAL); JACK MARTIN, *Bryn Mawr*; J. DAVID OGILBY, *Allegheny* (SP: ANGIOPLASTY); MICHAEL P. SAVAGE, *Jeff* (SP: INTERVENTIONAL); WILLIAM J. UNTEREKER, *CMC*

Dermatology
General

EDWARD BONDI, *UPMC*; KAREN K. DEASEY, *Bryn Mawr*; ALEXANDER E. EHRLICH, *Graduate*; PAUL R. GROSS, *Penna*; ALLAN HALPERN, *UPMC* (SP: PIGMENTED LESIONS); WARREN R. HEYMANN, *CMC*; HARRY J. HURLEY, *UPMC*; BERNETT L. JOHNSON, *UPMC* (SP: VITILIGO); CAROLINE S. KOBLENZER, *UPMC* (SP: PSYCHO-CUTANEOUS DISEASE); JAMES J. LEYDEN, *UPMC*; ALAIN H. ROOK, *UPMC* (SP: CUTANEOUS LYMPHOMA); RICHARD L. SPIELVOGEL, *Allegheny*; MARIE O. UBERTI-BENZ, *Presby*

Cosmetic

LEONARD DZUBOW, *UPMC* (SP: MOHS, LASERS); ALEXANDER EHRLICH, *Graduate*; STEVEN GREENBAUM, *Jeff* (SP: MOHS); PAUL R. GROSS, *Penna*; DEBRA GROSSMAN, *UPMC* (SP: MOHS, LASERS); NATHAN HOWE, *Allegheny* (SP: MOHS); JAMES LEYDEN, *UPMC* (SP: ACNE); SUSAN TAYLOR, *Penna*

Hair Transplantation

LEONARD DZUBOW, *UPMC*; THOMAS GRIFFIN, *Graduate*; DAVID W. LOW, *UPMC* (SP: PLASTIC SURGERY)

Emergency Medicine

STEPHANIE ABBUHL, *UPMC*; WILLIAM BAXT, *UPMC*; MICHAEL CHANSKY, *CMC*; LAURENCE GAVIN, *Presby*; FREDERIC KAUFFMAN, *Temple*; DOUGLAS MCGEE, *Einstein*; ROBERT MCNAMARA, *Allegheny*; DAVID K. WAGNER, *Allegheny*; JOSEPH ZECCARDI, *Jeff*

Endocrinology

DAVID M. CAPUZZI, *Allegheny* (SP: LIPIDS); DOMINIC F. CORRIGAN, *Abington*; SOL EPSTEIN, *Einstein* (SP: OSTEOPOROSIS); JOSEPH S. FISHER, *Holy Redeemer*; ELIHU GOREN, *Chestnut Hill* (SP: DIABETES); JOHN G. HADDAD, *UPMC*; GHADDA HADDAD, *CMC*; ANTHONY JENNINGS, *Presby* (SP: THYROID DISEASES); ALLAN D. MARKS, *Temple* (SP: METABOLISM, HYPERTENSION); STEVEN NAGELBERG, *Allegheny*; LESLIE ROSE, *Allegheny* (SP: DIABETES); PETER J. SNYDER, *UPMC*

Diabetes

SETH BRAUNSTEIN, *UPMC*; WILLIAM W. FORE, *Wills*; JEFFREY MILLER, *Jeff*; STANLEY SCHWARTZ, *UPMC*

Family or General Practice

IRWIN BECKER, *Germantown*; BARRY R. COOPER, *Abington*; HARRY FRANKEL, *Graduate*; WARREN B. MATTHEWS, *Abington*; MARC MCKENNA, *Chestnut Hill*; ALEXANDER R. PEDICINO, *Holy Redeemer*; ROBERT PERKEL, *Jeff*; ANN E. REILLY, *Paoli*; NEIL SKOLNIK, *Abington*; GEORGE VALKO, *Jeff*; RICHARD C. WENDER, *Jeff*

Gastroenterology
Diagnostic

WILLIAM M. BATTLE, *Jeanes*; DONALD O. CASTELL, *Graduate* (SP: ESOPHAGEAL DISEASE); SIDNEY COHEN, *Temple* (SP: ESOPHAGEAL AND MOTILITY DISORDERS); JULIUS DEREN, *UPMC* (SP: INFLAMMATORY BOWEL DISEASE); ANTHONY J. DIMARINO JR., *Jeff*; SUSAN GORDON, *Jeff*; DAVID A. KATZKA, *Graduate*; WILLIAM H. LIPSHUTZ, *Penna* (SP: ESOPHAGEAL AND INFLAMMATORY BOWEL DISEASE); MICHAEL LUCEY, *UPMC* (SP: HEPATOLOGY); RICHARD MENIN, *Einstein*; GARY NEWMAN, *Lankenau*; STEVEN PEIKIN, *CMC*

Therapeutic

CRAIG ARONCHICK, *Penna*; MARTA DABEZIES, *Temple* (SP: ENDOSCOPIC ULTRASOUND); STEVEN A. EDMUNDOWICZ, *Jeff*; MARK JACOBS, *Delco Memorial*; WILLIAM LONG, *UPMC*; LARRY MILLER, *Temple* (SP: ENDOSCOPIC ULTRASOUND)

Geriatrics

CHRISTINE ARENSON, *Jeff*; BARBARA BELL, *Abington*; THOMAS A. CAVALIERI, *Kennedy Memorial*; MARY ANN FORCIEA, *UPMC*; DAVID GALINSKY, *Lankenau*; TODD H. GOLDBERG, *Einstein*; JERRY C. JOHNSON, *UPMC*; BRUCE KINOSIAN, *UPMC*; RISA LAVIZZO-MOUREY, *UPMC*; MARTIN LEICHT, *Temple*; KAREN NOVIELLI, *Jeff*; JOEL POSNER, *Allegheny* (SP: EXERCISE, NUTRITION); BRUCE SILVER, *Lankenau*

Ob/Gyn
General

EILEEN ENGLE, *Doylestown* (GYN, MENOPAUSE); JOSEPH FERRONI, *Paoli*; DAVID GOODNER, *Allegheny* (GYN); MARVIN R. HYETT, *Jeff* (GYN); RONALD M. JAFFE, *CMC* (GYN); DREW MELLEN, *Penna* (OB); OWEN MONTGOMERY, *Allegheny*; RICHARD NEMIROFF, *Penna*;

Joel I. Polin, *Abington*; Deborah Schrager, *Penna*; Beverly M. Vaughn, *Penna*; Robert Weinstein, *UPMC*; Victor Zachian, *Penna*

High-Risk Pregnancy

Ronald Bolognese, *Penna*; Frank J. Craparo, *Abington*; Alan E. Donnenfeld, *Penna* (sp: genetics); Linda K. Dunn, *Abington*; Andrew G. Gerson, *Lankenau*; Joel I. Polin, *Abington*; Nancy S. Roberts, *Lankenau*; Neil Silverman, *Jeff*; Stephen Smith, *Abington*; Ronald Wapner, *Jeff* (sp: genetics); Stuart Weiner, *Penna*

Infertility

Jerome H. Check, *CMC*; Stephen L. Corson, *Penna*; Christos Coutifaris, *UPMC*; Martin F. Freedman, *Abington*; Luigi Mastrioanni, *UPMC*; William H. Pfeffer, *Lankenau*; Jay F. Schinfeld, *Abington* (sp: lupus); Steven J. Sondheimer, *UPMC*

Gynecological Surgery

Marvin H. Terry Grody, *Temple* (sp: urogynecology & pelvic reconstruction); Richard Isenberg, *Penna*

Gynecological Oncology

Matthew Boente, *Fox Chase*; John A. Carlson Jr., *Jeff*; Charles Dunton, *Jeff*; Enrique Hernandez, *Allegheny*; W. Michael Hogan, *Fox Chase*; Charles E. Mangan, *Penna*; Mark Morgan, *UPMC*; Joel Noumoff, *Crozer-Chester*; Thomas F. Rocereto, *CMC*; Stephin C. Rubin, *UPMC*

Laparoscopy/Hysteroscopy

Stephen L. Corson, *Penna*; Benjamin Gocial, *Penna*; Francis L. Hutchins Jr., *Graduate*; Martin Weisberg, *Jeff*; Mark Woodland, *Penna*

Hematology-Oncology

Isadore Brodsky, *Allegheny*; Ronald Cantor, *Jeff*; Robert L. Comis, *Jeff*; H. James Day, *Abington*; John R. Durocher, *Penna*; Paul Engstrom, *Fox Chase*; Kevin R. Fox, *UPMC* (sp: breast cancer); John H. Glick, *UPMC*; Donna Glover, *Jeff*; Jack Goldberg, *CMC*; Du Pont Guerry, *UPMC* (sp: melanoma); Daniel G. Haller, *UPMC*; David H. Henry, *Graduate*; Sheldon Lisker, *Graduate*; John S. Macdonald, *Temple* (sp: gi); Kenneth F. Mangan, *Temple* (sp: bone marrow); Jose Martinez, *Jeff*; Bernard A. Mason, *Graduate*; Michael Mastrangelo, *Jeff*; Robert F. Ozals, *Fox Chase* (sp: ovarian cancer); Lynn Schuchter, *UPMC* (sp: melanoma); Edward A. Stadtmauer, *UPMC* (sp: bone marrow); Joseph Treat, *UPMC* (sp: lung cancer)

Infectious Diseases

Michael Braffman, *Jeff*; P.J. Brennan, *UPMC*; R. Michael Buckley, *Penna*; Neil Fishman, *UPMC* (sp: antibiotics); Stephen J. Gluckman, *UPMC*; Bennett Lorber, *Temple*; Rob Roy MacGregor, *UPMC* (sp: aids); Carl W. Norden, *CMC*; Jerome Santoro, *Lankenau*; David Schlossberg, *Episcopal*; Peter Spitzer, *Bryn Mawr*

Internal Medicine

Bonnie Lee Ashby, *Bryn Mawr*; Michael J. Baime, *Graduate*; Richard J. Baron, *Chestnut Hill*; Diane Barton, *CMC*; Michael Cirigliano, *UPMC*; Gary W. Crooks, *UPMC* (sp: vascular disease & hypercholesterolemia); Roger B. Daniels, *Penna*; Thomas De Berardinis, *Lankenau*; Gary W. Dorshimer, *Penna*; Bradley W. Fenton, *Penna*; Hal S.

HOCKFIELD, *Abington*; FREDERICK JONES, *UPMC*; ISRAEL H. LICHTENSTEIN, *Jeanes* (SP: INFECTIOUS DISEASE); GENO J. MERLI, *Jeff* (SP: VASCULAR DISEASE); HOWARD A. MILLER, *Allegheny*; PAUL M. ROEDIGER, *Abington*; MARIE A. SAVARD, *Penna* (SP: WOMEN'S HEALTH); GAIL B. SLAP, *UPMC* (SP: ADOLESCENT MEDICINE); THORNE SPARKMAN JR., *UPMC*; ELLEN TEDALDI, *Temple*; JOHN L. TURNER, *Graduate* (SP: AIDS); ED VINER, *CMC*

Nephrology

JAMES F. BURKE, *Jeff*; PEDRO FERNANDEZ, *VA*; GARY S. GILGORE, *Montgomery*; MARTIN GOLDBERG, *Temple*; ROBERT A. GROSSMAN, *UPMC*; SIDNEY KOBRIN, *UPMC*; JOHN D. KOETHE, *Penna*; BRENDA R.C. KURNIK, *CMC*; MICHAEL R. RUDNICK, *Graduate*; MILES H. SIGLER, *Lankenau*; ROBERT A. SIROTA, *Abington*; KEITH SUPERDOCK, *Lankenau*; BRENDAN P. TEEHAN, *Lankenau*; RAYMOND R. TOWNSEND, *UPMC* (SP: HYPERTENSION); ALAN G. WASSERSTEIN, *UPMC*

Neurology

ROBERT D. AIKEN, *Jeff* (SP: BRAIN TUMORS); ARTHUR ASBURG, *UPMC*; RODNEY D. BELL, *Jeff* (SP: CEREBROVASCULAR); THOMAS BOSLEY, *Penna* (SP: NEURO-OPHTHALMOLOGY); MARK J. BROWN, *UPMC* (SP: EMG); SHAWN BYRD, *UPMC* (SP: ELECTRODIAGNOSTICS); CHRISTOPHER M. CLARK, *UPMC* (SP: MEMORY DISORDERS); DAVID G. COOK, *Penna*; H. BRANCH COSLETT, *Temple* (SP: COGNITIVE DISORDERS); MARK D'ESPOSITO, *UPMC* (SP: COGNITIVE DISORDERS); JUNE FRY, *Allegheny* (SP: SLEEP DISORDERS); STEPHEN M. GOLLOMP, *Lankenau* (SP: MOVEMENT DISORDERS); LEONARD GRAZIANI, *Jeff* (SP: PEDIATRICS); JEFFREY GREENSTEIN, *Temple* (SP: NEURO-IMMUNOLOGY); TERRY HEIMAN-PATTERSON, *Jeff* (SP: NEUROMUSCULAR); HOWARD HURTIG, *Graduate*; LAWRENCE KERSON, *Montgomery* (SP: NEURO-OPHTHALMOLOGY); FRED LUBLIN, *Jeff* (SP: MS); MARK MOSTER, *Einstein* (SP: NEURO-OPHTHALMOLOGY); DAVID PLEASURE, *CHOP*; ERIC RAPS, *UPMC*; DAVID ROBY, *Jeannes*; DONALD SCHOTLAND, *UPMC* (SP: NEUROMUSCULAR); PAUL SCHRAEDER, *CMC* (SP: EPILEPSY); DONALD SILBERBERG, *UPMC* (SP: MS); STEPHEN SILBERSTEIN, *Germantown* (SP: HEADACHES); MICHAEL SPERLING, *Graduate* (SP: EPILEPSY); MATTHEW STERN, *Graduate* (SP: PARKINSON'S)

Ophthalmology
General

ROBERT BAILEY JR., *Chestnut Hill*; SYLVIA BECK, *Allegheny*; DION EHRLICH, *Abington*; ZORAIDA FIOL-SILVA, *Wills* (SP: CONTACT LENSES); MARVIN GREENBAUM, *Scheie*; EDWARD JAEGER, *Wills*; LOUIS KARP, *Penna*; MICHAEL KAY, *Wills*; W. REED KINDERMAN, *Wills*; DAVID KOZART, *Scheie*; JAMES NACHBAR, *Wills*; MICHAEL NAIDOFF, *Wills*; CHARLES NICHOLS, *UPMC*; RICHARD PRINCE, *Holy Redeemer*; ROBERT REINECKE, *Wills* (SP: PEDIATRIC); RICHARD TIPPERMAN, *Lankenau*; T. RAMSEY THORP, *Chestnut Hill*; VINCENT YOUNG, *Einstein*

Cataracts

RAYMOND ADAMS, *Wills*; DANIEL KANE, *Wills*; STEPHEN LICHTENSTEIN, *Lankenau*; HERBERT NEVYAS, *Allegheny*; STEVEN SIEPSER, *Montgomery*; MYRON YANOFF, *Allegheny*

Cornea

ELISABETH COHEN, *Wills*; PETER R. LAIBSON, *Wills*; STEPHEN ORLIN, *Scheie*; IRVING RABER, *Wills*

Glaucoma

MARLENE MOSTER, *Lankenau*; JODY PILTZ-SEYMOUR, *UPMC*; GEORGE SPAETH, *Wills*; ELLIOT WERNER, *Allegheny*; RICHARD WILSON, *Wills*

Neuro-Ophthalmology
THOMAS M. BOSLEY, *Penna*; STEVEN L. GALETTA, *UPMC* (SP: NEUROLOGY); MARK MOSTER, *Einstein*; PETER J. SAVINO, *Wills*; ROBERT C. SERGOTT, *Lankenau*

Ocular Oncology
JAMES J. AUGSBURGER, *Wills*; CAROL L. SHIELDS, *Wills*; JERRY A. SHIELDS, *Wills*

Ophthalmic Plastic Surgery
MARC S. COHEN, *Wills*; JOSEPH C. FLANAGAN, *Wills*; SUSAN M. HUGHES, *Wills*; JAMES A. KATOWITZ, *CHOP*; MARLON MAUS, *Wills*; DAVID B. SOLL, *Frankford*; MARY A. STEFANYSZYN, *Wills*; (SP: ORBITAL TUMORS); ALLAN E. WULC, *Abington*

Refractive Surgery
FREDERIC B. KREMER, *Graduate*; JAMES G. NACHBAR, *Wills*; IRVING RABER, *Lankenau*; CHRISTOPHER J. RAPUANO, *Wills*

Retina and Vitreous
WILLIAM BENSON, *Wills*; GARY C. BROWN, *Wills*; ALEXANDER BRUCKER, *Scheie*; JAY FEDERMAN, *Allegheny*; DAVID FISCHER, *Wills*; RICHARD GOLDBERG, *Wills*; ALBERT MAGUIRE, *Scheie*; ARUNAN SIVALINGAM, *Wills*; WILLIAM TASMAN, *Wills*

Otolaryngology
JOSEPH ATKINS, *Penna* (SP: HEAD AND NECK); DOUGLAS BIGELOW, *UPMC*; (SP: CRANIAL BASE SURGERY); RICHARD HAYDEN, *Allegheny* (SP: HEAD AND NECK); GLENN ISAACSON, *St. Chris*; WILLIAM KEANE, *Jeff* (SP: HEAD & NECK); DAVID KENNEDY, *UPMC* (SP: SINUS); DONALD C. LANZA, *UPMC*; FRANK MARLOWE, *Allegheny*; WILLIAM POTSIC, *CHOP*; CHARLES L. ROJER, *Abington*; MAX RONIS, *Temple*; ROBERT SATALOFF, *Jeff* (SP: NEUROTOLOGY, VOICE CARE); HARVEY SILBERMAN, *Jeanes*

Pathology
BARBARA ATKINSON, *Allegheny* (SP: CYTO); HERBERT AUERBACH, *Abington*; FREDERIC BARR, *UPMC* (SP: MOLECULAR); HUGH BONNER, *Chester County* (SP: HEMO); EDISON CATALANO, *CMC* (SP: HEMO); HARRY COOPER, *Fox Chase* (SP: GI); MARY CUNNANE, *Penna* (SP: CYTO); DAVID ELDER, *UPMC* (SP: MELANOMA); PRABODH GUPTA, *UPMC* (SP: CYTO); PETER FARANO, *Holy Redeemer*; RICHARD JACOBY, *Jeff* (SP: DERMO); TILDE KLINE, *Lankenau* (SP: CYTO); VIRGINIA LIVOLSI, *UPMC*; LESLIE LITSKY, *UPMC* (SP: PULMONARY); FRANCIS MCBREARTY, *Lankenau*; ARTHUR PATCHEFSKY, *Fox Chase*; LUCY RORKE, *CHOP*; EMANUEL RUBIN, *Jeff* (SP: LIVER); MIN SOHN, *Graduate* (SP: GI); JOHN TOMASZEWSKI, *UPMC* (SP: KIDNEY); JAMES WHEELER, *UPMC* (SP: GYN)

Physical Medicine
ERNEST BARAN, *Nazareth* (SP: ELECTRODIAGNOSTICS); FRANCIS J. BONNER JR., *Graduate* (SP: OSTEOPOROSIS); JOHN DITUNNO, *Jeff*; MARK ELLEN, *UPMC* (SP: SHOULDERS); ALBERTO ESQUENAZI, *Moss*; GARY GOLDBERG, *Moss* (SP: BRAIN INJURY); GERALD HERBISON, *Jeff* (SP: REHAB); NATHANIEL MAYER, *Einstein* (SP: BRAIN INJURY); JOHN MELVIN, *Moss* (SP: DISABILITY EVALUATION); FRANCIS NASO, *Jeff* (SP: CARDIAC REHAB); JUDITH PETERSON, *Jeff* (SP: PAIN MANAGEMENT); KEITH ROBINSON, *UPMC* (SP: COGNITIVE AND GERIATRIC); CURTIS SLIPMAN, *UPMC* (SP: NONSURGICAL NECK AND BACK); WILLIAM STAAS JR., *Magee*; JAY SIEGFRIED, *Lankenau* (SP: REHAB); V. THEERASAKDI, *Abington* (SP: GAIT AND MOTOR CONTROL)

Psychiatry

SALMAN AKHTAR, *Jeff*; HOWARD BAKER, *Institute* (SP: ADHD); KENNETH COHEN, *Belmont*; WILLIAM DUBIN, *Belmont* (SP: GERIATRICS); PHILIP ESCOLL, *Institute* (SP: PSYCHOANALYSIS); DAVID FINK, *Institute/Jeff* (SP: MPP); PAUL FINK, CHARTER FAIRMOUNT; ELIO FRATTAROLI, *private practice*; GREGG GORTON, *Jeff*; IRA HERMAN, *UPMC* (SP: COGNITIVE); RICHARD KLUFT, *Institute/Jeff* (SP: MPP); SYDNEY PULVER, *Institute*; LAWRENCE REAL, *Belmont* (SP: SCHIZOPHRENIA); STEPHEN SCHWARTZ, *Jeff*; BRADLEY SEVIN, *Penna*; JAMES STINNETT, *UPMC*; TROY THOMPSON II, *Jeff*; ROBERT TOBOROWSKY, *Penna* (SP: FORENSICS); MICHAEL VERGARE, *Einstein* (SP: GERIATRICS); EDWARD VOLKMAN, *Einstein* (SP: SCHIZOPHRENIA)

Child/Adolescence

PAUL AMBROSINI, *Allegheny* (SP: DEPRESSION); MARYANNE DELANEY, *Allegheny*; JOSEPHINE ELIA, *Allegheny* (SP: ADHD); DAVID ELLIS, *Institute*; SELMA KRAMER, *Jeff*; RICHARD MALONE, *Allegheny* (SP: AUTISM); HENRI PARENS, *Jeff*; ANTHONY ROSTAIN, *CHOP* (SP: ADHD/LEARNING DISABILITIES); JOEL SCHWARTZ, *Abington*; ELLEN SHOLEVAR, *Temple*; G. PIEROOZ SHOLEVAR, *CMC*; WALTER H. TROFFKIN, *Einstein*

Eating Disorders

SUSAN ICE, *Belmont*; LAURENCE B. MILLER, *Renfrew*; MICHAEL PERTSHUK, *Friends*; BARBARA WINGATE, *UPMC*

Family Therapy

ELLEN M. BERMAN, *UPMC*; HOWARD DICHTER, *Belmont*; ROBERT GARFIELD, *Allegheny*; MARTIN GOLDBERG, *Institute*; JOHN SARGENT, *Child Guidance*; OSCAR R. WEINER, *Allegheny*

Geriatric

GARY GOTTLIEB, *Friends*; DAVID GREENSPAN, *Institute* (SP: DEPRESSION); IRA R. KATZ, *UPMC*; ANAND KUMAR, *UPMC*; MARTHA LITTLE, *Abington*; BARRY ROVNER, *Wills/Jeff*; BARBARA A. SCHINDLER, *Allegheny*; RUTH STEINMAN, *Institute*; JOEL E. STREIM, *UPMC*

Substance Addiction

KEVIN P. CAPUTO, *Crozer-Chester*; CHARLES GIANNASIO, *Abington*; DONALD GILL, *Institute*; MICHAEL J. MCCARTHY, *Institute*; JOSEPH VOLPICELLI, *UPMC*; GEORGE WOODY, *UPMC*

Psychopharmacology

WILLIAM BALL, *UPMC* (SP: DEPRESSION); BURR EICHELMAN, *Temple*; ALAN M. GRUENBERG, *Institute/Jeff*; LASZLO GYULAI, *UPMC* (SP: BI-POLAR); MARTIN ROSENSWEIG, *Institute*; JOHN M. RUSK, *Bryn Mawr* (SP: ADHD); EDWARD SCHWEIZER, *UPMC*; RICHARD F. SUMMERS, *Institute*; STEVEN TARGUM, *Crozer-Chester*; THEODORE WEISS, *Lankenau*; HYONG UN, *Institute*; HARRY ZALL, *Institute* (SP: MOOD DISORDERS)

Pulmonary Medicine

MICHAEL CASEY, *Penna*; GERARD CRINER, *Temple*; PAUL EPSTEIN, *Graduate*; STANLEY FIEL, *Allegheny* (SP: CYSTIC FIBROSIS); JAMES FISH, *Jeff*; LEE GREENSPON, *Lankenau*; MICHAEL GRIPPI, *UPMC*; JOHN HANSEN-FLASCHEN, *UPMC*; ROBERT KOTLOFF, *UPMC*; MICHAEL LIPPMANN, *Einstein*; EUGENE LUGANO, *Penna*; HAROLD I. PALEVSKY, *UPMC*; DONALD PETERSON, *Lankenau* (SP: SLEEP DISORDERS); MELVIN R. PRATTER, *CMC*; S. DAVID SCOTT, *Jeff*; RICHARD SNYDER, *Abington*; DANIEL STERMAN, *UPMC*; MICHAEL UNGER, *Penna* (SP: LASER BRONCHOSCOPY)

Radiology
Diagnostic
Abass Alavi, *UPMC* (sp: nuclear medicine); Marc Banner, *UPMC* (sp: urology); Bernard Birnbaum, *UPMC* (sp: abdominal); Emily Conant, *Jeff* (sp: breast); Murray Dalinka, *UPMC* (sp: musculoskeletal); Stephen Feig, *Jeff* (sp: breast); Warren Gefter, *UPMC* (sp: chest); Seth Glick, *Allegheny* (sp: GI); Barry Goldberg, *Jeff* (sp: ultrasound); Robert Grossman, *UPMC* (sp: kidney); Ziv Haskal, *UPMC* (sp: interventional); Richard Herzog, *UPMC* (sp: MRI); Robert Hurst, *UPMC* (sp: interventional neuro); Ami Iskandrain, *Allegheny* (sp: cardiac nuclear medicine); Alfred Kurtz, *Jeff* (sp: ultrasound); Igor Laufer, *UPMC* (sp: GI); Marc Levine, *UPMC* (sp: GI); Wallace Miller, *UPMC* (sp: chest); Vijay Rao, *Jeff* (sp: head and neck); Mitchell D. Schnall, *UPMC* (sp: MRI); Mark Schweitzer, *Jeff* (sp: musculo-skeletal); Michael Soulen, *UPMC* (sp: interventional); Daniel Sullivan, *UPMC* (sp: breast); Robert Zimmerman, *CHOP* (sp: neuro)

Oncologic
Luther Brady, *Allegheny*; Lawrence Coia, *Fox Chase* (sp: GI); Barbara Fowble, *Fox Chase* (sp: breast); John Glassburn, *Penna*; Joel Goldwein, *UPMC* (sp: pediatric); Gerald Hanks, *Fox Chase* (sp: prostate); Lydia Komarnicky, *Jeff*; Rachelle Lanciano, *Fox Chase* (sp: GI, GYN); William Powlis, *Crozer-Chester* (sp: lymphoma); Melvyn Richter, *Abington*; Lawrence Solin, *UPMC* (sp: breast); Jeffrey Wenger, *CMC* (sp: breast); Richard Whittington, *UPMC* (sp: GI/GYN)

Rheumatology
Martin Bergman, *Taylor*; Raphael J. Dehoratius, *Jeff* (sp: lupus); Bruce Freundlich, *Graduate*; Gary Gordon, *Lankenau*; Bruce Hoffman, *Allegheny*; Sergio Jimenez, *Jeff* (sp: scleroderma); Warren Katz, *Presby*; Antonio Reginato, *CMC*; Barry Schimmer, *Penna*; Ralph Schumacher, *UPMC*; Frederick Vivino, *Presby* (sp: sjögrens syndrome)

Surgical Specialists

Cardiac/Thoracic
Mark Adkins, *Einstein* (sp: cardiac); Joseph Bavaria, *UPMC*; Herbert Cohn, *Jeff* (sp: thoracic only); Anthony Delrossi, *CMC* (sp: thoracic aneurisms); Verdi DiSesa, *Allegheny*; Richard Edie, *Jeff*; Timothy J. Gardner, *UPMC*; Scott Goldman, *Lankenau*; W. Clark Hargrove, *Allegheny* (sp: valves); Larry Kaiser, *UPMC* (sp: thoracic only); James Sink, *Allegheny*; Michael D. Strong III, *Allegheny*

Colon/Rectal
Scott D. Goldstein, *Jeff*; Gerald Marks, *Allegheny*; Joseph Nejman, *Abington*; Mark Pello, *CMC*; Robin Rosenberg, *Allegheny*; Stephen Silver, *Delco Memorial*

General Surgery
Patricia Bailey, *Chestnut Hill*; Daniel T. Dempsey, *Temple*; Robert Fried, *Paoli*; Robert Minor, *West Jersey*; Jon Morris, *UPMC* (sp: laparoscopic); David Paskin, *Penna*; Ernest Rosato, *UPMC*; Francis Rosato, *Jeff*; David Rose, *Bryn Mawr* (sp: laparoscopic); Joel Roslyn, *Allegheny*, (sp: GI); Alan Schuricht, *Penna* (sp: laparoscopic)

Breast Cancer

Marcia Boraas, *Jeanes*; Tom Frazier, *Bryn Mawr*; Anne L. Rosenberg, *Jeff*; Dahlia Sataloff, *Graduate*; Gordon F. Schwartz, *Jeff*; Robert G. Somers, *Einstein*; Michael Torosian, *UPMC*

Oncology Only

Burton L. Eisenberg, *Fox Chase*; Douglas Fraker, *UPMC*; Chris Pezzi, *Abington*

Neurosurgery

David Andrews, *Jeff* (SP: BRAIN TUMORS); Leonard Bruno, *Allegheny*; Stephen Dante, *Penna*; Eugene S. Flamm, *UPMC* (SP: VASCULAR); Thomas Gennarelli, *Allegheny* (SP: BRAIN TUMORS); H. Warren Goldman, *Jeff*; Paul Marcotte, *UPMC* (SP: SPINE); Raj Narayan, *Temple* (SP: HEAD TRAUMA); Michael O'Connor, *Graduate* (SP: EPILEPSY); Robert Rosenwasser, *Jeff* (SP: CEREBROVASCULAR/INTERVENTIONAL); Frederick Simeone, *Jeff* (SP: MICRO); Leslie Sutton, *CHOP*; Eric Zager, *UPMC* (SP: PERIPHERAL NERVE)

Organ Transplant
Heart

Michael Acker, *UPMC*; Verdi J. Disesa, *Allegheny*; Valluvan Jeevanandam, *Temple*; James B. McClurken, *Temple*; Rohinton Morris, *Allegheny*

Lung

Joseph Bavaria, *UPMC*; Larry Kaiser, *UPMC*

Kidney/Pancreas

Francisco Badosa, *Einstein*; Clyde Barker, *UPMC*; Kenneth Brayman, *UPMC*; Stephen Dunn, *St. Chris*; David Laskow, *Allegheny*; Michael Moritz, *Jeff* (KIDNEY ONLY); Ali Naji, *UPMC*

Liver

Stephen Dunn, *St. Chris*; Michael Moritz, *Jeff*; Cosme Manzarbeitia, *Einstein*; Ali Naji, *UPMC*; Kim Olthoff, *UPMC*; Abraham Shaked, *UPMC*

Orthopedics
General

Christopher Born, *CMC* (SP: TRAUMA); Michael Clancy, *Temple*; William Delong, *CMC* (SP: TRAUMA); Malcolm Ecker, *Chestnut Hill* (SP: SCOLIOSIS); John Esterhai Jr., *UPMC* (SP: NONUNION FRACTURES); Robert Good, *Bryn Mawr* (SP: SHOULDERS, HIPS, KNEES); Michael Gratch, *Abington* (SP: SPINE); John Gregg, *CHOP*; Frederick Kaplan, *UPMC* (SP: OSTEOPOROSIS); Mary Ann Keenan, *Einstein* (SP: NEUROMUSCULAR); Richard Lackman, *Allegheny* (SP: ONCOLOGY)

Foot and Ankle

Paul Angotti, *Abington*; Michael S. Downey, *Presby*; Ira Fox, *CMC*; Paul Hecht, *Allegheny*; Kieran Mahan, *Presby*; Paul R. Quintavalle, *West Jersey* (SP: DIABETES); Keith L. Wapner; *Allegheny*

Hands

John M. Bednar, *Jeff* (SP: WRIST ARTHROSCOPY); F. William Bora Jr., *UPMC*; Randall

CULP, *Jeff*; WILLIAM KIRKPATRICK, *Bryn Mawr*; BONG SIK LEE, *Graduate*; MARK NISSENBAUM, *Abington*; A. LEE OSTERMAN, *Jeff*; LAWRENCE H. SCHNEIDER, *Jeff*; JOHN S. TARAS, *Jeff*

Joints
ROBERT BOOTH, *Penna* (SP: KNEES); JOHN FENLIN JR., *Jeff* (SP: SHOULDERS); ROBERT FITZGERALD, *UPMC* (SP: INFECTIONS); WILLIAM HOZACK, *Penna* (SP: HIP AND KNEE REVISIONS); ERIC HUME, *Jeff* (SP: HIPS AND KNEES); NORMAN JOHANSON, *Temple* (SP: HIPS AND KNEES); PAUL LOTKE, *UPMC*; RICHARD ROTHMAN, *Penna* (SP: HIPS); MARVIN STEINBERG, *UPMC* (SP: HIPS); GERALD WILLIAMS JR., *UPMC* (SP: SHOULDERS)

Spine
TODD ALBERT, *Penna*; RICHARD BALDERSTON, *Penna*; RANDAL BETZ, *Temple*, JEROME COTLER, *Jeff*; DENNIS DRUMMOND, *CHOP*; ALEXANDER VACCARO, *Jeff*

Sports Medicine
FREDERICK BALDUINI, *Graduate* (SP: JOINT RECONSTRUCTION); ART BARTOLOZZI, *Penna* (SP: KNEE & SHOULDER); MICHAEL CICCOTTI, *Penna*; NICHOLAS DINUBILE, *Delco Memorial* (SP: ARTHROSCOPIC SURGERY, INJURY REHAB); VINCENT DI STEFANO, *Graduate*; WILLIAM EMPER, *Bryn Mawr* (SP: SHOULDERS & KNEES); JOHN GREGG, *CHOP*; LAWRENCE MILLER, *Lankenau* (SP: KNEES & SHOULDERS); PEKKA MOOAR, *Allegheny* (SP: TRAUMA); BRIAN SENNETT, *Allegheny*; JOSEPH TORG, *Allegheny*

Plastic and Cosmetic Surgery
Facial/Cosmetic
JAMES FOX, *Jeff* (SP: BREASTS); HERBERT KEAN, *Jeff* (SP: NOSES); PAUL KIM, *Brandywine*; JULIUS NEWMAN, *Graduate*; R. BARRETT NOONE, *Bryn Mawr*; HARVEY M. ROSEN, *Penna* (SP: MAXILLOFACIAL); RICHARD SCIPIONE, *Graduate* (SP: NOSES); LINTON WHITAKER, *UPMC*

Liposuction
RICHARD L. DOLSKY, *Mercy Catholic*; ZAKI S. FTAIHA, *Graduate*; DAVID W. LOW, *UPMC*; R. BARRETT NOONE, *Bryn Mawr*

Reconstructive
LENORA BAROT, *CMC*; SCOTT P. BARTLETT, *UPMC* (SP: CRANIOFACIAL); ARTHUR BROWN, *CMC* (SP: CONGENITAL DEFORMITIES); MARK GRANICK, *Allegheny* (SP: HEAD AND NECK); JOSEPH F. KUSIAK, *Fox Chase* (SP: ONCOLOGY); DON LAROSA, *UPMC*; AMIT MITRA, *Temple* (SP: HANDS); JOHN MOORE JR., *Jeff*; DENNIS MONTEIRO, *Graduate*; J. BRIAN MURPHY, *Bryn Mawr*; R. BARRETT NOONE, *Bryn Mawr*; HARVEY ROSEN, *Penna*; LINTON WHITAKER, *UPMC*

Trauma Surgery
COLLIN E.M. BRATHWAITE, *Crozer-Chester*; ROBERT F. BUCKMAN JR., *Temple*; PATRICK M. REILLY, *UPMC*; STEVEN E. ROSS, *CMC*; MICHAEL F. ROTONDO, *UPMC*; C. WILLIAM SCHWAB, *UPMC*; STANLEY Z. TROOSKIN, *Allegheny*; JEROME J. VERNICK, *Jeff*

Urology
DEMETRIUS BAGLEY, *Jeff* (SP: ENDO-UROLOGY); P. KENNETH BROWNSTEIN, *Jeff*; JOHN DUCKETT, *CHOP*; LEONARD GOMELLA, *Jeff* (SP: CANCER); RICHARD GREENBERG, *Fox Chase* (SP: CANCER); PHILIP HANNO, *Temple* (SP: FEMALE UROLOGY, SEXUAL DYSFUNCTION); S. BRUCE MALKOWICZ, *UPMC* (SP: CANCER); TERRENCE MALLOY, *Penna*; JOEL MARMAR, *CMC*

(SP: MALE INFERTILITY); S. GRANT MULHOLLAND, *Jeff*; KEITH VAN ARSDALEN, *UPMC* (SP: STONES); ALAN WEIN, *UPMC* (SP: VOIDING DISFUNCTION); KRISTENE WHITMORE, *Graduate* (SP: FEMALE UROLOGY)

Vascular Surgery

HENRY BERKOWITZ, *Presby* (SP: AORTIC ANEURISM); KEITH CALLIGARO, *Penna*; ANTHONY CARABASI, *Jeff* (SP: CEREBRAL VASCULAR); JEFFREY CARPENTER, *UPMC*; ANTHONY J. COMEROTA, *Temple*; PETER MCCOMBS, *Abington*; ANDREW ROBERTS, *Allegheny*; STANTON SMULLENS, *Jeff* (SP: CAROTID ARTERY); MICHAEL WEINGARTEN, *Crozer-Chester* (SP: WOUND CARE)

Note: Many doctors on the list are affiliated with more than one hospital. Research assistance by Scott Ball, Kathleen Cooney, Laura Goodman, Ann Grant, Farah Lipitz, Marc Lombardi, Christina Macauly, Robyn Post and Julia Ricciuti.

If you're thinking about having laser eye surgery, or cataract removal, here're a few reasons why you ought to consider what we, at Kremer Laser Eye Center, can offer...

- The unique **LASER-K**[sm] procedure that can often eliminate the need for glasses or contacts and can offer a **faster recovery time** and **greater comfort.**
- In addition to treating **nearsightedness** and **farsightedness**, **LASER-K**[sm] can **simultaneously treat astigmatism.**
- **More experience** in performing refractive eye surgery than anyone else in the region – over fifteen years.
- **Cataract removal without stitches or injections.**
- **Cosmetic eye laser surgery.**
- Cornea, retina and glaucoma treatment.
- A state-of-the-art Center, **directed by a doctor named as a "Top Doc"** in May 1996 issue of *Philadelphia Magazine* and staffed by experienced and caring professionals.

We'll be glad to answer all of your questions and give you any information you require without obligation about the most advanced procedures available today. **All it takes is a phone call.**

1-800-694-3937

Philadelphia • Hatboro • King of Prussia Kutztown • Pottstown

KREMER LASER EYE CENTER

Trust your eyes to experience.

CHAPTER 6

Centers of Excellence

The best all-in-one facilities for special problems from headaches to heart disease, sports medicine to sleep disorders

I've been diagnosed with Parkinson's disease and told I'll need care and management for the rest of my life. Where's the best place to get it?

My five-year-old eats only three foods. Is there somewhere I can take him to be checked for an eating disorder?

We've had five miscarriages and been told nothing is wrong—they just say to keep trying. Is there a center for people with our problem?

Mom is depressed and seems out of it. Who does the best geriatric assessments?

The doctor can't explain this dizziness that's driving me crazy. How can I find out if I've got something treatable?

At some point in our lives, almost all of us will need some kind of special medical treatment. In that event, we should be thankful we're going to get sick in Philadelphia. This region has some of the country's finest doctors practicing at nearly 100 hospitals—five of which ranked in *U.S. News and World Report*'s 1994 list of America's best hospitals. But the abundance of options can make informed choices confusing.

While many health organizations are suddenly focused on measuring quality care, their numerical assessments of clinical outcomes and mortality rates provide only limited guidance to the average consumer. Ditto for the barrage of advertising that seems to sell hospitals as slickly as cars. These days nearly every hospital boasts a marketing department that packages its services. A favored gimmick is the creation of The Center for ... In reality, many of these so-called centers turn out to be little more than a title slapped on a group of specialists doing nothing special in a suite of gray and mauve offices.

These marketing ploys are hard to distinguish from the real McCoys—places that fulfill the true definition of a center of excellence. What exactly does that mean? In our opinion, the standard is a one-stop shopping headquarters for a particular problem, whether a headache or a hip replacement. The center should be staffed by reputable senior-level people and its examinations performed by experts, not trainees. It should offer a wide scope of support and auxiliary services, be engaged in important research and involved in educational outreach. When high-tech equipment matters, there should be no question that they've got the latest. Another criterion is the ease of getting an appointment. If you have to be a friend of the pope to get in without a six-month wait, forget it.

To separate the bogus from the best, we solicited suggestions from hundreds of physicians on *Philadelphia Magazine*'s top doctors list and asked area hospitals to name their top centers. Many of the responses were followed up with site visits and personal interviews. From this process, we're now able to issue our report card on the outstanding treatment centers, from adolescent health care to wounds that won't heal.

It's not surprising that most of our selections come from university medical centers, because they have the funding and resources to support centers of excellence. That doesn't mean there aren't fine services available at community hospitals, too, where convenience and familiarity with the doctors may be important personal considerations. If, for example, you live in Jenkintown, there's no reason to ignore the in vitro fertilization clinic or the cardiac program at Abington Hospital.

Although managed care has narrowed the options for many of us, it hasn't totally eliminated the notion of choice. When your life and your health are on the line, why not the best?

Adolescent Medicine

Adolescent Clinic of Children's Hospital
34TH STREET AND CONVENTION BOULEVARD,
PHILADELPHIA (215-590-3537)

Teenagers frequently think they're too old for a pediatrician but are embarrassed to talk to their mom's doctor about birth control. This broad-based, nationally recognized clinic bridges that gap, providing a personal physician for 2,500 patients ages 12 to 19. "If you look at what kills kids—HIV, suicide, violence, car accidents—75 percent is related to behaviors," says Dr. Kenneth Ginsburg. "So we're sensitive to the total environment. By picking up depression in a kid, we might prevent a later drug problem." For patients who prefer a more private setting, the clinic works closely with Teen Health Associates, a CHOP faculty practice.

ALS (Lou Gehrig's Disease)

ALS Clinical Services Center
ALLEGHENY UNIVERSITY HOSPITALS, CENTER CITY
(FORMERLY HAHNEMANN UNIVERSITY HOSPITAL),
1427 VINE STREET, PHILADELPHIA (215-762-6890)

The obvious link between Lou Gehrig's disease and baseball wasn't the only reason the Phillies raised $1.4 million for this clinic over the past several years. Allegheny's center, which set the standard for long-term management of ALS and is one of only nine programs certified by the national ALS Association, can help with every problem the ALS patient is likely to encounter—from breathing to diet to navigating the insurance maze. The center is also involved in experimental drug trials and clinical research.

Balance Disorders

The Balance Center
UNIVERSITY OF PENNSYLVANIA MEDICAL CENTER, FIVE SILVERSTEIN, 3400 SPRUCE STREET, PHILADELPHIA (215-662-6017)

Serious inner-ear problems have traditionally been among the most perplexing medical mysteries—which is what makes this new center so valuable. The medically diverse staff of 18 figures out the cases that others can't: bizarre vertigo found to be the result of Lyme disease, persistent ear stuffiness that turned out to be caused by a benign tumor, recurrent dizziness connected to an autoimmune disease that was detected only by a sophisticated protein test available nowhere else in the city.

Birth Defects

Craniofacial Clinic
CHILDREN'S HOSPITAL OF PHILADELPHIA, 34TH STREET AND CIVIC CENTER BOULEVARD, PHILADELPHIA (215-590-2208)

"What I like most about working here," says nurse coordinator Patty Shultz, "is that we see so many of these kids as babies and often get to know them all the way through their teen years." They are kids like Joey, born with a cleft in his face from his eyes to his mouth. The Furlong, Pennsylvania, youngster first had surgery at six months; operations timed to his growth continued over the next decade. Along the way, he had access to this unique clinic's legion of experts—top-flight plastic, reconstructive and neurosurgeons, a psychologist, an anthropologist (to chart bone growth), a social worker, a pediatrician, an orthodontist, a geneticist, an audiologist, a speech pathologist and a paramedical cosmetician—in other words, every human resource imaginable to help kids like Joey look and feel normal.

Cerebral Palsy Clinic
CHILDREN'S SEASHORE HOUSE, 3405 CIVIC CENTER BOULEVARD, PHILADELPHIA (215-895-3835)

For the bewildered parents of a child born with CP, this affordable consultation service is a godsend. It furnishes case management to 200 families under a Pennsylvania state grant that allows it to accept any payment insurance will cover. Children undergo a thorough examination by a team of specialists who then meet to determine treatment—everything from suggestions about appropriate wheelchairs to the right drugs and diet to be implemented by the child's physician and school. Patients return periodically for an update and can call the clinic for advice at any time. Patients from other states are seen on a fee-for-service basis.

Cystic Fibrosis Center
St. Christopher's Hospital for Children,
Erie Avenue at Front Street, Philadelphia
(215-427-5183)

In just 20 years, the average life expectancy of a child born with this fatal genetic disease has increased from 13 to 29 years. Much of that is due to drug advances, but just as important is the expert medical management offered at clinics like this one—the third-largest CF center in the United States. The 375 young patients treated here each year benefit from an active research program; top pulmonologists, nurses and physical and respiratory therapists; nutrition counseling; social work; informal support groups; and formal education programs. Many patients have been inspired to pursue careers in the health field.

Bone Marrow Transplants

Bone Marrow Transplant Center
Allegheny University Hospitals, Center City
(formerly Hahnemann University Hospital),
Broad and Vine streets, Philadelphia
(215-762-4695)

When Hahnemann did the Delaware Valley's first bone marrow transplant in 1976, it was highly experimental. Some 600 patients later, it's become the treatment of choice for certain leukemias and lymphomas and the last hope for advanced metastatic breast cancer. Patients, who spend several weeks undergoing the intensive procedure, have rooms with a stunning view of the city and the support of a veteran medical, nursing and psychological team. Allegheny Center City offers both autologous (using one's own bone marrow) and allogeneic (using the marrow of a brother or sister) transplants. But it is the only hospital in the city—and one of just a dozen nationwide—doing transplants of bone marrow from a matched but unrelated donor.

Other bone marrow transplant centers of excellence:

Bone Marrow and Stem Cell Transplant Program, University of Pennsylvania Medical Center, 3400 Spruce Street, Philadelphia (215-662-7909). Autologous and allogeneic transplants with a specialty in innovative stem cell purging techniques; last year conducted 130 autologous transplants, the highest volume in the region.

Bone Marrow Transplant Program, Temple University Hospital, 3400 North Broad Street, Philadelphia (215-707-2847). Both autologous and allogeneic blood stem cell and bone marrow transplants; currently performing more than 80 transplants per year.

Cooper Hospital/University Medical Center, One Cooper Plaza, Camden, N.J. (609-963-3572). Innovative transplant program involving 50 patients a year.

Brain Injury

Bryn Mawr Rehab
414 Paoli Pike, Malvern (610-251-5400)

Drucker Brain Injury Center
MossRehab, 1200 Tabor Road, Philadelphia (215-456-9700)

Helping one of the 750,000 Americans with serious brain injury return to self-sufficiency is a long, arduous process requiring a broad team of professionals—the kind found at both Drucker and Bryn Mawr. Bryn Mawr's 141 beds and 186-acre suburban site allow it to offer luxuries like aquatic, equestrian and horticultural therapy. Drucker, located in a 152-bed facility in Philadelphia's Olney section, is directed by Dr. Nathaniel Mayer, a true pioneer in the field, and has the advantage of being adjacent to Albert Einstein Medical Center for emergency medical needs.

Breast Cancer

Breast Cancer Program
University of Pennsylvania Cancer Center,
6 Penn Tower, 3400 Spruce Street, Philadelphia (215-349-5024)

After a slight "thickening" was detected in her left breast, Princeton's Cecile was bounced from doctor to doctor. One took a mammogram and said not to worry. Another performed lumpectomies and recommended a double mastectomy. Finally, Cecile came to Penn, where under the Breast Cancer Program's weekly Breast Cancer Evaluation Center, she met with surgeons, a medical oncologist and a breast radiation specialist, and had a counseling session. On her very next visit, she got the good news: It looked as if radiation in her hometown combined with periodic chemotherapy at Penn would do the trick. "I'm sure they do the same thing all the time," a healthy Cecile says two years later. "But they made me feel unique." And there's more to recommend Penn's program: Dr. John Glick is a giant in the field, and Dr. Barbara Weber, a key participant in the search for the "breast cancer gene," has set up one of the country's first programs to test women from families with a high incidence of the disease for the presence of the genetic mutation.

The Breast Cancer Program at Fox Chase
Fox Chase Cancer Center, 7701 Burholme Avenue, Philadelphia (215-728-6900)

Fox Chase Cancer Center's Margaret Dyson Family Risk Assessment Program, directed by medical oncologist Mary Daly, was the first in the area to provide genetic counseling for families at high risk for breast and ovarian cancer.

Fox Chase has also begun testing for the breast cancer gene and, like Penn, has a full complement of geneticists, technicians and genetic counselors to make sure this tricky business is handled accurately and sensitively. The program also boasts the skills of radiation oncologist Dr. Barbara Fowble and pathologist Dr. Arthur Patchefsky, both of whom have national reputations, and places a strong emphasis on research, enabling women to participate in important long-range clinical trials.

Albert Einstein Breast Cancer Center
5401 Old York Road, Philadelphia (215-456-7383)

Einstein's is another top-drawer comprehensive breast cancer program, with all the latest diagnostic equipment, a highly coordinated team approach to evaluation and treatment, physical therapy, counseling and genetic-based family risk assessment (the actual DNA work is done at Penn). Einstein is particularly active in outreach, regularly staging workshops to educate and empower its patients.

Thomas Jefferson University Hospital
111 South 11th Street, Philadelphia (215-955-4500)

Jeff is noteworthy for its star mammographer, Dr. Stephen Feig, and two of the city's top breast surgeons, Dr. Anne Rosenberg and Dr. Gordon Schwartz. The latter won international acclaim for a research project in which he administered chemo prior to lumpectomy and radiation, significantly improving outcomes.

Burns

Nathan Speare Regional Burn Treatment Center
Crozer-Chester Medical Center, Upland, Pa.
(610-447-2000)

Since its inception in 1973, the Nathan Speare Regional Burn Treatment Center has been a national and local leader in the arena of burn care and research. The center's co-directors lecture worldwide, and the staff performs hours of free community service teaching burn prevention. As the long-reaching effects of managed care enter the realm of burn treatment, Crozer-Chester Medical Center has created the Burn Wound Care Center, an ambulatory burn care facility adjacent to the Speare Center that provides easy access to comprehensive outpatient wound care. Through daily wound care and patient education, the Burn Wound Care Center—staffed by surgeons and nurses who work within the Speare Center itself—provides a multidisciplinary approach to cost-efficient burn wound supervision without lowering the quality of patient care.

Stuart J. Hulnick Burn Center
St. Christopher's Hospital for Children,
Erie Avenue at Front Street, Philadelphia
(215-427-5323)

Fire and burn accidents are the third-leading cause of death for children under 18. So, when five-year-old Tommy Foggy of Philadelphia suffered severe burns after he played with matches and his clothes caught on fire, he was lucky to be brought to St. Christopher's. The hospital has the only pediatric burn center between Boston and Washington, D.C. Approximately 150 children are admitted to the five-bed center every year. Tommy underwent extensive skin grafts, and after discharge he spent weeks in a pressure garment custom-sewn for him by a hospital volunteer—the kind of child-first extra that helps earn this center its reputation.

Cancer

The National Cancer Institute in Washington designates just 26 hospitals nationwide as Comprehensive Cancer Centers. For approval, a hospital must excel in three areas: patient care (in both diagnosis and treatment), research and medical education. In Philadelphia, only the University of Pennsylvania Medical Center and Fox Chase Cancer Center have been deemed part of that select group.

University of Pennsylvania Cancer Center (1-800-383-UPCC) is particularly strong in breast (See "Breast Cancer," above), gynecological, head, neck and lung cancer, melanoma and neuro-oncology.

Fox Chase (215-728-6900) is a leader in prostate, lung, head and neck, gastrointestinal, breast and gynecological cancer and sarcomas.

Cosmetic Medicine

The Edwin and Fannie Gray Hall Center for Human Appearance
PENN TOWER, 3400 SPRUCE STREET, PHILADELPHIA
(1-800-789-7366)

"If we were a gimmick," Hall Center founder Dr. Linton Whitaker says, "we'd have died off by now." Indeed, after the seven years the center has devoted to removing wrinkles, smoothing over pockmarks and shrinking thunder thighs, teaching hospitals across the country have replicated the Hall Center's concept. In an attractive office suite, 18 specialists split their time between reconstructive surgery, cosmetic improvements and engaging in lively—and fruitful—give-and-take. Like the plastic surgeon who recently learned of a material he could use to rebuild eye sockets from a discussion with an oral surgeon on the team about a new process for creating jawbone.

Diabetes

Diabetes Center for Children
CHILDREN'S HOSPITAL OF PHILADELPHIA, 34TH STREET AND CIVIC CENTER BOULEVARD, PHILADELPHIA
(215-590-3172)

The staff here talks a lot about "empowerment." While it designs and monitors individual treatment plans, its main goal is moving the 800 young diabetics who visit the center annually away from physician- to family-focused care. Led by Dr. Lester Baker, the American Diabetes Association 1994 Clinician of the Year, the endocrinologists, nurse practitioners, nutritionists and psychotherapists help families gain the information, coping skills and confidence they need to juggle endless decisions about insulin quantities, food intake and physical activity. An added plus are the research programs that provide access to the latest technology for measuring blood levels, improving control and preventing complications.

Eating Disorders

Eating Disorders Program
FRIENDS HOSPITAL, 4641 ROOSEVELT BOULEVARD, PHILADELPHIA (215-831-4840)

A thirtysomething, 350-pound man with a long history of compulsive gambling and overeating who feels his life is out of control; a distraught, bright teenage girl who has been in and out of hospitals for depression, drug abuse and bulimia; a 40ish working woman who's been anorexic off and on since her teens. These are just some of the patients enrolled here under the supervision of Dr. Michael Pertschuk, the psychiatrist who, during 12 years at Graduate Hospital, originated the "multi-level" approach to seeing eating-disorder patients all the way through recovery using hospitalization, day treatment and intensive outpatient therapy. Now he's moved to this magnificent 100-acre campus with a team of professionals expert in a range of healing treatments, from individual and family work to movement and art therapy.

Weight and Eating Disorders Program
UNIVERSITY OF PENNSYLVANIA MEDICAL CENTER, 3600 MARKET STREET, SUITE 738, PHILADELPHIA (215-898-7316)

Thousands of Philadelphians swear that this weight-loss program, directed by eating-disorder authorities Dr. Thomas Wadden and Dr. Albert Stunkard, is the one that successfully taught them how to eat to live instead of the other way around. Participants can choose either a private or a small-group program emphasizing changes in weight and behavior, backed by the services of a ten-person staff skilled in nutrition, psychiatry/psychology, general medicine and exercise. In the late 1970s this group pioneered the combination of medicine (fenfluramine) and lifestyle modification that is so popular today.

Pediatric Center for Dysphagia and Feeding Management
CHILDREN'S SEASHORE HOUSE, 3405 CIVIC CENTER BOULEVARD, PHILADELPHIA (215-895-3803)

"Don't worry, she'll outgrow it." That's what their pediatrician kept telling Jennifer and Leo Powers while their daughter, Jenna, continued to spit, scream and gag at every feeding. After two years, Jenna's diet consisted of sucking on a few bites of peanut-butter-and-jelly sandwich. Finally, the Roxborough couple brought her to this center, where doctors found she had the common digestive disorder called reflux, prescribed medication to ease her physical symptoms and put her in the hospital for more than three weeks to teach her how to eat, helping her progress from puréed to chopped to solid foods. Most of the 300 kids seen here each year don't require hospitalization. But whether they are just picky eaters who subsist on a menu of macaroni and cheese or toddlers who've been kept alive on feeding tubes, this cheerful-looking center is equipped to defuse the problem.

Epilepsy

Comprehensive Epilepsy Center
THE GRADUATE HOSPITAL, 1800 LOMBARD STREET, PHILADELPHIA (215-893-2322)

Back in the '70s and '80s, this was the only place in the Mid-Atlantic doing surgery to remove epileptic tissue from the brain. Today, it remains a major internationally recognized center for what's become an accepted method of controlling seizures, performing nearly 100 operations annually. The center offers complete outpatient care for people with epilepsy, using both conventional and investigational drugs, sophisticated diagnostic services including inpatient 24-hour video EEG monitoring and MRI, a women and family planning program, an epilepsy surgery program, counseling and psychological care, social support and community education. Graduate's center is also deeply involved in research and all the other recent advances gradually taming this once-frightful disease.

Eyes

Wills Eye Hospital
900 WALNUT STREET, PHILADELPHIA (215-928-3000)

Founded in 1832 as the nation's first hospital devoted solely to eye care, Wills was in on the very genesis of ophthalmology as a medical specialty. A quarter of the 300-member staff consistently appear on national best-doctor lists, and the entire institution has been the only hospital listed in its category for the past five years by *U.S. News and World Report*. Among the million patients treated here in recent years have been a famous American painter, a U.S. senator and a cardinal.

Gastroenterology

GI Division
UNIVERSITY OF PENNSYLVANIA MEDICAL CENTER, 3400 SPRUCE STREET, PHILADELPHIA (215-349-8222)

Though it has long boasted an excellent GI program, over the past few years Penn has assembled some of the top subspecialists in the country, including noted experts in liver transplants, inflammatory bowel disease and pancreatic diseases, as well as a former National Institutes of Health physician who is one of only two doctors on the East Coast offering a noninvasive breath test for the bacteria now believed to cause most ulcers. Furthermore, Dr. Peter Traber, the chief of the division, is himself heading up a new multidisciplinary clinic for GI cancers. Among other cutting-edge services offered by Traber's clinic is DNA testing for the roughly 10 to 20 percent of all colon cancer cases thought to be genetic in origin.

GI Section
TEMPLE UNIVERSITY HOSPITAL, 3401 NORTH BROAD STREET, PHILADELPHIA (215-707-3435)

When a close relative of mine needed a definitive answer that her recurrent chest pain and nausea were the result of a digestive, not heart, problem, her doctor sent her here. Like Penn, Temple has its share of national experts in such areas as liver disease and endoscopic ultrasound, but it's perhaps best known for the wealth of GI experience contained inside its walls. Dr. Sidney Cohen and Dr. Robert Fisher have a combined 50 years in diagnosing and treating the full range of ailments afflicting the gut. Particularly if the problem has to do with motility (like nausea or cramping) or functional GI disorders (like irritable bowel syndrome or chronic constipation), many Philadelphians wouldn't feel comfortable seeking help anywhere else.

Geriatrics

One of the biggest frustrations for the elderly is finding quality coordinated care. In our mind, an excellent geriatric center brings together medical, psychological, social, nursing and rehabilitative services for patients who are certain to have multiple needs requiring very different levels of care. A top-notch center should be prepared to handle both a relatively robust senior citizen like Bob Dole and a patient ready for the nursing home.

The huge **Philadelphia Geriatric Center**, 5301 Old York Road, Philadelphia (215-456-2900), covers the entire map of senior concerns: assisted housing in either a nursing home or retirement community, rehab, medically supervised fitness, a consultation and diagnostic center, counseling for caregivers, adult day care, a comprehensive geriatric medical practice and a home-health-service program. This is the model for total senior care, one system that can truly see seniors through the rest of their lives.

In a more specialized vein, the **Wills Geriatric Psychiatry Program** at 9th and Walnut streets, Philadelphia (215-928-3021), combines the bright, classy setting of the renovated eighth floor of the eye hospital with the geriatric psychiatry expertise of Thomas Jefferson University. The staff is particularly sensitive to depressions triggered by too many medications or poor nutrition.

The **ACE (Acute Care of Elders) Unit** at Presbyterian Medical Center of the University of Pennsylvania Health System (215-662-8197) is one of only four programs in the entire country specially designed, both architecturally and philosophically, for acutely ill patients over 65. What makes the ACE Unit unique is its multidisciplinary team approach, carried out by staff members who have received special training and education in care for the elderly. Opened in 1994, it occupies a full floor that has been tastefully redecorated with age-appropriate furniture and lighting.

Hands

The Philadelphia Hand Center, P.C.
901 WALNUT STREET, PHILADELPHIA (1-800-971-HAND)

When the weekend warrior who works down the hall from me jammed his ring finger playing basketball, the doctors here gave him exercises and special tape to keep his time on the sidelines to a minimum. When the famous rock guitarist could no longer strum out his ear-shattering chords for all the pain in his right hand, he came here to get it healed before a world tour. The doctors at The Philadelphia Hand

Center routinely treat members of the Philadelphia Eagles, Flyers and Phillies, as well as other elite athletes, but you don't have to be a star to go there. From shoulder to pinky, from routine sprain to dire emergency, there is little the Hand Center can't do. Under the dire category, its salvage rate for reattaching lost limbs is 92 percent—22 percent higher than the national average. And under a category affecting a steadily growing number of white-collar workers, the center has helped to pioneer a new arthroscopic surgery for carpal tunnel syndrome that's been getting people back to their keyboards faster with less swelling and discomfort.

Headaches

Comprehensive Headache Center
GERMANTOWN HOSPITAL, ONE PENN BOULEVARD, PHILADELPHIA (215-843-5070)

While 40 million people in the United States are plagued by chronic headaches, only a tiny minority ever seek help. That's too bad, considering that this 12-year-old center has a success rate of 85 percent. Co-directed by Dr. Stephen Silberstein, editor of the definitive textbook in the field, the center spends an entire day evaluating each patient before starting an individual program of one or more of the latest biologically based approaches to reducing the frequency and severity of headache pain. Behavior modification, physical therapy, medication, biofeedback and diet all regularly come into play, often with remarkable results.

Heart

The Heart Hospitals
ALLEGHENY UNIVERSITY HOSPITALS, CENTER CITY (FORMERLY HAHNEMANN UNIVERSITY HOSPITAL), BROAD AND VINE STREETS, PHILADELPHIA (215-762-3221); AND ALLEGHENY UNIVERSITY HOSPITALS, EAST FALLS (FORMERLY MEDICAL COLLEGE OF PENNSYLVANIA HOSPITAL), 3300 HENRY AVENUE, PHILADELPHIA (215-842-6000)

The concept of a hospital within a hospital, dedicated solely to the care and recovery of cardiac patients, was introduced at Hahnemann University Hospital (now known as Allegheny University Hospitals, Center City) in 1993. The result has been a highly successful and growing program encompassing everything from cardiac catheterizations to heart transplants to a surgical unit that does more cardiac procedures than any other local facility.

Now Allegheny University Hospitals, East Falls (formerly Medical College of Pennsylvania Hospital) has used the Heart Hospital model to expand on its own well-established cardiac programs. It has added to its team of cardiac specialists, with the majority of physicians from the Philadelphia Heart Institute joining the faculty of the Allegheny University of the Health Sciences (formerly MCP/Hahnemann). Allegheny East Falls constructed new cardiac patient units, renovated patient areas, and added and updated cardiac cath and electrophysiology labs. The Heart Hospitals also offer expanding state-of-the-art cardiac preventive and rehab programs in locations in Philadelphia, Montgomery and Bucks counties.

Temple University
3401 North Broad Street, Philadelphia
(215-707-4733)

The ads say "In matters of the heart, choose Temple." And if the matter involves any sort of cardiac transplant, we concur. Site of the Delaware Valley's first heart transplant in 1984, Temple put more new hearts into desperately ill adults last year than any other hospital in the country. It is one of a select number of facilities using battery-operated mechanical hearts to buy time for people waiting for donated organs. The transplant and mechanical heart programs allow Temple to reduce the risk of conventional heart surgery for high-risk patients. And it's one of just a handful of places that do valve replacements using human valves, eliminating the need for the anti-rejection drugs required with mechanical and pig valves.

Infertility

An explosion in technology over the past ten years has enabled top infertility centers to do some amazing things. The procedures are costly—$6,000 to $12,000 per try—and the chance of success hardly ever above 50-50. Still, the three programs we've singled out have had as much success as anywhere with the most eye-popping new procedures the field has to offer.

Philadelphia Fertility Institute/ Pennsylvania Reproductive Associates
Pennsylvania Hospital, 800 Spruce Street, Suite 786, Philadelphia (215-829-5095), and 5217 Militia Hill Road, Plymouth Meeting (610-834-1140)

Dr. Stephen Corson, author of the popular book *Conquering Infertility: A Guide for Couples*, leads a staff of 54 that has produced nearly 1,000 births in the past ten years. This is the only local center that will find couples a woman to carry their baby and one of only a few with an anonymous egg-donor program. With the incorporation of a successful micromanipulation program, which includes Intro-Cytoplasmic Sperm Injection (ICSI) and Assisted Hatching, PRA offers the full spectrum of state-of-the-art therapies for male and female infertility.

Infertility and Reproductive Medicine Program
University of Pennsylvania Medical Center, 106 Dulles, 3400 Spruce Street, Philadelphia (215-662-2951), and the Merion Building, 700 South Henderson Road, King of Prussia (610-662-7712)

Led by Dr. Luigi Mastroianni, an international star who's trained most of the city's other top infertility specialists, Penn's was one of only six infertility centers in the country recently chosen by the National Institutes of Health as a Reproductive Medicine Unit. Five of its six physicians are in *Best Doctors in America*. They established the first in vitro fertilization (IVF) program in this area and pioneered laparoscopic surgery.

Cooper Institute for In Vitro Fertilization
8002E GREENTREE COMMONS, MARLTON, N.J.
(609-751-5575)

Maverick Dr. Jerome Check runs one of the area's largest IVF programs. His most recent landmark: triplets born from a technique called IXIS, in which a father's sperm is injected directly into a mother's egg.

Maternity Services

The Birthing Suite
PENNSYLVANIA HOSPITAL, 800 SPRUCE STREET, PHILADELPHIA (215-829-8000)

These days more women want to have their babies delivered by a midwife but are still nervous about what happens if something goes wrong. This center solves that dilemma with one of the few natural-birthing suites in the country located just a short gurney ride from a full-service hospital delivery room. In most instances, of course, women deliver right in the suite itself, a cozy nest of two spacious bedrooms with stereos, rockers, birthing chairs, a bathroom with a jacuzzi to ease labor pain and a kitchen. The staff of midwives is highly skilled, with more than 85 years of experience among them. And it may hold the record for the most people to participate in a birth—an extended family of 27.

High-Risk Obstetrics Program
PENNSYLVANIA HOSPITAL, 800 SPRUCE STREET, PHILADELPHIA (215-829-8700)

While for most women pregnancy is marred mainly by morning sickness and bearable discomfort, some fetuses and expectant mothers require highly sophisticated care. This exemplary program offers the best state-of-the-art technology for everything from routine maternal age-related complications to life-threatening emergencies stemming from a congenital heart defect. Its portable monitoring equipment travels to satellite offices throughout the region.

MOM (Making Options for Motherhood)
THOMAS JEFFERSON UNIVERSITY HOSPITAL, 834 CHESTNUT STREET, SUITE 300, PHILADELPHIA (215-955-5000)

For a disabled woman, the fears and worries about having and caring for a child are magnified tenfold. Enter MOM, the country's only program that specifically addresses the needs of disabled pregnant women and new mothers with social services as well as occupational therapy, home visits and wheelchair-friendly scales and examining tables. It was started in 1992 with a grant from the March of Dimes after a mother-to-be with spina bifida made the Jeff staff aware of how little support was available for women like her.

The Pregnancy Loss Center
Thomas Jefferson University Hospital,
1015 Chestnut Street, Suite 1017, Philadelphia
(215-955-2507)

Dr. Susan Cowchock started this center in 1983 when she realized how fragmented the treatment was for couples suffering recurring miscarriages. Since then, she and her staff have seen close to 3,000 couples, who are drawn from all over the United States by the center's 70 percent successful birthrate. They bring problems of genetic errors, malformed uteruses, abnormal ovulation and even abnormal immune response to their pregnancies. A typical case was the 40-year-old woman who'd endured seven immune-induced miscarriages in her second marriage despite having successfully conceived a child in her first. She was immunized with her husband's white blood cells and delivered a healthy, ten-pound girl.

Movement Disorders
The Parkinson's Disease and Movement Disorders Center
The Graduate Hospital, 1800 Lombard Street,
Philadelphia (215-545-8406)

It makes sense that of the handful of centers in the world performing pallidotomy and deep brain stimulation—surgeries that, as a result of improved brain mapping techniques, have brought remarkable relief to some Parkinson's and tremor patients—Graduate's program would be one. Graduate has long been both a first place to turn and a source of last resort for patients with neurological diseases like Parkinson's, Huntington's chorea, dystonia and Tourette's syndrome. Its active research program is currently running eight clinical drug trials, while its workshops and support activities continue to remind patients and caregivers that, as bad as such an illness may be, they needn't feel they're alone.

Multiple Sclerosis
The Jefferson MS Comprehensive Clinical Center
9th and Chestnut streets, Suite 420, Philadelphia
(215-955-8118)

Amid the uncertainty of living with multiple sclerosis, Jeff's comprehensive MS center has been at least one thing thousands of patients could count on. The center encourages its patients—many of whom literally never know from one step to the next when an attack might occur that lands them in a wheelchair—to lean on their neurologist here as their primary physician and the referral source for all their medical and psychological needs. But in recent years the Jeff center has also provided something else: first crack at some of the first-ever treatments for MS. Betaseron, the landmark drug approved three years ago by the Food and Drug Administration, was originally tested here in 1986, and the center is actively involved in clinical trials of other drugs now. None of the new treatments is considered a "cure." But at a place whose greatest gift to its patients used to be its steadying hand, there's now reason to offer them hope for a relatively normal life.

Orthopedics

The Rothman Institute
PENNSYLVANIA HOSPITAL, 800 SPRUCE STREET, PHILADELPHIA (215-829-3458)

When you do more hip and knee replacements than any other place in the country, you get pretty good at it. Both Walter Annenberg and a Saudi Arabian prince chose to have their hips replaced at Dr. Richard Rothman's pioneering center. The first in Philadelphia to do hips, and one of the first in the United States to use a plastic greenhouse-shaped operating room that's now an industry standard for reducing infection, the Rothman Institute boasts a track record that, if anything, has grown more impressive over the years. A recent study, for example, showed that compared to four other area medical centers, the costs here were $12,000 to $30,000 lower than at all but one other hospital, while Rothman's patients got better the fastest, with the lowest complication rate.

Limbs With Restricted Motion Program
MOSSREHAB, 1200 WEST TABOR ROAD, PHILADELPHIA (215-456-9693)

This program, offered through MossRehab and Albert Einstein Medical Center, takes on neuro-orthopedic cases others have given up on. Matthew, of Flemington, New Jersey, was 15 when a car he was a passenger in hit a tree, leaving his right arm and leg severely bent. He could neither walk nor cut the food on his plate until three rounds of surgery and countless hours of rehab at MossRehab allowed him to get around with a walker and eat on his own. Einstein's Dr. Mary Ann Keenan wrote the only textbook on surgery for spastic disorders such as cerebral palsy, and physiatrists Dr. Nathaniel Mayer and Dr. Albert Esquenazi are national figures in brain injury and gait disorders, such as having a locked knee or walking bent to one side.

Pain

Neuro-Implant Center
1015 CHESTNUT STREET, SUITE 1400, PHILADELPHIA (215-955-2364)

Chronic pain or spasticity that fails to respond to any other treatment can sometimes be alleviated by an operation championed by Jefferson neurosurgeon Dr. Giancarlo Barolat. In a surgical procedure he has performed on an unparalleled 800 patients, Barolat implants a battery-operated device about the size of a pocket watch in the abdomen and a tiny electrode on the spinal cord. Emitting an electrical signal that interferes with unwanted messages sent by nerves to the brain, the system improves 65 percent of patients and creates nothing short of a miracle in some.

Pediatric Transplants

Pediatric Transplant Institute
ST. CHRISTOPHER'S HOSPITAL FOR CHILDREN,
ERIE AVENUE AT FRONT STREET, PHILADELPHIA
(215-427-5000)

This institute is a nationally recognized leader in the field of pediatric organ transplantation. Surgeons at St. Christopher's perform pediatric heart, liver and kidney transplants, and they are proud to hold the best record of successful pediatric transplants in the region. A multidisciplinary team—including a pediatric transplant surgeon, cardiologist or nephrologist, specially trained nurses, nutritionist, social worker, psychiatrist and child life therapist—provides comprehensive care to transplant patients.

In 1971, surgeons at St. Christopher's performed the first pediatric kidney transplant in the region. Fourteen years later, surgeons at the hospital performed the first pediatric liver transplant and first pediatric heart transplant in the region; in 1987 St. Christopher's became the site of the first combined pediatric kidney/liver transplant performed in the Delaware Valley.

Since that time, surgeons here have continued to make transplant history. The liver transplant team, under the direction of Dr. Stephen Dunn, has been at the cutting edge of two new types of liver transplants. The first is living related donor transplants, in which a portion of a parent's liver is transplanted into a critically ill child, where it regenerates. In addition, Dunn and his team have performed split-liver transplants, in which a cadaver liver is divided and transplanted into two children.

Scleroderma

Scleroderma Center
THOMAS JEFFERSON UNIVERSITY HOSPITAL, 10TH AND
WALNUT STREETS, PHILADELPHIA (215-955-5042)

Scleroderma and its close cousin Raynaud's phenomenon are connective-tissue diseases characterized by progressive hardening of the skin and multiple internal organs. Their typical victims are women between the ages of 30 and 50, like the local woman who in a period of a few months went from feeling perfectly healthy to being told by her primary physician that she had scleroderma and had perhaps eight months to live. Fortunately, she came to Dr. Sergio Jimenez's large, internationally recognized center for a second opinion and was given a medication that had been introduced here. Fifteen years later, she's still coming by for periodic monitoring.

Sleep Disorders

If your chronic insomnia is related to an organic problem, a good night's sleep may be as close as the nearest sleep-disorder center. After a thorough physical examination, you'll probably be asked to bunk down in a sleep lab for a night or two hooked up to electrodes so that a proper diagnosis can be made. The differences between the centers is negligible, since the American Sleep Disorder Association sets rigid standards for approval. The following facilities have earned ASDA accreditation:

Allegheny University Hospitals, East Falls (formerly Medical College of Pennsylvania) (215-842-4250)
Crozer-Chester Medical Center (610-447-2689)
Lankenau Hospital (610-645-3400)
Lower Bucks Hospital (215-785-9751)
Thomas Jefferson University Hospital (215-955-6175)
University of Pennsylvania Medical Center (215-662-7300)

Spinal Cord Injury

The Regional Spinal Cord Injury Center of the Delaware Valley
132 SOUTH 10TH STREET, PHILADELPHIA (215-955-6579)

This joint venture of Thomas Jefferson University Hospital and Magee Rehabilitation is one of 18 centers in the nation offering long-term support to victims of spinal-cord injuries. The center provides acute care and rehabilitation and conducts cord-injury research.

Sports Medicine

Sports Medicine Program
TEMPLE UNIVERSITY HOSPITAL, BROAD AND TIOGA STREETS, PHILADELPHIA (215-221-2111; CALL FOR OTHER LOCATIONS IN FORT WASHINGTON, NORTHEAST PHILADELPHIA AND MARLTON, N.J.)

Of the many fine sports-medicine programs in the region, this one, led by Dr. Ray Moyer, helped to pioneer the specialty and still treats more high school, college and weekend athletes than any other local practice. In addition to having a full complement of all the latest rehab gizmos, the center is backed by the services of a top-flight hospital. So if the real cause of that back pain turns out to be rheumatoid arthritis, not a strenuous tennis match, it's likely to be detected most quickly here.

Center for Continuing Health
MONROE OFFICE CENTER, CITY AVENUE AND PRESIDENTIAL BOULEVARD, PHILADELPHIA (215-878-1234), AND HILLMAN MEDICAL CENTER, 2116 CHESTNUT STREET, PHILADELPHIA (215-568-4080)

The latest research confirms that exercise in the golden years is the best antidote to the ravages of aging. Of course, Medical College of Pennsylvania geriatrician Dr. Joel Posner and his staff see the evidence of that every day. One of Posner's favorite elderly exercisers was an 83-year-old woman who came to him after three years in the program and abruptly announced she was quitting. Having started out sedentary and depressed, she now felt so wonderful she was moving to Florida to enjoy the rest of her life. All participants undergo a rigorous checkup before embarking on an individualized routine supervised by a staff that includes a physician, physician's assistant, physical therapist and several certified trainers.

Stroke

Young Stroke Program
BRYN MAWR REHAB, 414 PAOLI PIKE, MALVERN
(610-251-5655)

Of the half-million people who suffer strokes annually, about 5 percent are under age 45. Here at Bryn Mawr Rehab the staff has developed an agenda for dealing with the young stroke patient's special needs. Instead of just relearning how to do things like feed and dress themselves, patients here are just as likely to relearn to feed and dress a dependent child, drive a car and get back up to speed at work.

Taste and Smell Disorders

Monell/Jefferson Chemosensory Clinical Research Center
909 WALNUT STREET, PHILADELPHIA (215-955-5652)

Ben Cohen, of Ben and Jerry's ice cream fame, doesn't smell too good. He says his sense of taste is pretty much shot too. So it wasn't too surprising last year when he had a physician friend contact this highly regarded NIH-funded research center to see if it could help. Dr. Beverly Cowart, who took the call, said Cohen's problems could be related to his chronic sinus and allergy conditions; she suggested he try a steroid nasal spray and passed on the name of another research center closer to B&J's Vermont headquarters—in other words, the same kind of advice Monell's staff dispenses to hundreds of lesser-known noses and palates every year. Though only about 20 percent of all cases in this emerging field are treatable, for people who suffer in silence with these bizarre afflictions, it's often a great relief just to know that they're not crazy. Besides, Monell can frequently make suggestions that at least enable them to compensate for their problems—say, by enhancing the tactile quality of their food to make up for a loss of taste. Of course, on that score Ben Cohen was way ahead of Cowart. How do you think his ice cream got to be so chunky and chewy?

Urology

The Bladder Health Center
THE GRADUATE HOSPITAL, 1800 LOMBARD STREET, SUITE 602, PHILADELPHIA (215-893-2710)

In the course of a year, Sharon saw 14 different doctors about the excruciating burning in her vagina. She was told she might have, among other things, a yeast infection, irritable bowel syndrome, genital warts, anxiety and AIDS. Then by chance she saw Dr. Kristene Whitmore on a local talk show, made an appointment and was diagnosed with interstitial cystitis, a surprisingly common inflammatory bladder disease. That rarest of breeds, a female board-certified urologist, Whitmore founded this center to bring a sensitive, creative approach to solving women's bladder problems. In treating incontinence, for example, she'll sometimes try dietary changes, acupuncture, biofeedback, surgery, collagen injections and even electrical gadgets she calls "my toys" to strengthen pelvic muscles.

Women's Health
Center for Women's Health
MONROE OFFICE CENTER, CITY AVENUE AND
PRESIDENTIAL BOULEVARD, PHILADELPHIA
(215-581-6267)

This program exceeds what's offered at most of the plant-filled, mauve-carpeted places advertised as "women's centers." To begin with, the carpet is blue. Center directors Dr. Carol Fleischman and Dr. Ann Honebrink and their staff have taken the radical step of combining traditional gynecology with all the services of a primary physician. On a typical checkup, a woman gets a pelvic exam, hormone counseling, Pap smear, lifestyle counseling and a general physical. Mammography and ultrasound are available on site. In short, women get all their basic health needs met under one roof, with appropriate referrals made when necessary.

Wounds
Wound Care Center
THE GRADUATE HOSPITAL, 1740 SOUTH STREET,
PHILADELPHIA (215-893-7655)

The longest nonhealing wound treated here had oozed for nearly half a century. Typically suffering from diabetes, arterial disease or pressure ulcers, many patients arrive at this sleek contemporary office suite with a sense of hopelessness, having been told their wounds will never heal. But within six months of treatment, frequently with a special topical solution made of growth factor from the patients' own blood, 70 percent of them are cured. Even the New Jersey man whose gaping wound on the back of his right heel hadn't healed for 45 of his 68 years.

Wound Healing Clinic
PAOLI MEMORIAL HOSPITAL, 255 WEST LANCASTER
AVENUE, PAOLI (610-648-1212)

The majority of patients seen for specialized care here have wounds resulting from an underlying chronic medical condition, such as diabetes, neuropathy, arthritis, chronic venous insufficiency, peripheral arterial disease, autoimmune disease and factors associated with immobility. Patients visit the clinic weekly, where careful monitoring of the wound is coupled with attentive care.

Section

Choosing a Hospital

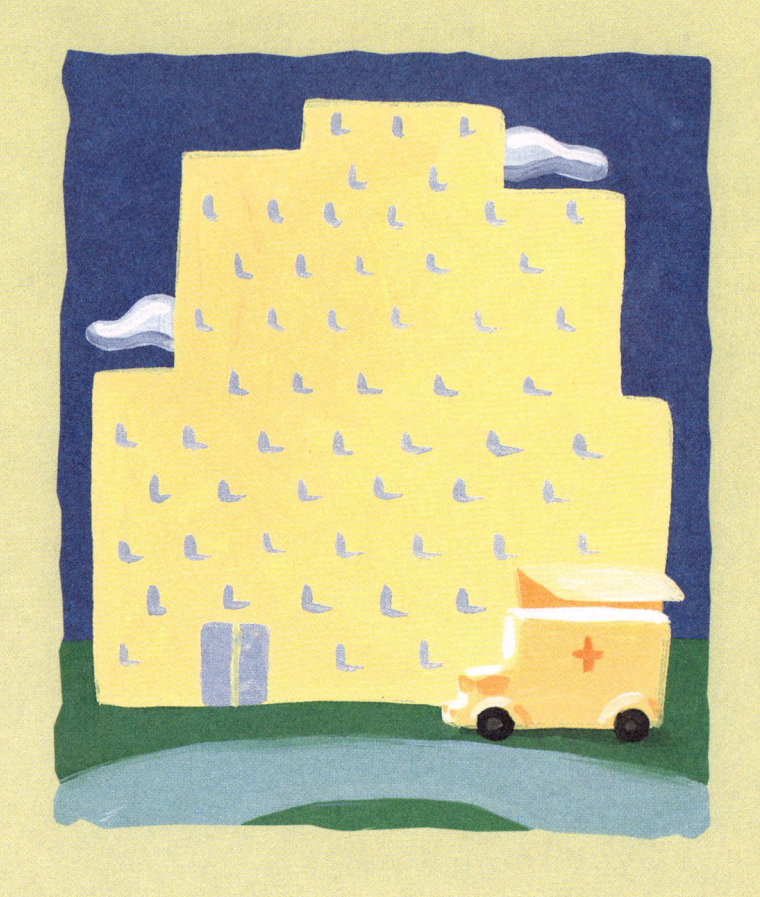

Three

Chapter 7
Inside Story
The lowdown on diagnostic techniques

Chapter 8
Check It Out Before You Check In
Mini-profiles of area hospitals

Chapter 9
Emergency!
What to do when time is critical

WE'VE CHANGED OUR NAME!

Medical College of Pennsylvania and Hahnemann University Hospital System is now

ALLEGHENY UNIVERSITY HOSPITALS

We're now — **Allegheny University Hospitals, Bucks County**
— **Allegheny University Hospitals, Center City**
— **Allegheny University Hospitals, East Falls**
— **Allegheny University Hospitals, Elkins Park**

We're a system of adult hospitals and medical practices, working together with St. Christopher's Hospital for Children, and extending from Center City to the suburbs — places you've trusted for generations. Our new names are a pledge of our commitment to continue to lead the way in finding newer and better ways to heal — and of our belief that the best is yet to be.

For more information or to make an appointment with an Allegheny physician, call

1-800-PRO-HEALTH[SM]
(1-800-776-4325)

ST. CHRISTOPHER'S HOSPITAL FOR CHILDREN

ALLEGHENY UNIVERSITY HOSPITALS

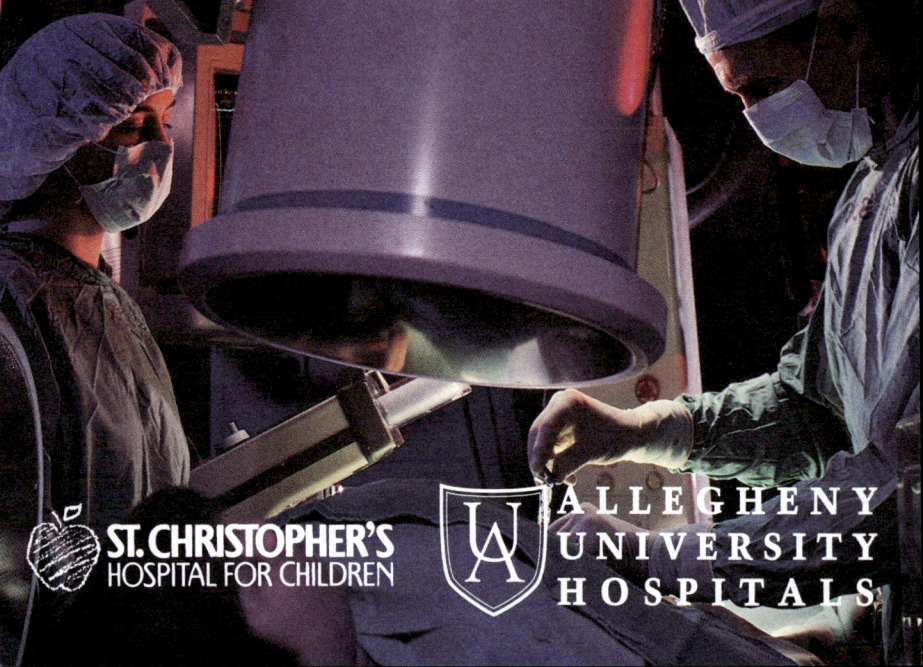

CHAPTER 7

Inside Story

A glossary of the many techniques used to see inside the body

Wilhelm Roentgen, a German physicist, holds the distinction of having been the first man to get under anybody's skin. In 1895, while experimenting with the cathode ray, Roentgen accidentally generated electromagnetic radiation so energetic it could pass through virtually any substance and make an impression on a plate painted with a photographic emulsion. One of the first "pictures" he took was of the bones in his wife's hand. He called it an X-ray because of its mysterious nature. Within a year, doctors all over the world were taking X-ray pictures.

Before that, the knife was the only tool for seeing inside the human body. Doctors would use their hands and ears to locate internal problems, and when their probing and tapping indicated trouble, they had no alternative to cutting open the patient to see what was wrong. By then, it was often too late. The X-ray provided a window into a previously invisible world, and enabled doctors to diagnose all kinds of problems at the crucial early stages. Amid all the excitement, nobody realized how dangerous X-rays were—until people working with them began to die from overexposure. From that point on, the search was launched to find safer ways to reveal the body's intricacies.

From the crude still photos of bones that were early X-rays, radiology has progressed to the stage today where it's possible to view the heart and brain in action. It's a world Roentgen would hardly recognize. Here are explanations of some of its latest techniques.

CT scans: A slice of life

More than anything else, medical imaging owes its spectacular advancement to computers—and to Godfrey Hounsfield, a British scientist who worked for a British conglomerate that also produced records for the Beatles. While working on a project that involved the use of X-rays and electronic music, he began toying with other applications for bytes and rads. His inventiveness was later combined with the research of a mathematician. The result was computerized axial tomography, popularly known as the CT scan—the first practical application of the marriage of computers and X-rays. He and the mathematician won the Nobel Prize in medicine for creating a way to take cross-sectional pictures of the body from head to toe.

What made these pictures so amazing was their unique perspective. Before the CT scan, X-rays could photograph only through the front or side of the body, frequently showing organs superimposed on each other, which made accurate readings difficult. But these new pictures seemed to dissect the body without a knife, depicting body parts in thin, individual cross-sections, each as clearly defined as a drawing in a biology textbook.

For the patient, the procedure is quite painless. You report to the hospital or imaging center as an outpatient, and soon find yourself lying on a table in a brightly lit room, with the part of your body to be examined placed in the hole of what looks like a huge metal doughnut. A physician sometimes begins the scan by injecting a contrast solution into your bloodstream through a vein at the end of your elbow. This solution affects how much X-ray will be absorbed, and also enhances certain features of the final image. A computer uses the information on the amount of X-ray being transmitted through the tissue and translates it into numbers, from which it makes a picture. In just seconds, images of your lung or brain or stomach, one slice after the other, appear on a computer screen. Not only is there an outline of the suspicious organ, but a sense of its density as well.

In rare instances someone gets a severe allergic reaction to the contrast solution. More typical symptoms are nausea, hives, a warm flush or an unpleasant metallic taste, though most people experience nothing more annoying than the prick of the injection itself. The side effects can be pretty much eliminated with newer non-ionic contrast materials that are safer but more expensive. If you're allergic, you might want to ask about them.

CT scans aid in evaluating inflammatory diseases and tumors by showing their exact size, their location and whether they are solid or filled with fluid. In the case of tumors, these can be important clues to whether a growth is benign or malignant. CT scans are also useful for checking the extent of an injury or infection. Where X-rays would show only a bone fracture, a more exacting CT scan could reveal internal bleeding or cuts on an organ.

The CT scan has recently been improved with the Spiral CT, which dramatically reduces exam time and provides improved image quality. Instead of acquiring images one slice at a time, the new scanner (which looks like a regular CT) takes images of the entire volume, spiraling along the body sections at high speed. The entire chest or abdomen is imaged in one breath-hold.

Magnetic resonance imaging: May the force be with you

Although scientists have managed to reduce the dosage of radiation from X-rays, their dream has long been to find a way to see inside the body without using any ionizing radiation at all. Now that's possible, with a procedure that depends entirely on magnetic force.

Magnetic resonance imaging (MRI) first appeared as a laboratory technique for chemical analysis in the '30s, when it became known that parts of every cell had magnetic properties. Forty years later, researchers learned that normal and abnormal tissues respond differently in a magnetic field. In the '80s, technology advanced to the point where it became possible to translate these differences into a picture. The "camera," if you will, is a piece of high-tech machinery that looks like a giant tunnel and exerts a magnetic force as high as 30,000 times the power of the earth's magnetic field. When a patient lies on a bed inside this tunnel, the intense magnetic force causes a portion of the protons in the body to line up in certain patterns. During this process of spinning and aligning, the protons give off energy signals that can be measured by a radio frequency receiver and assembled into photographic images. Pictures can be made from many different planes: side to side, front to back, and head to toe, to name just a few. The images are actually cross-sections, like slices in a loaf of bread, and some machines can take as many as an image per second.

You may have seen advertisements for MRIs where it isn't necessary for the patient to lie inside a tunnel. These open-sided units, which are an alternative for obese or claustrophobic patients, use a lower magnetic field than the original high-field units—and the stronger the field, the better quality the image. Though the cost to the patient is the same, says Dr. Mitchell Schnall, director of MRI at the University of Pennsylvania Medical Center, "you do sacrifice significant scan quality." You'll see a lot of these units around, because they can be bought for $800,000, versus $2 million for a tunnel unit.

Other than the slight discomfort of lying quietly inside a tunnel, MRI patients have reported no ill effects from the procedure. Any alteration to the body's molecules is slight and transient. According to Dr. Stanley Baum, chairman of radiology at UPMC, studies have indicated that there is no known magnetic strength that has shown any biological effect on cells or chromosomes. MRI produces pictures of striking anatomical clarity and images of things never seen before, such as changes in bone marrow and the stages of a hemorrhage. Tumors show up very clearly, along with ligaments, tendons and cartilage, which makes this an excellent tool for diagnosing sports injuries. Today MRIs are starting to be used to look at heart problems and catch early breast cancers even sooner than mammography. And an offshoot called MRA—magnetic resonance angiography—can look into the blood vessels and pinpoint small clots or aneurysms without the risk of a more invasive angiogram. This diagnostic information has many applications in vascular disease.

Angiography: Just dyeing to see you

Like any other heavily trafficked highway, the body's blood vessels frequently need repair. Our rich, fatty diets produce plaque that collects in certain spots and creates roadblocks to impede the smooth flow of blood. Moreover, as we age, the elasticity of the roadbed itself diminishes and vessels harden and narrow, and sometimes sections need replacing. With the development of angiography—a kind of X-ray photography of blood vessels—it's possible to do quite sophisticated medical roadwork.

The angiographer's tools include long thin plastic catheters, guide wires that slide inside them and a colorless contrast solution—popularly referred to as dye—that mixes with the blood and blocks enough X-rays to create an image. Using these instruments, doctors can locate a clogged artery in the heart, pinpoint a blockage causing severe leg cramps or check whether the brain is being sufficiently nourished with blood.

The procedure begins with a small puncture (in the groin, arm or neck) to insert the catheter. These pliable tubes come in a variety of lengths and widths, and often have special curves or hooks on the ends designed to fit particular arteries. By twisting and turning the guide wire, an angiographer manipulates the catheter up one blood vessel and into another. He is directed by a fluoroscope, a device that uses a weak X-ray to display the route the angiographer is following on a TV monitor. (Years ago, some shoe stores had fluoroscopy machines so customers could check the fit by viewing their feet inside their new shoes.) When the angiographer reaches the spot he wants to examine, he withdraws the wire and injects the contrast solution through the catheter. It squirts out of the far end directly into the blood vessel, and a rapid series of X-ray pictures maps the solution's path.

Angiograms are performed without anesthesia, and patients generally experience little discomfort other than a warm flush from the contrast solution. But there are genuine concerns every time a doctor puts a catheter into a blood vessel, especially when these vessels are already weakened by disease. Excessive bleeding is one possible complication. An extreme example was the 83-year-old woman with unusually hard arterial walls that simply wouldn't seal when the catheter was removed. After several hours of continued bleeding, she had to be taken to the operating room, where the vessel was stitched shut. A more common risk is the chance a blood clot will dislodge, shut off the blood supply and cause a stroke.

Interventional radiology: Critical openings and closings

The practitioners of this delicate art refer to what they do as surgery without a scalpel. With techniques related to those used in angiograms, they are able to reach places deep within the body and correct conditions that once would have demanded a trip to the operating room—or in some cases, would have been untreatable. The interventional radiologist uses a variety of visual tools such as fluoroscopy, ultrasound, CT scan and even MRI to guide him as he threads his tubes and wires to the site of the problem.

Generally the work falls into three categories. The first is opening up blood vessels blocked by fatty plaque or bile ducts and ureters blocked by a stone, a tumor or scar tissue. By far the most common procedure in this category is the balloon angioplasty, where a tiny catheter with a balloon on the end is threaded through the artery to the impasse. When inflated, the balloon flattens out the plaque and clears the passage. The problem in the past with balloon angioplasties was something called re-stenosis—which basically means the roadblocks tended to come back. To fight that reoccurrence, a metal stent is now inserted after the balloon to act as a scaffolding to keep the opening from closing.

The second category does just the opposite by closing leaks in blood vessels that are hemorrhaging from trauma or bleeding ulcers. Tiny balloons or metal coils are delivered to the site of the leak and left in place to plug it. Lately this procedure has been used to obstruct vessels that feed cancerous tissue, in effect cutting off the blood supply so the cancer can't grow. It's generally tried with liver cancer.

The third application is to remove certain kinds of fluids such as the infected gook of an abscess, urine from an obstructed kidney or bile from an obstructed liver. A tube is inserted through the skin to the spot where the problem lies and drains the area. A CT scan helps guide the tube and keep it from damaging critical organs. In the past, the removal of this material would have required an operation.

The brainy folks at the University of Pennsylvania Medical Center are doing amazing things inside the head at the Interventional Neuro Center. They can pass micro-size catheters into the brain, not only for diagnostic purposes but also to treat aneurysms and tumors. Their tools enable them to seal off or open up vessels that are inaccessible through surgery.

A new and very exciting development may save some people from the destruction of an acute stroke. In a method similar to what's used in the emergency treatment of some heart attacks, the neuro-interventional radiologists at UPMC have the ability to unblock even the tiniest arteries in the brain with a clot-dissolving drug called urokinase. Clots prevent arteries from delivering oxygen, causing death by starvation to the part of the brain they feed. That results in the loss of speech or motor function, typical of stroke victims. If the clot can be disintegrated and the blood supply quickly restored, the brain cells will suffer little or no damage. "This is an incredible advance in the treatment of stroke," says Dr. Robert I. Grossman, chief of neuroradiology at UPMC. "You can take a person who has had a major stroke and by reversing the process, restore him to normal function and productive life."

Unfortunately, the window of applicability is very short—roughly six hours. It is critical that someone showing the symptoms of a stroke—difficulty speaking, weakness or paralysis of a limb—be taken to Penn immediately.

Ultrasonography: From submarines to problem pregnancies

Submarines are tracked by sending sound waves through the ocean's depths. In medicine, the same principle allows doctors to monitor everything from a fetus developing in the womb to the degree of damage to a heart valve. Unique pictures are produced from harmless high-frequency sound waves passing over certain areas of the body. The returning signal varies with the density of the tissue it hits. A computer measures that variance—how long it takes the sound to bounce back, as well as how much of it returns. The digital information gleaned from the reflected sound gets translated into a shadowy image.

This noninvasive screening device is widely used in perinatology, the care of unborn babies, since X-rays are far too dangerous to be used during pregnancy. Doctors are now able to study the fetus in its own little world. Is it the normal size for its stage of development? Is there any abnormal bleeding? Are all four chambers of the heart present? With the advent of ultrasound, doctors have reduced the number of stillbirths by diagnosing an absence of critical amniotic fluid and delivering a baby early who would otherwise starve to death. If ultrasound should reveal that a fetal bladder isn't emptying properly, doctors can insert a needle to drain the fetal urine and prevent damage to the unborn's kidney. Ultrasound has also cut the risk of amniocentesis, an important test for birth defects that requires drawing fluids from the womb. In the past, doctors occasionally harmed the fetus when they inserted the needle. With the help of the ultrasound, these accidents can be averted.

In adults, ultrasound routinely diagnoses certain heart problems that previously could be confirmed only with the riskier procedure of cardiac catheterization. Using a technique called Doppler echocardiography, doctors can watch heart valves opening and closing, see the direction and speed of blood flowing from chamber to chamber, and determine whether there are any leaks or structural defects.

The test is painless. The patient lies on a table while an operator passes what looks like a small flashlight over the heart. The sound waves it emits produce an electrical signal that is translated by computer into moving images on a TV screen. A whooshing sound that accompanies the picture tells an experienced listener how much a valve has actually narrowed. Echocardiography is particularly successful in diagnosing heart-valve problems, the cause of one out of seven open-heart surgeries in America. Many surgeons use it in the operating room to make certain their valve repairs have completely plugged the leak.

Doppler ultrasound is now available in color, which has opened new avenues for examining other parts of the body. It can give information about the kidneys, detect early ectopic pregnancies and illuminate the body's vascular roadways. Through different colors and different gradations of a single color, it shows both the structure of blood vessels and the speed of blood flow. Color Doppler ultrasound in the vagina is a good screening device to identify before surgery whether ovarian growths are malignant or benign.

Nuclear medicine: The magic bullet approach

Despite the ominous implications of its name, nuclear medicine is a relatively safe and inexpensive way to detect certain abnormalities that don't stand out on traditional X-ray pictures. Actually, it's just the reverse of standard X-ray technique. Instead of using machines outside the body to fire radiation through it, nuclear medicine works from the inside out, by sending off very low-level radiation generated by a solution injected into the body.

The field came to prominence after World War II, when research on atomic weapons yielded information about radioactivity that had applications beyond the military. From the men who made bombs, medicine learned how to combine chemicals with radioactive isotopes and study the effect these chemicals have on living tissue. In adapting radioactivity to mapping organs in action, the science of nuclear medicine was born.

First, a solution laced with radioactive isotopes is injected into the bloodstream. Then a special camera, equipped with a crystal that picks up these signals, translates them into an image. With this technique, doctors can see if a transplanted kidney is functioning properly, or whether a thyroid gland is behaving normally. The presence or absence of the tracer indicates whether there's a problem, and also determines the extent of any damage.

Currently, more than 30 kinds of nuclear scans are done routinely in most area hospitals, to diagnose problems such as blood clots in the lung or cirrhosis of the liver. A scan of the spine will tell if cancer has spread, since bones are a common secondary site for the disease. When doctors want to know how fast a stomach empties in a patient with gastric problems, they might feed that patient scrambled eggs seasoned with a tracer, and take a series of images to see how quickly the isotope disappears. A gallium scan, normally used to detect inflammation or infection, has been helpful in diagnosing AIDS through a characteristic lung infection. Another type of isotope that concentrates in dead heart tissue can identify where a heart attack took place, as well as the amount of tissue affected. Even blood flow can be measured radioactively.

Nuclear scans are commonly used in stress tests. The patient walks on a treadmill to build up his heart rate. Toward the end of the exercise period, he's injected with a radioactive isotope that immediately travels to the heart muscle and reveals whether a normal amount of blood is coursing through.

Except for the prick of the needle to inject the isotope solution, nuclear scans are no more painful than X-rays. Allergic reactions are rare; the isotopes are nontoxic, and the most commonly used isotopes have an average half-life of only six hours—which means they are gone from the body faster than the average meal.

PET scans: Windows on the body at work

Most of the machines that peer into the body take what might be called architectural pictures, the kind that show the basic structure of human parts. The advent of positron emission tomography—the PET scan—made it possible to leap from anatomy to function, to see living organs in action. Want to know what happens in the brain when we smell a flower or read a book, when we get upset or have a seizure? Or what happens when our heart doesn't get enough oxygen? PET scans can supply answers like these without invading the body.

Traditionally, researchers who studied the living brain relied on tests done with electrodes, or on whatever was revealed before their eyes when they cut open the body's think tank. Now they can get a wealth of information by injecting nontoxic chemicals laced with radioactive tracers into the bloodstream, then measuring how and where these chemicals are absorbed. By pairing glucose (a chemical that acts in the brain like gas in a car) with a tracer that emits measurable gamma rays, doctors can map the way the brain metabolizes its various fuels. PET studies have shown with precision what parts of the brain process high and low sounds, what regions react to feelings of anxiety and how memory loss due to a stroke differs from that resulting from Alzheimer's disease.

Fewer than 20 hospitals across the country are doing PET research, because the radioactive isotopes usually need to be manufactured in costly cyclotrons right on the hospital grounds. (Penn has one of them.) Some of the isotopes have a half-life of just 30 seconds and can't be transported. PET scans pose relatively little danger to patients. Depending on the test, the chemical compounds are either injected or inhaled, and the pictures are taken by machinery that looks similar to that used in CT scans.

PET scans are opening up all kinds of hidden secrets. For instance, we can now identify certain areas of damaged brain cells in stroke victims, because they do not absorb glucose or oxygen. By following whether these areas resume activity, doctors can chart the course of recovery. Such monitoring could eventually lead to an understanding of why some people recover from strokes, and perhaps make it possible to initiate recovery where it doesn't occur spontaneously. With patients suffering from seizures, PET scans can pinpoint the exact area in the brain responsible for triggering the attacks—a flaw not always revealed on standard brain-wave tests. Once identified, the abnormal tissue can sometimes be removed, and the seizures will disappear. PET studies of schizophrenics have shown a pattern of glucose metabolism markedly different from that in normal brains. These findings support the biochemical theory of mental illness, and could be instrumental in identifying its causes.

Another fruitful arena for the PET scan is in the diagnosis and treatment of cancer. It provides information useful in evaluating the disease, determining prognosis and differentiating scar tissue from diseased tissue following chemotherapy. For example, because active tumors gobble up glucose, doctors can measure glucose intake with a PET scan and use that information to evaluate how effective chemotherapy is, and whether to step it up or stop it.

PET scans are also gaining a place in cardiac care, because they are able to show blood flow into the heart muscle with greater accuracy than traditional thallium scanning. This information is valuable in deciding whether to proceed with heart surgery.

For researchers in particular, PET scans provide a priceless opportunity to bypass animal models and study a variety of human conditions as they occur in their natural settings. Their potential is virtually unlimited, because the number of available radioactive tracers has increased in a decade from a few to a few hundred. Compared to still photography, the PET scan is like a movie that will provide medicine with endless living studies of the way our marvelous engine works.

All these modern imaging techniques have one thing in common: They are all digital. Image data is now acquired under computer control; the images are created and processed in a computer and are often stored there as well. Today, these images can be "written" to film by use of a laser camera (a device much like a laser printer, except that it uses film instead of paper) and viewed on a light box just like ordinary X-rays. It is also possible to display the images on a high-resolution monitor to avoid the time-consuming and expensive steps of printing, distributing and eventually storing the film. This new process of picture acquisition, storage (or archiving), and communication to the display is called PACS.

Because of the digital nature of these images, they can be distributed via standard computer networks, enabling images to be transmitted to a surgeon in the operating room or a consultant in a remote clinic.

New methods of taking X-ray images digitally (a chest X-ray, for example) are being added to the PACS system. Soon, radiology departments will be filmless. All image data will be stored in large computer archives, which will be available quickly for radiologists and clinicians. This new technology provides a number of benefits: faster interpretations, rapid transmission of images to appropriate physicians, easy comparison with prior studies and a surefire way to eliminate lost and missing films.

Endoscopy: Following the body's pathways

While technologies like CT and MRI take an overall look at the body and how it functions, the field of endoscopy takes a peek inside the body's various systems.

Endoscopy examines interiors with a long, flexible fiber-optic tube. A gastroenterologist performs a colonoscopy to examine the inside of the colon; the pulmonologist performs a bronchioscopy to look at the bronchial tract. Endoscopy provides fine detail about the inner walls of the body's pathways, explains Dr. Igor Laufer, chief of gastrointestinal radiology at the University of Pennsylvania Medical Center. If we view the entire body as a map, he explains, endoscopy is a noninvasive way to explore all the major highways.

Though endoscopy has been around for about half a century, it wasn't until about 25 years ago with the advent of flexible fiber-optics that endoscopy became a viable option. Flexible fiber-optics allow greater maneuverability of the endoscope, which can wind its way through the curved contours of the colon, for example. En route, a magnified image is projected from the endoscope for the physician to view during the procedure, which can also be recorded on videotape for later consultation.

Gastrointestinal endoscopy constitutes the largest share of this technology. There are three major applications. First, in terms of diagnosis, a physician can inspect the inner lining of the gastrointestinal tract for growths, ulcers or changes in the interior. Secondly, endoscopy can be used for therapeutic functions. During a routine sigmoidoscopy (examination of the lower third of the colon, called the sigmoid, via a long, flexible fiber-optic tube) or colonoscopy (examination of the entire colon), small forceps can be inserted through the fiber-optic tube to perform a tissue biopsy or remove polyps for a pathologist's inspection, says Laufer. The third application of endoscopy involves endoscopic retrograde cardiological pancreatography (ERCP), either to diagnose abnormalities of the bile ducts or provide therapeutic relief by widening strictures or draining clogged tubes.

Gastrointestinal endoscopy, which is usually performed while the patient is under mild sedation, has been credited with drastically reducing the number of colon surgeries, as well as detecting colon cancer at an early stage, says Laufer. Roughly 5 million to 10 million of these procedures are performed annually. New on the horizon is an endoscopic ultrasound (EUS), where an ultrasound probe travels into the stomach through the endoscope to examine the wall of the gastrointestinal tract, the pancreas and its pathways for abnormalities and obstructions.

If your specialist suggests surgery, be sure to ask whether there is a noninvasive, or nonsurgical, method to get this same information or achieve the same therapeutic results, cautions Laufer. For instance, in many patients with cancer in the gastrointestinal tract, the combination of endoscopy, cross-sectional imaging and barium exams will be adequate to determine whether surgery is required. Radiologic or endoscopic techniques can also be used in treating many conditions, such as strictures of the gastrointestinal tract or biliary (bile-related) tree.

There are costs and risks associated with endoscopy (perforating the intestine or complications from sedation), so when a diagnostic endoscopic exam is recommended, you should ask whether the same or similar information can be obtained from barium radiologic studies (use of a white, radio-opaque substance that casts a shadow on X-rays as it passes through the gastrointestinal tract).

CHAPTER 8

Check It Out Before You Check In

Mini-profiles of area hospitals

It's hard to turn on the television or pick up a magazine these days without being confronted with an advertisement for a hospital. In the competitive field of health care, hospital marketing has burgeoned into big business. Americans spend more than $200 billion for hospital care—more than $1,000 for every man, woman and child in the country. No wonder hospitals are selling their services the way stores sell clothes and appliances. Since hospitals have entered the consumer marketplace, you, the buyer, need information to be a wise comparison shopper. That's why we compiled the following hospital profiles. We did not rate or evaluate individual hospitals. Rather, we let them present themselves as they'd like to be seen. Some hospitals chose not to answer everything we asked, particularly in regard to costs. If you want to know more, ask them directly.

Be aware that the more expensive hospitals do not necessarily provide better care. The costliest hospitals are likely to be teaching institutions, because of the added expense of maintaining academic programs. In general, use the hospital charges listed in these profiles as benchmark figures, because what you see is not usually what you pay. Like the sticker price on an automobile, hospital costs wind up being discounted and negotiated, especially by insurers. Hospitals are frequently reimbursed at reduced rates by insurance companies, HMOs, Medicare and Medicaid. And some people pay nothing at all. In 1992, area hospitals provided $147.7 million in free care.

Pennsylvanians are fortunate in that the state's Health Care Cost Containment Council gathers, analyzes and gives away, free of charge, an immense amount of information about area hospitals, ranging from mortality rates to costs to how many back operations a particular place has done. You can get copies of the council's Hospital Effectiveness Report by calling 717-232-6787 or by writing to the Council at 225 Market Street, Suite 400, Harrisburg, PA 17101.

The best doctors

in the Delaware Valley practice at the University of Pennsylvania Medical Center ... according to *American Health* magazine, which recognized "The Best Doctors in America" and named more doctors who practice at Penn than any other local institution.

The best hospital

in the Delaware Valley is the Hospital of the University of Pennsylvania ... ranked by *U.S. News & World Report* as best in the Delaware Valley in 13 key specialties. That's more top rankings than all other local hospitals combined. And HUP was the only hospital in Pennsylvania, New Jersey and Delaware recognized in the recent national performance survey of *100 Top Hospitals*.

The best health system

in the Delaware Valley is the University of Pennsylvania Health System. Our system includes 184 doctors recognized by *Philadelphia* magazine as "Top Docs," more than any other system.

The best choice

It all adds up to the best health care in the Delaware Valley, and it's available to your family by calling **1-800-789-PENN.** The University of Pennsylvania Health System. Best at what counts. Best when it counts.

UNIVERSITY OF
PENNSYLVANIA
HEALTH SYSTEM

The future of medicine.℠

Not surprisingly, the council's reports have been criticized by both doctors and hospitals. They complain the statistics don't reflect the difficulty of the cases they admit or the severity of the patient's illness. Doctors caution that publishing mortality rates for individual surgeons may make some of them stop operating on really sick patients, to improve their performance records. The council says its studies are adjusted to compensate for these differences. Bear in mind when you're interpreting these kinds of data that the success of any surgery depends on a variety of factors, including the patient's health, the surgeon's and the anesthesiologist's skill, the cleanliness of the hospital, the attention of the nursing care and the overall quality of the support staff. Studies suggest that you're more likely to live and less likely to have complications when you undergo a given procedure at a hospital where that procedure is done with a frequency approaching 200 cases a year. For more information, call the Delaware Valley Hospital Council at 215-735-9695.

A note: Hospitals were asked to complete a standard form, but not all provided information for every category we requested. In the interest of space, we have eliminated from each profile any category for which we weren't given information.

Codes

- overnight facilities for families
- pastoral care
- hospice care
- barber
- patient advocate
- smoke-free environment
- teaching hospital
- **E** emergency room
- prepayment for deductible required

Philadelphia

Albert Einstein Medical Center

5501 OLD YORK ROAD, PHILADELPHIA; 215-456-7890, 1-800-EINSTEIN (*physician referral/health information*). DOCTORS ON ACTIVE STAFF: 660 (*82% board-certified*). NUMBER OF BEDS: 600. RNs PER BED: 1.16. SEMIPRIVATE ROOM COST: $970. PRIVATE ROOM COST: $1,170. ACCREDITATION: JCAHO, ACS, PTSF, ACR.

Sample charges for surgical services including ancillary and supplies: coronary bypass without cardiac cath, $84,134; back and neck procedures without complication, $16,567; vaginal delivery, $6,320; prostate removal, $12,373; standard local anesthesia, $225; hourly operating-room charge, $2,351 (first hour); preadmission testing, $773 (average).
Special surgical units: heart surgery, surgical intensive care, organ transplants.
Special intensive care units: surgical, medical, pediatric, neonatal.

Base cost for emergency room visit: $110.
Also available in ER: trauma, Fast Track, psychiatric emergency services.
Ob/gyn programs: Healthy Beginnings Plus, A Better Start, high-risk obstetrics, Menopause Program.
Specialized treatment programs: Heart Center, Women's Heart, Cancer Center, High-Risk Breast Program, Center for Orthopedic Sciences, Center for Organ Transplantation, psychiatry (with Belmont Center for Comprehensive Treatment), geriatric medicine.
Physical rehab services: physical, occupational and speech therapy (MossRehab is part of Einstein and provides intensive medical rehab services).
Outpatient centers: Einstein Plaza Olney in Philadelphia's Olney section for primary health-care services; Einstein Center One in Northeast Philadelphia for primary and specialty care, radiology and cancer treatment; Einstein Plaza Jenkintown for primary and specialty care; The Imaging Center of Elkins Park for comprehensive radiology services; Prime Health for geriatrics in Northeast Philadelphia.

Allegheny University Hospitals, Center City (formerly Hahnemann University Hospital)

BROAD AND VINE STS., PHILADELPHIA; 215-762-7000, 1-800-PRO-HEALTH (*physician referral*). DOCTORS ON ACTIVE STAFF: 585. NUMBER OF BEDS: 636. ACCREDITATION: JCAHO, CAP, AABB, ACGME, ACR. MEMBER OF ALLEGHENY HEALTH, EDUCATION AND RESEARCH FOUNDATION.

Special surgical units: Heart Failure/Cardiac Transplant Center, Dedicated Kidney and Pancreas Transplant Care Unit, medical/surgical ICUs.
Special ER services: Level I Regional Resource Trauma Center, university MedEvac helicopter, 24-hour registered nurse triage, self-contained radiology section, cardiac resuscitation area, minor treatment area, psychiatric emergencies.
Ob/gyn programs: general obstetrics and gynecology, well-woman care, gynecologic oncology, high-risk obstetrics; reproductive endocrinology and infertility; genetic counseling; Level III NICU; LDRs, midwifery services; childbirth, breastfeeding, sibling and grandparent classes; prenatal testing; pelvic floor dysfunction and incontinence care.
Specialized treatment programs: numerous treatment programs in specialty and subspecialty areas. Programs include cardiac catheterization, electrophysiology, echocardiography, nuclear cardiology, cardiovascular and coronary care ICU, Dental Center, dialysis unit, geriatric assessment, Bone Marrow Transplant Unit, Foot and Ankle Center, Brain Tumor Center, Bone Tumor Center, Center for Neurosciences, Sleep Disorders Center, Travel Health Center, Breast Health Center, Pain Management Center, Home Health Care.
Physical rehab services: cardiovascular rehab; sports medicine; occupational, physical and speech therapy; Prosthetics Clinic; ALS Clinic.

Outpatient health and wellness programs: Executive Health and Wellness Center, Business Medicine (occupational/employee health).

Allegheny University Hospitals, East Falls (formerly Medical College of Pennsylvania Hospital)

3300 HENRY AVE.; 215-842-6000, 1-800-PRO-HEALTH (*physician referral*). DOCTORS ON ACTIVE STAFF: 695. NUMBER OF BEDS: 465. ACCREDITATION: JCAHO, CAP, AABB, ACGME, ACR. MEMBER OF ALLEGHENY HEALTH, EDUCATION AND RESEARCH FOUNDATION.

Special surgery units: cardiothoracic, medical/surgical ICUs.

Special ER services: Level I Regional Resource Trauma Center, university MedEvac helicopter, 24-hour registered nurse triage, self-contained radiology section, minor treatment area, psychiatric emergencies, toxicology.

Ob/gyn programs: general obstetrics and gynecology, Center for Women's Health, gynecologic oncology, high-risk obstetrics; reproductive endocrinology and infertility; genetic counseling; Level III NICU; new state-of-the-art maternity unit with LDRs; midwifery services; childbirth, breast-feeding, sibling and grandparent classes; prenatal testing; pelvic floor dysfunction and incontinence care.

Specialized treatment programs: numerous treatment programs in specialty and subspecialty areas. Programs include adult cystic fibrosis, Lung Health Center, Center for Women's Health, Center for Continuing Health, cardiac catheterization, electrophysiology, echocardiography, nuclear cardiology, cardiovascular and coronary care ICU, Spine Center, Center for Neurosciences, Dental Center, dialysis unit, geriatric assessment, Lipid Disorders Center, Mid-Atlantic Regional Epilepsy Center, Sleep Disorders Center, Travel Health Center, Center for the Study and Treatment of Anxiety, Caring Together, Home Health Care.

Physical rehab services: cardiovascular and pulmonary rehab, sports medicine; occupational, physical and speech therapy.

Outpatient health and wellness programs: Center for Continuing Health (fitness for people over 50); diabetes education; smoking cessation; prostate cancer support group; Advantage Passport (a program of health information and benefits for people 55 and older); Advantage for Women (a program of health information and benefits for women of all ages); Business Medicine (occupational/employee health).

Chestnut Hill Hospital

8835 GERMANTOWN AVE., PHILADELPHIA; 215-248-8200, 215-248-8069 (*physician referral*). DOCTORS ON ACTIVE STAFF: 196 (*98% board-certified*). NUMBER OF BEDS: 200. RNs PER BED: 1.03. ACCREDITATION: JCAHO, ACGME, CAP, PDH, ACR, AABB.

Special surgical units: outpatient surgical center.

Base cost for ER visit: $83.

Ob/gyn programs: family-centered maternity care, antenatal testing, perinatology, labor/delivery/recovery rooms, childbirth education, neonatology affiliation.

Specialized treatment programs: family practice center, dialysis, endoscopy, ICCU, CICU, ICU, cardiac rehab, pain management, breast disease, vascular disease, Hospital HomeCare, radiation oncology center, cancer care, cardiology services.

Physical rehab services: physical, occupational, speech therapy.

Outpatient health and wellness programs: Parents' Inc., childbirth education, sibling preparation, maternity exercise, Our First, cardiac rehab, diabetes, smoking cessation, speakers bureau, CPR, Senior CHEC, blood pressure, various cancer screenings and support groups, comprehensive health risk assessment program.

Children's Hospital of Philadelphia

34TH ST. AND CIVIC CENTER BLVD., PHILADELPHIA; 215-590-1000, 1-800-TRY-CHOP (*for referrals*). DOCTORS ON ACTIVE STAFF: 260 (*99% board-certified*). NUMBER OF BEDS: 304. RNs PER BED: 2.4. SEMIPRIVATE ROOM COST: $775. PRIVATE ROOM COST: $825. ACCREDITATION: JCAHO, ABP.

Surgical charges: not applicable.

Special surgical units: fetal surgery, transplants (heart, lung, heart/lung, liver, kidney and bone marrow), cardiothoracic, craniofacial, craniofacial reconstruction, neurosurgery, urology, orthopedics.

Base cost for an ER visit: $110.

Special ER services: Level I trauma service, six isolation rooms for patients with infectious diseases, trauma resuscitation room, modern radiology suite, decontamination room.

Specialized programs: fetal diagnosis and treatment, Growth Center, pain management, sleep disorders, Diagnostic Center, attention deficit/hyperactivity disorders, hemangioma, lipid heart, obesity clinic, cystic fibrosis, scoliosis, sports medicine, orthopedics, dyslexia testing, neurofibromatosis, sickle-cell anemia, hemophilia, neuro-oncology, Pediatric Regional Epilepsy Program, electroencephalography, neuromuscular program, psychiatric unit, spina bifida, trauma program, neonatal and pediatric follow-up, bone marrow transplantation.

Special treatment units: oncology, surgical (trauma and short-stay), medical (diabetes and asthma, cardiology), cardiac intensive care unit, newborn/infant center, pediatric ICU (acute, intermediate and isolation), Infant Transitional Unit. Provides physical rehab services through the Children's Seashore House.

Episcopal Hospital

100 East Lehigh Ave., Philadelphia; 215-427-7000. Doctors on active staff: 313 (*64% board-certified*). Number of beds: 275. RNs per bed: .71. Semiprivate and private room cost: $830. Accreditation: JCAHO, AABB, ACS, CAP.

Special surgical units: laparoscopic cholecystectomy, neurosurgery, cardiothoracic, colorectal, laser.
Base cost for an ER visit: $78.
Special ER services: rape crisis center, drug overdose program.
Ob/gyn programs: prepared childbirth classes; maternal/infant care; neonatal intensive care unit; Women, Infants and Children; cocaine outreach services.
Specialized treatment programs: substance abuse, dialysis, dental (pediatric), industrial medicine, Beacon House (residential facility for female drug abusers), cardiac rehab, asthma center, ophthalmology, diabetic foot center.
Physical rehab services: physical and occupational therapy; work hardening and Back School; Pain Management Center; medical and dental outpatient pediatrics; cardiovascular diagnostic and therapeutic procedures such as cardiac catheterization, electrophysiology studies, bypass surgery, stress testing, angioplasty, laser surgery and pacemaker implants; Memory Disorder Center; Mammography Center; Coumadin Clinic.
Outpatient health and wellness programs: prenatal classes, fitness/circuit training, nutritional counseling service, community outreach screening programs.

Frankford Hospital

Frankford campus: Frankford Ave. and Wakeling St., Philadelphia; 215-831-2000. Torresdale campus: Knights and Red Lion roads, Philadelphia; 215-612-4000, 215-612-4888 (*physician referral for both campuses*). Doctors on active staff: 596 (*77% board-certified*). Number of beds: 344. RNs per bed: .96. Private room cost: $1,979. Accreditation: JCAHO, AABB.

Special surgical units: endoscopy suite, ambulatory surgery centers, laparoscopy.
Base cost for ER visit: $74.
Special ER services: Level II Trauma Center, Fast Track.
Ob/gyn programs: family-centered maternity program, Women's Health Center, gynecologic oncology, perinatology, neonatology, home visit program, Healthy Beginnings Plus.
Specialized treatment programs: health center clinics for low-income families, radiation oncology, inpatient detox, outpatient drug and alcohol counseling and treatment, pain clinic, wound care program, inpatient rehabilitation unit.
Physical rehab services: physical therapy (in- and outpatient), Work Hardening, home care rehab, Work Health (occupational medicine).
Outpatient health and wellness programs: diabetes education, exercise classes,

weight management, nutritional counseling, CPR, first aid, cholesterol and blood pressure screening, maternity fitness and breast-feeding classes, cardiopulmonary rehab program.

Germantown Hospital and Medical Center

ONE PENN BLVD., PHILADELPHIA; 215-951-8000. DOCTORS ON ACTIVE STAFF: 215 (*92% board-certified*). NUMBER OF BEDS: 226. RNS PER BED: .90. ROOM COST (*all private*): $887.50. ACCREDITATION: JCAHO, CAP, AABB, ACR.

Sample charges for surgical services: back and neck procedures without complication, $14,500; vaginal delivery, $7,400; prostate removal, $10,200; hourly operating-room charge, first half-hour $1,654, each additional half-hour $954; preadmission testing, $650.

Base cost for ER visit: $203.

Special ER services: Fast Track.

Ob/gyn programs: Healthy Beginnings Plus, childbirth education and free adjusting-to-parenthood classes, Women's Health Center, physician and midwifery birth care.

Specialized treatment programs: skilled nursing facility, Ambulatory Infusion Center, Comprehensive Headache Center, Women's Health Center, human cartilage transplantation, Northwest Medical Practice (for those who are uninsured or underinsured).

Physical rehab services: physical therapy, occupational therapy, speech pathology and audiology, Ergometer, Kinetron II, Fitron, treadmill, Biodex.

Outpatient health and wellness programs: Living Well Health (free and reduced-cost services); blood pressure and cholesterol screenings; Easy Breathers Club; breast self-exam instruction; screenings for diabetes, glaucoma, prostate cancer, hearing and colorectal cancer. Passport to Health is a senior membership program with Center in the Park, free speakers bureau, Care-A-Van (reduced-cost transportation).

Graduate Health System City Avenue Hospital

4150 CITY AVE., PHILADELPHIA; 215-871-1000, 1-800-GRAD-LINE (*physician referral*). DOCTORS ON ACTIVE STAFF: 422 (*71% board-certified*). NUMBER OF BEDS: 210. RNS PER BED: 1.2. SEMIPRIVATE ROOM COST: $550. PRIVATE ROOM COST: $600. ACCREDITATION: AOA, CAP, AABB.

Special surgical units: surgical short procedure unit, carbon dioxide and Yag laser, laparoscopic procedures, sinus endoscopy with video capabilities.

Base cost for ER visit: $70. Level II emergency services available for minor traumas and fractures.

Ob/gyn programs: family-centered maternity care with certified midwives and

obstetricians, parenting, perinatology, neonatology, infertility, advanced laparoscopic surgery, childbirth education, certified nurse-midwifery.
Specialized treatment programs: inpatient mental health, podiatry, pediatrics, TMJ clinic, medical short procedures unit for outpatient chemotherapy, pain management, autologous blood donations, ICU, CCU, telemetry.
Physical rehab services: in- and outpatient physical therapy, outpatient audiology and speech pathology.

Graduate Health System Parkview Hospital

1331 East Wyoming Ave., Philadelphia; 215-537-7400, 1-800-GRAD-LINE (*physician referral*). Doctors on active staff: 410 (*75% board-certified*). Number of beds: 200. RNs per bed: 1.1. Semiprivate room: $600. Private room: $680. Accreditation: AOA.

Special surgical units: laparoscopic procedures, sinus endoscopy with video capabilities.
Base cost for ER visit: $90.
Special ER services: fully equipped cast room with orthopedic specialists available 24 hours, cardiac treatment, trauma treatment, thromolytic therapy.
Ob/gyn programs: full-service obstetrics with labor, postpartum and nursery on same floor; optional rooming-in; modified mother-infant care; classes in sibling and grandparent preparation, childbirth education and breast-feeding.
Specialized treatment programs: dialysis, skilled nursing, pediatrics, ICCU, pulmonary care unit, telemetry unit, short procedure unit, minor surgery, chemotherapy, medical detox.
Physical rehab services: in- and outpatient occupational, physical and speech therapy.
Outpatient health and wellness programs: family and parenting courses; CPR; skin cancer, blood pressure, prostate, diabetes and cholesterol screenings.

The Graduate Hospital

18th and Lombard sts., Philadelphia; 215-893-2000, 1-800-GRAD-LINE (*physician referral*). Doctors on active staff: 294 (*84% board-certified*). Number of beds: 330. RNs per bed: 1.4. Semiprivate room cost: $1,150. Private room cost: $1,180. Suite cost: $1,255. Gourmet food service: $16.75 per day. Accreditation: JCAHO, ACGME, ACR, PDH, AABB.

Special surgical units: open-heart, musculoskeletal tumor surgery, neurosurgery for epilepsy and Parkinson's disease, colon and rectal surgery, surgical oncology, gynecologic oncology, same-day surgery, laser and laparoscopic surgery.
Base cost for ER visit: $102.
Gynecological services emphasize organ preservation and include a range of surgical procedures, including total laparoscopic hysterectomies.

Specialized treatment programs: Arthritis Center, Bladder Health Center, Bloodless Care Program, Cancer Program, Cardiac Care Unit, Cerebral Blood Flow Lab, Comprehensive Epilepsy Center, kidney dialysis (inpatient and outpatient), Intra-Operative Radiation Therapy (IORT), medical stress management program, Medical/Surgical ICU, Nutritional Support Unit, Musculoskeletal Tumor Service, Neurological ICU, Occupational Therapy, Parkinson's Disease and Movement Disorders Center, Physical Therapy, Phase I cardiac rehab, radiation therapy, speech therapy, Stem Cell Transplantation Program, TMJ service, Vascular Blood Flow Laboratory, Wound Care Center. Graduate also operates a Human Performance and Sports Medicine Center in Wayne (610-688-6767).

Jeanes Hospital

7600 CENTRAL AVE., PHILADELPHIA; 215-728-2000, 215-728-2033 (*Women's Healthline*), 215-728-2100 (*Seniors' Healthline*). DOCTORS ON ACTIVE STAFF: 171 (*87% board-certified*). NUMBER OF BEDS: 188. RNs PER BED: 1. SEMIPRIVATE ROOM COST: $1,243. PRIVATE ROOM COST: $1,315. ACCREDITATION: JCAHO, PDH, CAP.

Sample charges for surgical services: back and neck procedures without complication, $11,546; vaginal delivery, $5,811; prostate removal, $11,202; standard local anesthesia, $54.75; hourly operating-room charge, $1,530; preadmission testing, $256.50.
Special surgical units: orthopedics, cancer care.
Base cost for ER visit: $80.25.
Special ER services: Level II general emergency department.
Ob/gyn programs: LDR rooms; whirlpools during labor; Level II NICU; perinatology; videophone to show infant to long-distance loved ones; childbirth education; UNITE; women's health; sibling, infant care, and breast-feeding class; maternity exercise; physical therapy for expectant and new mothers.
Specialized programs: adult day health care center, diagnostic imaging center, home health.
Physical rehab services: occupational, physical and speech therapy; audiology; cardiac and pulmonary rehab.
Outpatient health and wellness programs: blood pressure screenings, support groups, smoking cessation, speakers bureau, diabetes, Parkinson's exercise group, nutritional counseling, Lifestrides for adults over 50, arthritis aquatics.

Methodist Hospital

2301 SOUTH BROAD ST., PHILADELPHIA; 215-952-9000, 215-BROADST (*physician referral*). DOCTORS ON ACTIVE STAFF: 254 (*85% board-certified*). NUMBER OF BEDS: 289. RNs PER BED: 1.3. ACCREDITATION: JCAHO, PDH, DVHC.

Special surgical units: rapid recovery surgical center, short procedure unit, car-

diac cath lab, G.I. procedure unit.
Special ER services: Chest Pain Emergency Center, Fast Track.
Ob/gyn programs: Family Birth Center, neonatal ICU, antenatal testing services, laparoscopic gynecological surgery.
Physical rehab services: physical and occupational therapy, speech pathology, cardiac rehab (affiliated with Magee Rehabilitation).
Outpatient health and wellness programs: smoking cessation, weight loss, nutrition counseling, free patient transport van, free screenings and wellness lectures.

Misericordia Hospital

5301 CEDAR AVE., PHILADELPHIA; 215-748-9000, 1-800-422-8815 (*physician referral*). DOCTORS ON ACTIVE STAFF: 414. NUMBER OF BEDS: 286. ACCREDITATION: AABB, CAP, JCAHO, PDH, PDW.

Special surgical units: same-day surgery unit, surgical ICU.
Base cost for ER visit: $72.
Special ER services: 24-hour staffing by board-certified emergency medicine physicians; hyperbaric oxygen therapy; trauma; toxicology; Fast Track for non-life-threatening injuries.
Ob/gyn programs: women's services; midwifery; Family Birthing Center featuring labor, delivery, recovery and postpartum suites; Family Life Program series (parenting and childbirth education); breast-feeding instruction.
Specialized treatment programs: detox, inpatient pregnancy detox, acute dialysis, psychiatric crisis, vascular lab, Iris V. Henderson Cancer Center (linear accelerator); CT; medical imaging (general radiology, mammography); nuclear medicine; ultrasound; skilled nursing facility; pain management program.
Outpatient health and wellness programs: ambulatory care (ob/gyn, pediatrics, surgery); diagnostic cardiology; laboratory; audiology; Community Outreach Health Links (community health-care support); weight loss; cancer, blood pressure, cholesterol, lung and glaucoma screenings; infant and adult CPR training; Mercy Community Health Team mobile health van; Older Adult Club (nutrition support); cardiovascular risk reduction program; low-cost mammography and breast cancer early-detection program; smoking cessation; cancer support groups; social service support for parents and teens; AIDS Community Committee (HIV/AIDS education).

Nazareth Hospital

2601 HOLME AVE., PHILADELPHIA; 215-335-6000, 215-335-6690 (PHYSICIAN REFERRAL). DOCTORS ON ACTIVE STAFF: 326 (*81% board-certified*). NUMBER OF BEDS: 387. ACCREDITATION: JCAHO, PDH, CAP, AABB, AMA.

Special surgical units: short procedure unit.
Ob/gyn programs: Women's Health Center, NICU, rooming-in, childbirth classes, perinatal testing, sibling classes.
Specialized treatment programs: emergency services, mental health, perinatal testing, heart testing, high-risk pregnancy clinic.
Physical rehab services: 19-bed inpatient unit focusing on the needs of stroke and orthopedic patients; IndustriCare occupational health services; outpatient physical, occupational and speech therapy.
Outpatient health and wellness programs: Testing, surgery, cardiac rehab, pulmonary rehab, radiation therapy. Free van service for all outpatient services.

North Philadelphia Health System

DOCTORS ON ACTIVE STAFF: 150 (*50% board-certified*). SEMIPRIVATE ROOM COST: $700. PRIVATE ROOM COST: $800. ACCREDITATION: JCAHO, AOA.

The 409-bed health system provides psychiatric services and care for the chemically dependent at Girard Medical Center, and medical, surgical and emergency care at St. Joseph's.

Sample charges for surgical services: prostate removal, $12,465; standard local anesthesia, $595; hourly operating room charge, $600.

Girard Medical Center

GIRARD AVE. AT 8TH ST., PHILADELPHIA; 215-787-2000, 215-787-CARE (*clinic, physician and general information*).

Specialized treatment programs: full behavioral medicine services including inpatient and outpatient psychiatry, dual-diagnosis program, and a dual-diagnosis service for Latino patients with bicultural, bilingual staff; complete drug and alcohol treatment center. Continuing Care Hospital of Philadelphia: The first extended acute care program in the Delaware Valley dedicated to patients needing longer-than-usual hospital stays and those who have multiple system failures. The facility also provides a ventilator-dependent reduction program.
Physical rehab services: physical, occupational and speech therapy (also at St. Joseph's).
Outpatient health and wellness programs: primary care, immunizations, travel care, nutrition, well baby care, drug and alcohol rehab.

St. Joseph's Hospital

16TH ST. AND GIRARD AVE., PHILADELPHIA; 215-787-9000, 215-787-CARE (*clinic, physician and general information*).

Special surgical units: short procedure unit.
Base cost for ER services: $140.
Special ER services: Fast Track (1-9 p.m.).
Outpatient health and wellness programs: full-service ambulatory care center including pediatrics, gynecology and plastic and reconstructive surgery.

Northeastern Hospital

2301 East Allegheny Ave., Philadelphia; 215-291-3000, 215-291-DOCS (*physician referral*). Doctors on active staff: 354. Number of beds: 231. Accreditation: ACR, AABB, JCAHO. A division of Temple University Health System.

Special surgical units: short-stay surgical program.
Special ER services: Heart Care, Chest Pain Center.
Ob/gyn: Women's Health Care Center offers family planning, comprehensive gynecologic services and care for patients with special financial needs.
Specialized treatment programs: Industrial Healthcare Center, Sports Medicine Center.
Outpatient health and wellness programs: extensive community education course selection.

Pennsylvania Hospital

800 Spruce St., Philadelphia; 215-829-3000, 215-829-6800 (*physician referral*), 215-829-KIDS (*pregnancy health line*). Doctors on active staff: 316 (*95% board-certified*). Number of beds: 739 (includes acute care and psychiatric facilities). Semiprivate room cost: $1,405. Private room cost: $1,590. Accreditation: JCAHO.

Special surgical units: Cardiac Surgery Suite, Vascular Surgery Suite, prostate cryosurgery, 14-room suite for surgery such as videoscopic, gynecologic oncology, neurosurgery, obstetrics and gynecology, ophthalmology, oral, orthopedics, otolaryngology, plastic/reconstructive, urology.
Base rate for ER visit: based on severity of injury: five levels of service ranging from $96 to $455.
Ob/gyn programs: area's largest obstetrics service, delivering 3,800 babies annually; antenatal testing unit; birthing suite (nurse-midwifery); childbirth education classes; Antepartum Unit; fetal therapy; home monitoring; high-risk obstetrics; infertility treatment; perinatal cardiology; postpartum disorders project; breast-feeding education and support; Joan A. Karnell Women's Cancer Center.
Specialized treatment programs: Special Care Unit, intensive care nursery, CCU, neurointensive unit, ICU, Sleep Disorders Laboratory, Neurosciences Center (including stroke center), Eichler Laser Center, Franklin Dialysis Center, Hall-Mercer Community Mental Health/Mental Retardation Center, Counseling Program (outpatient services for mental health and chemical dependency problems

of contracted companies). The Institute of Pennsylvania Hospital provides comprehensive in- and outpatient psychiatric treatment, including specialty services for substance abuse, eating disorders, dementia, depression and anxiety, and a women's mental health program. The Rothman Institute, one of the world's leading orthopedic centers, has performed more than 15,000 joint replacements. The Benjamin Franklin Clinic is the hospital's network of primary and specialty care providers.

Physical rehab services: physical therapy and rehab, occupational therapy, Skilled Care Center (addresses needs of patients during transitional period between stay in acute care hospital and return to daily living at home).

Outpatient health and wellness programs: HealthFirst (a physician referral and information service), Tel-Med, diabetes education, Travel Medical Service, nutrition counseling, free monthly seminars, speakers bureau, Child and Parent Center, childbirth education classes, Health Ways (a free program to address the needs of people 55 and older). Adult Day Health Center, the first hospital-based adult day care in Philadelphia, provides medically supervised care along with comprehensive rehab and recreational services for older adults. The Benjamin Franklin Center for Health offers comprehensive wellness and preventive medical services (including a cardiac rehabilitation and weight management program and exercise center).

Presbyterian Medical Center

39TH AND MARKET STS., PHILADELPHIA; 215-662-8000. DOCTORS ON ACTIVE STAFF: 337 (*82% board-certified*). NUMBER OF BEDS: 344. RNs PER BED: 1.6. SINGLE-BED ROOM COST: $975. ACCREDITATION: JCAHO, CAP.

Special surgical units: cardiothoracic, vascular, orthopedic, gastrointestinal, podiatric.

Specialized treatment programs: Acute Care of Elders (ACE) Unit; inflammatory bowel disease; angioplasty; coronary artery disease and arrhythmia management; outpatient cath; Penn Center for Musculoskeletal Medicine; Foot and Ankle Institute; inpatient psychiatric unit; addictions treatment and residential treatment for chronic mental illness; geropsychiatric services; cancer treatment and clinical research; women's imaging center; skilled nursing facility; home care and hospice.

Outpatient health and wellness programs: lipid research and risk reduction; repetitive stress injury center; dry mouth center; addiction counseling, education and support services; community outreach education programs on diabetes, hypertension, nutrition and general health; pastoral care.

Roxborough Memorial Hospital

5800 RIDGE AVE., PHILADELPHIA; 215-483-9900. DOCTORS ON ACTIVE STAFF: 166 (*76% board-certified*). NUMBER OF BEDS: 189. RNs PER BED: 1. SEMIPRIVATE ROOM COST: $651. PRIVATE ROOM COST: $704. ACCREDITATION: JCAHO, CAP, PDH, AABB, DPW.

Ob/gyn services: family planning, fertility procedures, prenatal and sibling classes.
Specialized treatment programs: breast prostheses, enterostomal therapy, skilled nursing facility, pain treatment, chest pain emergency center.
Physical rehab services: inpatient and outpatient physical, occupational and speech therapy; hand therapy; wound care clinic; work reconditioning.
Outpatient health and wellness programs: cardiac and pulmonary rehab; diabetes education; screenings for breast, colorectal and prostate cancer; community resource centers offering free weekly screenings and programs; CPR and smoking cessation classes; speakers bureau; monthly lectures; ElderMed program for those over 50; various support groups; babysitting course.

St. Agnes Medical Center

1900 SOUTH BROAD ST., PHILADELPHIA; 215-339-4100. DOCTORS ON ACTIVE STAFF: 199 (76% board-certified). NUMBER OF BEDS: 240; RNS PER BED: 1. ACCREDITATION: JCAHO, AOA, CAP.

Specialized treatment programs: St. Agnes Burn Treatment Center, comprehensive inpatient rehab, cardiac telemetry unit, renal dialysis center, adult day care center, cardiac care, ICU, TCU, minimally invasive surgery.
Special outpatient services: Work Care, IndustriCare, home care, rehab, Parish Nurse Program, physical capacity evaluations, pulmonary diagnostics, speech and hearing, cardiac rehab, electrodiagnostic lab, Women's Health Center.
Outpatient health and wellness programs: medically supervised/monitored exercise, adult fitness, aerobics, muscular conditioning, weight management, yoga, stress reduction, nutritional counseling, smoke cessation, free van service.

St. Christopher's Hospital for Children

ERIE AVE. AT FRONT ST., PHILADELPHIA; 215-427-5000. DOCTORS ON ACTIVE STAFF: 177 (90% board-certified). NUMBER OF BEDS: 183. RNS PER BED: 2. SEMIPRIVATE ROOM COST: $1,101. PRIVATE ROOM COST: $1,246. ACCREDITATION: JCAHO, ACGME, CAP, ADA, APOS. A MEMBER OF THE ALLEGHENY HEALTH, EDUCATION AND RESEARCH FOUNDATION.

Special surgical units: kidney, liver, heart and heart/lung transplantation; cardiothoracic surgery; burn surgery; neurosurgery; dental/oral, orthopedic, otolaryngological, plastic, craniofacial and reconstructive surgery; short procedure.
Base cost for ER visit: $101.
Special ER services: isolation rooms for patients with infectious diseases; trauma resuscitation room; decontamination room; dedicated suture and orthopedic casting room; trauma capabilities; 24-hour attending coverage; helipad; adolescent gynecology room.
Specialized treatment programs: Pediatric Transplant Institute (kidney, liver, heart and heart/lung); Stuart J. Hulnick Burn Center; NICU; Marian Anderson

Sickle-Cell Anemia Care and Research Center; Center for Cystic Fibrosis and Pulmonary Disease; Heart Center for Children; Orthopedic Center for Children; neurosciences services; gastroenterology and nutrition program; diagnostic referral service; family-centered HIV/AIDS program.

Physical rehab services: physical, occupational and speech therapy; audiology; scoliosis and spinal surgery; sports medicine.

Temple University Hospital

BROAD AND ONTARIO STS., PHILADELPHIA; 215-707-2000, 1-800-TEMPLE-MD (*physician referral*). DOCTORS ON ACTIVE STAFF: 494 (*100% board-certified*). NUMBER OF BEDS: 514. RNs PER BED: 1. SEMIPRIVATE ROOM COST: $1,355. PRIVATE ROOM COST: $1,423. GOURMET FOOD SERVICE: $23 PER DINNER. ACCREDITATION: JCAHO, CAP, PDH, PTCF, HCFA.

Sample charges for surgical services: coronary bypass without cardiac cath, $32,000; back and neck procedures without complication, $11,000; vaginal delivery, $4,500; prostate removal, $7,000; standard local anesthesia, $316; hourly operating-room charge, $1,770; preadmission testing, $650.

Special surgical units: heart, lung, bone marrow and kidney transplants; stereotactic radiosurgery; neurosurgical ICU; oncologic cryosurgery.

Base cost for ER visit: $173. Temple is a Level I Trauma Center and has a Psychiatric Emergency Center.

Ob/gyn programs: maternal-fetal medicine, gynecologic oncology, reproductive endocrinology, nurse-midwifery, Center for Women's Health, fetal testing, genetic counseling, perinatal cardiology, diabetes in pregnancy.

Specialized treatment programs: Center for Sports Medicine, multiple sclerosis, epilepsy, dialysis, oral surgery, Cancer Center, Comprehensive Breast Center, Ventilator Rehab Center. Temple also has a physical medicine and rehab unit.

Outpatient health and wellness programs: Nutrition Center, weight loss and stress management programs, pulmonary rehab, sports medicine.

Thomas Jefferson University Hospital

111 SOUTH 11TH ST., PHILADELPHIA; 215-955-6000, 1-800-JEFF-NOW (*hotline*). DOCTORS ON ACTIVE STAFF: 678. NUMBER OF BEDS: 717. ACCREDITATION: JCAHO.

Special surgical units: cardiothoracic, colorectal, Jefferson Surgical Center, short procedure unit, kidney and liver transplantation, hand surgery and urology suite.

Special ER services: Level I Regional Resource Trauma Center, Spinal Cord Injury Center, Neuroimplant Program, access through helicopter and JeffSTAT ambulance retrieval teams, access to stroke clinical trials, on-site trauma operating room, X-ray room, three trauma bays, patient testing lab, separate acute and intermediate care areas.

Ob/gyn programs: in-vitro fertilization, gynecologic oncology, abnormal Pap smears and cervical disease, high-risk pregnancy, reproductive endocrinology/fertility, ultrasound, Teenagers in Touch, MOM program for disabled women.
Physical rehab services: Regional Spinal Cord Injury Center; physical, occupational and speech therapy; Jefferson Comprehensive Rehabilitation Center; Work Fitness Program.
Outpatient health and wellness programs: Alzheimer's disease, amputee program, antenatal evaluation center, arts medicine, asthma, Back Center, biofeedback, Kimmel Cancer Center, Cardeza Foundation (hemophilia and sickle-cell centers), Children's Center for Cerebral Palsy and Neuromuscular Disorders, Weigh to Go, Smokestoppers, aerobics, Dining With Heart, free screening programs, seizure disorders, Comprehensive Rectal Cancer Center, corporate health, dietetics, drug and alcohol, dialysis, extracorporeal membrane oxygenation (for newborns), Enuresis Program, Familial Polyposis Registry, cardiac cath, stress testing, echocardiography, geriatric assessment, hand rehab, infant apnea, Jefferson Center for International Dermatology, medical genetics, Monell-Jefferson Taste and Smell, Multiple Sclerosis Comprehensive Clinical Center, NeuroMuscular Disease Clinic, Occupational and Environmental Medicine Clinic, Pain Center, perinatal addiction services, pigmented lesion, pregnancy loss, psychiatric clinic, psychosomatic treatment, Rape Center, scleroderma, sexual function, sleep disorders, sperm bank, SIDS, Tay-Sachs prevention, urodynamic testing.

The University of Pennsylvania Medical Center

3400 SPRUCE ST., PHILADELPHIA; 215-662-4000, 1-800-789-PENN (*Penn Physician Referral*). DOCTORS ON ACTIVE STAFF: 750 (*92% board-certified*). NUMBER OF BEDS: 725. RNs PER BED: 1.18. DOUBLE-BED ROOM COST: $1,121. PRIVATE SINGLE-BED ROOM COST: $1,235. ACCREDITATION: JCAHO, AABB, CAP, PDH, CARF, ACGME.

Special surgical units: cardiovascular surgery; surgical oncology; plastic surgery; oral and maxillofacial surgery; transplantation; state-of-the-art laparoscopic, endoscopic and thoracoscopic techniques.
Special ER services: Level I Trauma Center, Head Trauma Center, Radiation Emergency Center, Work Injury Evaluation Center.
Ob/gyn programs: infertility and in-vitro fertilization (one of six programs nationwide designated by the National Institutes of Health for research and state-of-the-art treatment); high-risk pregnancy; reproductive genetics; reproductive surgery including laparoscopic procedures; gynecologic oncology; Penn Health for Women, offering complete care at King of Prussia.
Specialized treatment programs: Penn has more than 200 specialty programs, clinics and laboratories. Among them are the University of Pennsylvania Cancer Center, one of 27 centers nationwide designated by the National Cancer Institute, which has more than 300 physicians and scientists specializing in cancer treatment,

research and education; Breast Cancer Risk Evaluation Program; Bone Marrow Transplant Program; Joint Reconstruction Center; Sports Medicine Center; Neurological Institute; Digestive and Liver Disease Center; Lung Center; Multi-Organ Transplant Center; Addictions Research/Treatment Center; Center for Human Appearance; Mood and Memory Disorders Clinic; Center for Cognitive Therapy; Weight and Eating Disorders Program; Center for Sleep Disorders; Institute for Human Gene Therapy.

Physical rehab services: Amputee Clinic; Back and Spine Center; stroke rehab; physical, hand and occupational therapy; trauma and transplant rehab; TMJ physical therapy.

Wills Eye Hospital

900 WALNUT ST., PHILADELPHIA; 215-928-3000 (*ophthalmology*), 215-928-3021 (*geriatric psychiatry*), 215-928-7000 (*neurosensory institute*). DOCTORS ON ACTIVE STAFF: 434 (*91% board-certified*). NUMBER OF BEDS: 115. RNS PER BED: 1.5. SEMIPRIVATE ROOM COST: $855. PRIVATE ROOM COST: $970. ACCREDITATION: JCAHO, PDH, ACGME, AMA, CAP.

Sample charges for surgical services: standard local anesthesia, $212; hourly operating room charge: $1,000.

Base cost for ER visit: $128.

Specialized ophthalmic treatment programs: services for contact lens, cornea, cataract and primary eye care; glaucoma; neuro-ophthalmology; oculoplastics and cosmetic surgery unit; oncology; pediatric ophthalmology; retina; low vision; Foerderer Center for the Study of Eye Movement Disorders in Children; refractive surgery unit; Center for Sports Vision; social service; ocular trauma center.

Specialized geriatric psychiatry treatment program: a 30-bed inpatient unit for the treatment of the unique psychiatric and neurological disorders of the older adult, such as memory loss, depression and dementia. The staff is composed of geriatric-trained psychiatrists and nurses, along with social workers, occupational and creative arts therapists, and mental health associates.

Specialized neurosensory treatment programs: gamma knife, stereotactic radiotherapy (linear accelerator) and interventional neuroradiology for the treatment of brain tumors, aneurysms, arteriovenous malformations, cerebrovascular abnormalities and other brain, neck and spine disorders.

Bucks County

Allegheny University Hospitals, Bucks County (formerly Bucks County Hospital)

225 NEWTOWN ROAD, WARMINSTER; 215-441-6600, 1-800-PRO-HEALTH (*physician referral*). DOCTORS ON ACTIVE STAFF: 178. NUMBER OF BEDS: 176. ACCREDITATION: JCAHO, CAP, PDH, ACR. MEMBER OF ALLEGHENY HEALTH, EDUCATION AND RESEARCH FOUNDATION.

Special surgical units: medical/surgical ICUs.
Special ER services: MedEvac access to Regional Resource Trauma Centers.
Ob/gyn programs: general obstetrics and gynecology; family-centered maternity services; state-of-the-art maternity unit; LDRPs; midwifery services; childbirth, breast-feeding, sibling and grandparent classes; prenatal testing.
Specialized treatment programs: behavioral services including substance abuse programs, adult and adolescent psychiatry and a psychiatric partial hospital program; family practice center; sports medicine and orthopedics; home health care; Sleep Disorders Center; dialysis.
Physical rehab services: Achievement Center for cardiac and pulmonary rehab; occupational, physical and speech therapy; adult fitness.
Outpatient health and wellness programs: SurgiCenter (ambulatory surgical procedures); Breast Center and breast cancer support groups and education; Diagnostic Imaging Center; Aqua Exercise and Water Walking programs; CPR, first-aid and childbirth education classes; Slim-a-Weigh with Exercise; variety of support groups and annual health screenings; Advantage Passport (a program of health information and benefits for people 55 and older); Advantage for Women (a program of health information and benefits for women of all ages); Business Medicine (occupational/employee health).

Delaware Valley Medical Center

200 OXFORD VALLEY ROAD, LANGHORNE; 215-949-5000, 215-946-5116 (*physician referral and general information*). DOCTORS ON ACTIVE STAFF: 291 (*80% board-certified*). NUMBER OF BEDS: 200. RNs PER BED: 1.2. ACCREDITATION: AABB, AOA, APMA, CAP, CPDH. DEPT. OF HHS, FDA, STATE BOARD OF OSTEOPATHIC MEDICAL EXAMINERS.

Special surgical units: cardiac cath lab, ambulatory surgery, laser, orthopedic, endoscopy, podiatry, neurosurgery, gynecology, oral-maxillofacial.
Special ER services: helipad, poison control center.
Ob/gyn programs: gynecological surgery.
Specialized treatment programs: cardiac and pulmonary rehab, occupational health, pain management, sleep disorders, cardiac telemetry, hemodialysis, home health care, family practice/primary care, wound care center, Behavioral Health Center for Older Adults, Transitions, The Skilled Care Center.
Physical rehab services: audiology, speech pathology, nerve conduction studies, physical and occupational therapy.
Outpatient health and wellness programs: CPR, first aid, diabetes and Lyme disease education; weight loss; nutritional counseling; senior citizen and youth programs; smoking cessation; cholesterol, blood pressure and other health screenings.

Doylestown Hospital
🛏 ✏ 🏥 🍴 ⚖ 🚫 E

ROUTES 202 AND 611, DOYLESTOWN, 215-345-2200. DOCTORS ON ACTIVE/ASSOCIATE STAFF: 167 (*82% board-certified*); NUMBER OF BEDS: 213; SEMIPRIVATE ROOM COST: $887; PRIVATE ROOM COST: $942; ACCREDITATION: JCAHO, CARF, PDH.

Sample charges for surgical services: back and neck procedures without complication, $17,764; vaginal delivery, $4,120; prostate removal, $13,034; standard local anesthesia, $269 per unit; operating-room charge first half-hour, $1,633 plus $312 each additional half-hour; preadmission testing, $468.
Base cost for ER visit: $99.
Special ER services: crisis intervention for mental health, 10 monitored beds for cardiac emergencies, ALS and PALS certified staff.
Ob/gyn programs: prenatal testing center (amniocentesis and CVS), educational programs, Baby Bracelets, visiting nurse program after delivery, labor, delivery, recovery, postpartum rooms.
Specialized treatment units: mental health, telemetry, critical care, cardiac cath lab, endoscopy, oncology nursing, rehab. Comprehensive cancer care available through a cooperative agreement with University of Pennsylvania Cancer Center.
Physical rehab services: physical, occupational, recreational and speech therapy; psychological services; hand therapy; brain injury program.
Outpatient health and wellness programs: CPR; diabetes education; first aid; cancer education; Dialogue with a Doctor physician lecture series; parenting and babysitting education; smoking cessation; stress reduction; blood pressure, cholesterol, diabetes and cancer screenings; senior wellness (exercise).

Grand View Hospital
🛏 ✏ 🏥 🍴 ⚖ 🚫 E

700 LAWN AVE., SELLERSVILLE; 215-453-4000, 215-453-9676 (*physician referral*), 1-800-752-2070 (*Cancer Answerline*), 1-800-752-3060 (*Women's Health Information Line*). DOCTORS ON ACTIVE STAFF: 240. NUMBER OF BEDS: 250. SEMIPRIVATE ROOM COST: $722. PRIVATE ROOM COST: $774. ACCREDITATION: JCAHO, ACR, PDH, CAP, ACS, AABB.

Special surgical units: ambulatory surgery (laparoscopy, radial keratotomy), surgical step-down unit.
Base cost for an ER visit: $200.
Special ER services: Advanced Life Support Program.
Ob/gyn programs: Women's Health Center, childbirth and sibling education, prenatal testing, preconception workshops.
Specialized treatment programs: sports medicine, cardiac rehab, incontinence, Community Cancer Center (member of the Jefferson Cancer Network), 20-bed skilled nursing facility, psych/detox unit.
Physical rehab services: physical, occupational and speech therapy; inpatient

orthopedic and medical rehab units; Orthopedic Brace and Appliance Center; industrial medicine; work hardening.

Outpatient health and wellness programs: CPR, first aid, choking safety, smoking cessation, cancer and blood pressure screenings, health education programs for schools, childhood asthma workshop, senior membership, free disease screenings, support groups, health lectures, speakers bureau, health fairs, child immunization clinic.

The Lower Bucks Hospital

501 BATH ROAD, BRISTOL; 215-785-9200. DOCTORS ON ACTIVE STAFF: 260 (*80% board-certified*). NUMBER OF BEDS: 320. RNS PER BED: 1.1. SEMIPRIVATE ROOM COST: $665. PRIVATE ROOM COST: $700. ACCREDITATION: JCAHO, AABB, CAP, ACR.

Sample charges for surgical services: back and neck procedures without complication, $2,577; vaginal delivery, $1,608; prostate removal, $1,590; standard local anesthesia, $76 per unit; hourly operating room charge, $1,027.
Special surgical units: Regional Eye Center, endoscopy, orthopedic.
Base cost for ER visit: $158.
Special ER services: advanced pediatric life support, Chest Pain Center.
Ob/gyn programs: Level II NICU; University Women's Center for Endocrinology, Infertility and Antenatal Testing; labor whirlpool; private postpartum wing; childbirth, sibling and VBAC classes; Motherwell fitness.
Specialized treatment programs: Jefferson radiation oncology, cardiac cath, 30-bed adult Mental Health Unit, sports medicine, pain management, member of the Jefferson Cancer Network.
Physical rehab services: speech, occupational, physical and hand therapy; Sports-Orthopedic Center; Athleticare (at Newtown Racquet and Fitness Club in Newtown, Bucks County, complete with an Aqua Ark for water therapy).
Outpatient health and wellness programs: stress, nutrition, cardiac rehab, senior health, smoking cessation, childbirth classes, CPR, first aid, health screenings, women's services. The Wellness Center offers nutritional programs, cholesterol screenings, speakers and conferences on health-related issues (215-788-8888).

St. Luke's Quakertown Hospital

1021 PARK AVE., QUAKERTOWN; 215-538-4500. DOCTORS ON ACTIVE STAFF: 175 (*95% board-certified*). NUMBER OF BEDS: 89. SEMIPRIVATE ROOM COST: $750. PRIVATE ROOM COST: $770. ACCREDITATION: JCAHO, CAP.

Surgical charges: No set fees; done based on time in the OR.
Ob/gyn programs: Healthy Beginnings, Women's Center, prenatal program.
Specialized treatment programs: psychiatry (including behavior disorders pro-

gram for traumatic brain injury victims), drug and alcohol rehab (adolescents and young adults), dialysis, skilled nursing facility, sub-acute care.
Physical rehab services: outpatient facility including pool therapy.
Outpatient health and wellness programs: diabetes education, cancer program, mammography and prostate screenings, monthly blood pressure and cholesterol screenings, community support groups.

St. Mary Medical Center

LANGHORNE-NEWTOWN ROAD, LANGHORNE; 215-750-2000, 215-741-6767 (TDD), 215-750-5888 (*physician referral*). DOCTORS ON ACTIVE STAFF: 293 (*87% board-certified*). NUMBER OF BEDS: 255. RNS PER BED: 1.4. ACCREDITATION: JCAHO, ACR, CARF, ACS, PTSF, AABB.

Special surgical units: cardiac cath lab; ambulatory surgery unit; Eye Center (cornea transplant); cosmetic/plastic, laser, orthopedic, oral-maxillofacial and videoscopic surgical procedures; laparoscopic suturing and skill improvement courses.
Special services: Regional Level II Trauma Center, ER services (urgent care/minor ER care); Dialysis Center; St. Mary Regional Cancer Center; outpatient diagnostic center; X-ray services (CAT scan, ultrasound, MRI on campus); Physical Medicine and Rehabilitation Center; cardiopulmonary rehabilitation; sleep lab; diabetes center.
Ob/gyn programs: LDR/birthing suites; Level II NICU; midwifery; expectant parent classes including getaway weekends and sibling classes; car-seat loaner program; Motherwell (exercise classes for expectant and new moms); "Contraction Connection" (beeper service for expectant parents), Mother Bachman Maternity Center (for disadvantaged women).
Outpatient health and wellness programs: Geriatric Assessment Program; Industricare (worksite health promotion); monthly senior seminars and blood pressure screening; Wellness Workshop, St. Mary Wellness and Sports Care Center; Home Health Services; Women's Diagnostic Center; St. Mary Children's Health Center (well and sick care for area children in need from birth to 18 regardless of family's ability to pay).

Chester County

Brandywine Hospital

201 REECEVILLE ROAD, COATESVILLE; 610-383-8000. DOCTORS ON ACTIVE STAFF: 138 (*86% board-certified*). NUMBER OF BEDS: 218. RNS PER BED: 1.3. ACCREDITATION: JCAHO, PTSF, AABB, CAP, NLN, ACS.

Special surgical units: surgical critical care, neurosurgery, plastic and reconstructive, outpatient surgery center.
Special ER services: Regional Trauma Center, Chest Pain Emergency Unit, Sky FlightCare helicopter.
Ob/gyn programs: private labor, delivery, recovery and postpartum and pediatric rooms; neonatal nursery; Healthy Beginnings Plus; prenatal clinic; maternity education including prepared childbirth, one-day Lamaze, sibling classes, infant care, active parenting series and babysitting certification program.
Specialized treatment programs: behavioral health services offering adult inpatient, geriatric partial hospitalization, crisis and assessment and psychiatric home health care; inpatient dialysis; Pain Control Center; dental clinic; cardiac catheterization lab; cardiac rehab; radiation oncology; occupational medicine.
Physical rehab services: physical, occupational, hand and speech therapy; sports medicine; industrial cardiopulmonary rehab.
Outpatient health and wellness programs: childbirth/parenting classes, CPR/first-aid training, diabetes education, family caregivers, trauma prevention and education, speakers bureau, health screenings, fitness evaluations/aerobics classes.

The Chester County Hospital

701 East Marshall St., West Chester; 610-431-5000. Doctors on active staff: 250. Number of beds: 250. RNs per bed: 1.76. Accreditation: JCAHO, NLN, CAP, AABB.

Special surgical units: endoscopy suite for diagnostic and surgical procedures, Ambulatory Care Center, cardiac cath lab.
Ob/gyn programs: 27-bed obstetrics unit with specially designed LDR rooms, Level II nursery, prenatal clinic, childbirth and sibling classes, genetic counseling, antenatal testing unit, sibling classes, Stork Alert, Childbirth Connection information line.
Specialized treatment programs: Occupational Health Center, critical care, Emergency Department, Cancer Program (with University of Pennsylvania Cancer Center).
Physical rehab services: Center for Health and Fitness, Center for Physical Therapy and Sports Medicine, Center for Cardiopulmonary Rehabilitation,
Outpatient health and wellness programs: wide range.

Paoli Memorial Hospital

255 West Lancaster Ave., Paoli; 610-648-1000, 610-648-1217 (physician referral). Doctors on active staff: 189 (*94% board-certified*). Number of beds: 208. Accreditation: JCAHO, CAP, PDH. Member of Jefferson Health System.

Special surgical units: short procedure unit, lithotripsy.

Ob/gyn programs: 8 LDRP suites, Perinatal Partners Program, Perinatal Testing Center, genetic counseling, infertility specialists.
Specialized treatment programs: cardiac cath lab; cardiopulmonary rehab, Center for Addictive Diseases (substance abuse); CT, MRI and ultrasound; neurodiagnostic and vascular lab; nuclear medicine; occupational medicine; Wound Healing Clinic. The Cancer Center at Paoli Memorial Hospital provides treatment in affiliation with Fox Chase Cancer Center and a grant coordinated with the University of Texas, MD Anderson Cancer Center; Comprehensive Breast Care Program and Family Risk Assessment Program.
Physical rehab services: cardiac rehab; physical, occupational and speech therapy.
Outpatient health and wellness programs: breast health awareness; children's programs; childbirth classes; developmental evaluation for school-age children; community education Care-a-Van providing health screenings; CPR classes; diabetes education; medical nutritional counseling; stress management; speakers bureau; various support groups.

Phoenixville Hospital

140 Nutt Rd., Phoenixville; 610-983-1000. Doctors on active staff: 123 (*93% board-certified*); number of beds: 143. Semiprivate room cost: $565. Private room cost: $675. Accreditation: JCAHO.

Base cost for ER visit: $125.
Special ER services: ALS-Medic 95 (physicians and staff certified in emergency care).
Ob/gyn programs: expectant parent course, early pregnancy, preconception care.
Specialized treatment programs: dialysis, pediatrics, oncology, Cancer Center, Maternity Pavilion.
Physical rehab services: physical therapy, cardiac rehab.
Outpatient health and wellness programs: community health education classes, Nutritional Resource Center, Healthy Birthing/Healthy Baby.

Southern Chester County Medical Center

1015 West Baltimore Pike, West Grove; 610-869-1000, 610-869-1111 (*Call-a-Nurse health information and physician referral*). Doctors on active staff: 64 (*85% board-certified*). Number of beds: 77. RNs per bed 1.25. Accreditation: JCAHO, PDH, CAP, AABB.

Special ER services: Mobile Medic 94 Advanced Life Support Unit.
Ob/gyn programs: physicians available.
Specialized treatment programs: cardiac rehab; nutrition counseling; sleep disorders center; Addiction Recovery Center; outpatient counseling services; Medicare-certified home care and hospice programs.

Physical rehab services: physical and occupational therapy, speech pathology. Outpatient health and wellness programs: Culinary Hearts; CPR, first-aid, basic-aid, babysitting and choking safety classes, diabetes education, occupational health.

Delaware County

Crozer-Chester Medical Center

One Medical Center Blvd., Upland; 610-447-2000, 610-447-6378 (*physician referral*). Doctors on active staff: 580 (*74% board-certified*). Number of beds: 708. Accreditation: ACS, PTSF, JCAHO, CARF, AOA.

Special surgical units: Short Procedure Unit, open-heart surgery, angioplasty, Nathan Speare Regional Burn Treatment Center, the John E. du Pont Trauma Center.
Ob/gyn programs: gynecologic oncology, antenatal assessment center, maternity center (12 LDR rooms and 14-bed intensive-care nursery), reproductive endocrinology and fertility center.
Specialized treatment programs: The Silberman Center, medical and social services for seniors; Center for Diabetes; Center for Headache Management; Sleep Disorders Center; Crozer Regional Cancer Center; Movement Disorders Center.
Physical rehab services: 45-bed rehab unit; Back Pain Center; Hand Center; Sports Medicine Center; Work Rehabilitation Center; full range of occupational and physical therapy, speech-language pathology, audiology and dysphagia services available on an outpatient basis.

Delaware County Memorial Hospital

501 North Lansdowne Ave., Drexel Hill; 610-284-8100. Doctors on active staff: 334 (*84% board-certified*). Number of beds: 257. Accreditation: JCAHO, PDH, CAP, ACS, AOA.

Special surgical units: outpatient surgery, endoscopy, laparoscopy, obstetrics, complete range of genito-urinary services, transitional care center.
Special ER services: paramedic unit.
Ob/gyn programs: prenatal; pregnancy; newborn; breast-feeding, birthing, parenting, exercise and child-care emergency classes; gynecologic oncology; reproductive endocrinology; parents' bereavement program; intensive care nursery; perinatal testing.
Specialized treatment programs: alcohol and addiction treatment, dialysis, Sports Medicine Institute, respiratory therapy/pulmonary rehab, cardiac cath, physical medicine and rehab, Delaware County Regional Cancer Center (affiliated with

Fox Chase Cancer Network), Hearing and Speech Center, Women's Diagnostic Center.

Physical rehab services: Stroke Club; amputee; activities of daily living; orthotics; prosthesis; occupational, physical and speech therapy; social work; hearing; specialized nursing.

Outpatient health and wellness programs: smoking cessation, stress management, CPR, babysitting courses, weight-loss program, nutrition, health and beauty seminar, ElderMed, screening programs.

Fitzgerald Mercy Hospital

1500 LANSDOWNE AVE., DARBY; 610-237-4000, 1-800-227-2575 (*physician referral*). DOCTORS ON ACTIVE STAFF: 414. NUMBER OF BEDS: 442. ACCREDITATION: AABB, CAP, JCAHO, PDH, PDW, CARF, ACGME.

Special surgical units: surgical ICU, short procedure unit.
Base cost for ER visit: $68.
Special ER services: FastCare (fast track for non-emergent injuries), toxicology, 24-hour staffing by board-certified emergency medicine physicians.
Ob/gyn programs: Family Birthing Center featuring 17 newly constructed labor, delivery, recovery and postpartum suites; midwifery; perinatology; Level II neonatal intensive care unit; Gamete Intra-Fallopian Transfer (GIFT) procedure for infertility; pre- and postpartum education; parent and family education and support group; lactation consultant.
Specialized treatment programs: Radiation Oncology Center (two linear accelerators and HDR Brachytherapy), LUNAR DEXA bone densitometer, cardiac cath, dialysis, Dornier Lithotripter 15/50 kidney stone treatment, psychiatry, psychiatric crisis, ultrasound, skilled nursing facility, CT, MRI, nuclear medicine, Mercy WorkCare occupational health program, Rehab After Work outpatient drug and alcohol rehabilitation, outpatient center, pain management program.
Physical rehab services: CARF-accredited physical rehab program, occupational therapy, cardiac rehab.
Outpatient health and wellness programs: medical imaging (general radiology, mammography), ambulatory care (ob/gyn, pediatrics, surgery), diagnostic cardiology, speech therapy, audiology, laboratory, Red Cross Autologous Blood Donor Center, nutrition services, cholesterol, blood pressure, diabetes, cancer screenings, infant CPR, *Mercy Community Health Team* mobile health van, diabetes and cancer support groups, diabetes education, speech, hearing and swallowing tests.

North Penn Hospital

100 MEDICAL CAMPUS, LANSDALE; 610-368-2100, 610-361-4848 (*physician referral and health information*). DOCTORS ON ACTIVE STAFF: 200 (*90% board-certified*). NUMBER OF BEDS: 150.

Special surgical units: short procedure unit.
Emergency services available: special trauma treatment rooms, on-site helipad.
Ob/gyn programs: Family BirthCenter, neonatal services, perinatology services, prenatal education.
Specialized treatment programs: North Penn Cancer Program (with Fox Chase Cancer Center), occupational health services.
Physical rehab services: physical therapy/sports medicine, occupational/speech therapy, respiratory care/pulmonary rehabilitation, Risk Profile Management (RPM) Program (cardiac fitness).
Outpatient health and wellness programs: community health education; parent and child skill-building; screenings for cancer, blood pressure, cholesterol and height and weight; first-aid, CPR (including pediatric and renewal), smoking cessation, mastectomy fitting and basic life support classes; Healthy Heart; Seniority Counts; diabetes education; variety of support groups.

Riddle Memorial Hospital

1068 West Baltimore Pike, Media; 610-566-9400. Doctors on active staff: 288 (*75% board-certified*). Number of beds: 251. RNs per bed: 1. Semiprivate room cost: $900. Private room cost: $950. Accreditation: JCAHO, PDH, ACS.

Special ER services: a team of specially trained board-certified physicians, nurses, paramedics and EMTs.
Ob/gyn programs: Birthplace (labor, delivery, recovery, postpartum in one room); Level II NICU; perinatology testing; Women's Imaging Center; childbirth education classes.
Specialized treatment programs: orthopedics; outpatient surgery; skilled nursing facility; ICU/CCU; member of the Jefferson Cancer Network; speech and hearing; occupational health; cardiac cath and rehab; sports aquatic program; home care; The Mirmont Treatment Center for substance abuse.
Physical rehab services: Riddle Rehabilitation Institute (physical therapy, back, neck and hand, work hardening).
Outpatient health and wellness programs: support groups; nutrition and weight management; cancer screenings; safe sitter, smoking cessation and CPR classes; community health education programs on various topics.

Taylor Hospital

175 E. Chester Pike, Ridley Park; 610-595-6000. Doctors on active staff: 183 (*78% board-certified*). Number of beds: 213. RNs per bed: .64. Private room cost: $990. Accreditation: JCAHO, CAP.

Specialized treatment programs: cardiovascular services (including cardiac cath

lab), oncology unit, emergency and ambulatory care.
Physical rehab services: physical therapy (inpatient and outpatient); occupational and recreational therapy; TCU (skilled nursing unit); speech pathology and audiology services.
Outpatient health and wellness programs: home health agency, cardiac rehab.

Montgomery County

Abington Memorial Hospital

1200 OLD YORK ROAD, ABINGTON; 215-576-2000. 215-576-MEDI (*physician referral*), 215-881-5750 (*ElderHelp*). DOCTORS ON ACTIVE STAFF: 490 (*91% board-certified*). NUMBER OF BEDS: 508. RNS PER OPERATING BED: 1.59. SEMIPRIVATE ROOM COST: $1,300. PRIVATE ROOM COST: $1,333. GOURMET FOOD SERVICE: $15 PER MEAL. ACCREDITATION: JCAHO, PTSF, ACGME, AMA, AABB, CAP, ACR.

Sample charges for surgical services: back and neck procedures without complication, $5,878; vaginal delivery, $1,985; prostate removal, $3,403; hourly operating-room charge, $1,587.
Special surgical units: neurosurgery, gynecology, plastic and reconstructive, vascular, fetal, ophthalmologic, dental, ambulatory surgery, mini-surgery, Surgical Trauma Unit, Abington Surgical Center.
Base cost for an ER visit: $89.
Special ER services: Level II Regional Trauma Center, Chest Pain Center.
Ob/gyn programs: family-centered maternity care, Level III Neonatal Intensive Care Unit, high-risk pregnancy and obstetrics, gynecologic oncology, genetic counseling, infertility services including in-vitro fertilization, Mother/Infant Unit, prenatal testing, amniocentesis, Maternal Observation and Monitoring (MOM) unit, PUBS, maternity education, sibling orientation, postpartum depression support group.
Specialized treatment programs: cardiac radio-frequency ablation therapy, cardiac catheterization, cardiac rehabilitation, CHAMPS (Children's Hospital/Abington Memorial Pediatric Service), Cardiac Diagnostic Center, Vascular Center, Pulmonary Rehabilitation Program and pulmonary diagnostic testing, pediatric ICU, hemodialysis, geropsychiatry, Fitness Institute, pain management, occupational medicine, high-dose chemotherapy with peripheral stem cell transplantation for cancer, stereotactic breast biopsy center, geriatric assessment, home health care, MRI Center, musculoskeletal unit.
Physical rehab services: 26-bed inpatient unit; Falls Prevention Clinic; geriatric rehab assessment; neuromuscular retraining; speech pathology and dysphagia; occupational, physical, and recreation therapy; stroke program; prosthetic/orthotic clinic; outpatient center.

Outpatient health and wellness programs: childbirth/parenting classes, Look Good, Feel Better (for women with cancer), Reach to Recovery (for breast cancer patients), CPR and first-aid training, diabetes education, smoking cessation, nutrition counseling, Eat Heart-y, Time Out for Men/Women, Abington Fitness Institute, ElderMed, van service for outpatient transportation, free or low-cost screenings and vaccination programs.

Allegheny University Hospitals, Elkins Park (formerly Elkins Park Hospital)

60 EAST TOWNSHIP LINE ROAD, ELKINS PARK; 215-663-6000, 1-800-PRO-HEALTH (*physician referral*). DOCTORS ON ACTIVE STAFF: 280. NUMBER OF BEDS: 280. ACCREDITATION: JCAHO, PDH, CAP, ACR. MEMBER OF ALLEGHENY HEALTH, EDUCATION AND RESEARCH FOUNDATION.

Special surgical units: medical/surgical ICUs.
Special ER services: MedEvac access to Regional Resource Trauma Centers.
Ob/gyn programs: general obstetrics and gynecology; high-risk obstetrics; family-centered maternity services including midwifery and neonatal services; childbirth, breast-feeding, sibling and grandparent classes; prenatal testing.
Specialized treatment programs: behavioral services including substance abuse programs; sports medicine and orthopedics; neurosurgery; home health care.
Physical rehab services: Achievement Center for cardiac and pulmonary rehab; physical therapy and adult fitness; occupational therapy; inpatient rehab unit; speech pathology.
Outpatient health and wellness programs: ambulatory surgical procedures; Breast Center and breast cancer support groups and education; diagnostic imaging and MRI services; CPR and first-aid classes; Slim-a-Weigh with Exercise; variety of support groups and annual health screenings; Advantage Passport (a program of health information and benefits for people 55 and older); Advantage for Women (a program of health information and benefits for women of all ages); Business Medicine (occupational/employee health).

Bryn Mawr Hospital

230 SOUTH BRYN MAWR AVE., BRYN MAWR; 610-526-3000, 610-526-4000 (PHYSICIAN REFERRAL). DOCTORS ON ACTIVE STAFF: 437 (*83% board-certified*). NUMBER OF BEDS: 283. ACCREDITATION: JCAHO, ACGME, AABB, ACR, CAP. PART OF THE JEFFERSON HEALTH SYSTEM.

Special surgical units: cardiothoracic, orthopedic, minimal-access, ambulatory and same-day surgery; SurgiCenter.
Ob/gyn programs: maternal/fetal medicine, labor/delivery/recovery unit, postpartum unit, newborn nursery, neonatal intensive care unit, neonatal developmental

follow-up, maternal and newborn transport, childbirth preparation classes, gynecologic surgery, infertility services.

Specialized treatment programs: inpatient and outpatient dialysis, inpatient psychiatry unit, dental clinic, eye clinic, pediatrics inpatient unit, intensive care unit, coronary care unit, cardiac catheterization labs, electrophysiology, Transitional Care Center, Arthritis and Orthopedic Center, Comprehensive Cancer Care Center, Community Clinical Oncology Program grant coordinated with the University of Texas, MD Anderson Cancer Center.

Physical rehab services: physical, occupational and speech therapy; pulmonary and cardiac rehab.

Outpatient health and wellness programs: monthly blood pressure screenings, StressSmart, adult and infant/child CPR, babysitting course, nutrition counseling, adult health fair, Life Without Diets, travelers advisory service, diabetes screening and counseling, childbirth preparation, cancer and cholesterol screenings, support groups.

Eagleville Hospital

100 Eagleville Road, Eagleville; 610-539-6000, 1-800-255-2019 (*out-of-state*). Doctors on active staff: 15 (*82% board-certified*); number of beds: 159; RNs per bed: .33; accreditation: JCAHO, PDH, PODAP.

Specialized treatment programs for adults 18 and over: Program for Employed Persons, a short-term intensive program for men and women; medically supervised detox; men's inpatient rehab program (focused on the special issues confronting chemically addicted men); women's inpatient rehab program (a multidisciplinary approach for chemically addicted women); Continuum, a partial hospitalization program.

A pioneer in the field of combined drug and alcohol treatment, Eagleville is the only hospital in Pennsylvania licensed exclusively for drug and alcohol rehabilitation. It has provided substance-abuse treatment for more than 27 years and is nationally recognized for quality care.

Holy Redeemer Hospital and Medical Center

1648 Huntingdon Pike, Meadowbrook; 215-947-3000. Doctors on active staff: 391 (*79% board-certified*). Number of beds: 283. RNs per bed: 1.3. Room cost: $1,397. Accreditation: JCAHO, ACR.

Sample charges for surgical services: back and neck procedures without complication, $12,829; vaginal delivery, $5,872; prostate removal, $11,517; standard local anesthesia, $66 per half-hour; hourly operating-room charge, $2,134.

Special surgical units: infertility (reproductive endocrinology), corneal trans-

plants, total joint replacements, reconstructive knee surgery, full endoscopic urology service.
Base cost for ER visit: $162.
Ob/gyn programs: maternal/fetal medicine, oncology, perinatology, prenatal education, reproductive endocrinology (infertility), lactation consultation, antenatal testing.
Specialized treatment programs: renal dialysis; cardiac cath lab; neonatology; neonatal follow-up clinic; telemetry; labor, delivery and recovery; outpatient retina; sports medicine; ambulatory surgery and care; regional pediatric center; critical care; wellness center.
Physical rehab services: physical therapy, occupational therapy, speech pathology, pediatric development clinic and rehab, EMG/NCV, psychological services, sports medicine, aquatic therapy.
Outpatient health and wellness programs: diabetes management program, speakers bureau, nutrition counseling, FreshStart smoking cessation program, fitness and exercise, education series for expectant families, health screenings, enterostomal therapy, Kids' Health Connection, pastoral counseling, asthma care training (ACT).

The Lankenau Hospital

100 LANCASTER AVE., WYNNEWOOD; 610-645-2000, 610-645-2001 (*physician referral*). DOCTORS ON ACTIVE STAFF: 319 (*90% board-certified*). NUMBER OF BEDS: 375. ACCREDITATION: JCAHO, ACGME, AABB, ACR, CAP, SDA. LANKENAU HOSPITAL IS PART OF THE JEFFERSON HEALTH SYSTEM.

Special surgical units: cardiothoracic, orthopedic, minimal-access surgery, ambulatory and same-day surgery; intensive care.
Ob/gyn programs: labor/delivery/recovery rooms, reproductive endocrinology, perinatology and Perinatal Testing Center, midwifery, childbirth education classes, antepartum unit, Level III neonatal intensive care unit, neonatal development follow-up program, osteoporosis management, gynecologic oncology, incontinence treatment, family planning clinic, infant bereavement counselor.
Specialized treatment programs: Breast Diagnostic Center, Sleep Disorders Center, Cancer Center, kidney transplant program, Transitional Care Center, cardiac catheterization lab, electrophysiology, inpatient and outpatient dialysis, neurodiagnostic lab, CT scan and high-resolution ultrasound, MRI, nuclear medicine, Community Clinical Oncology Program grant coordinated with the University of Texas, MD Anderson Cancer Center.
Physical rehab services: physical and occupational therapy, speech therapy/pathology, hand therapy, cardiac rehab, sports medicine rehab.
Outpatient health and wellness programs: free health lectures and screenings; Health Education Center for children; travelers advisory service; dietary/nutrition

counseling; fitness, exercise, diet and smoking cessation classes; diabetes education; support groups; Thrift Rx on site.

Mercy Haverford Hospital

2000 OLD WEST CHESTER PIKE, HAVERTOWN; 610-645-3600. DOCTORS ON ACTIVE STAFF: 180 (*99% board-certified*). NUMBER OF BEDS: 107. ACCREDITATION: AABB, JCAHO, PDH, CAP.

Specialized treatment programs: general medical/surgical, ICU/CCU, Short Procedure Unit, 24-hour ER, Substance Abuse Center (inpatient detox), Retina and Diabetic Eye Institute, Geriatric Assessment Program, Pain Management Program, Clinical Lab, diagnostic radiology, respiratory therapy.
Physical rehab services: orthopedic physical therapy, speech and occupational therapy (inpatient and outpatient).
Outpatient health and wellness programs: Diabetes education; cardiopulmonary rehab exercise program; free screenings for blood pressure, cholesterol and diabetes.

Montgomery Hospital Medical Center

1301 POWELL ST., NORRISTOWN; 215-270-2000. DOCTORS ON ACTIVE STAFF: 265. NUMBER OF BEDS: 269. RNs PER BED: .75. ACCREDITATION: JCAHO, ACS, CAP.

Special surgical units: cardiac catheterization, eye laser center.
Special ER services: hospital-based ambulance and paramedics, cardiac, trauma room.
Ob/gyn services: childbirth education, childbirth refresher, breast-feeding class, sibling preparation.
Specialized treatment programs: in- and outpatient psychiatry, dialysis, pediatrics, Cancer Center, obstetrics, Women's Imaging Center, eye laser center, bone densitometer.
Physical rehab services: cardiac and pulmonary rehab; Back School; physical, occupational and speech therapy.
Outpatient health and wellness programs: lifestyle lecture series; older adult programs; free screenings; exercise classes for osteoporosis, arthritis, pulmonary, cardiac and Parkinson's patients; support groups for cancer, diabetes, stroke, bereavement and pulmonary patients; annual wellness fair.

Pottstown Memorial Medical Center

1600 EAST HIGH ST., POTTSTOWN; 610-327-7000. DOCTORS ON ACTIVE STAFF: 250. NUMBER OF BEDS: 295. ACCREDITATION: JCAHO, ACR, ACP, ACS, AABB.

Special surgical units: endoscopy, interventional radiology suite, lithotripsy, pre-

admission surgical testing program.
Ob/gyn programs: Maternity and Women's Health Center; private labor, delivery and recovery rooms; prenatal clinic; telephone support program; women's health care seminars.
Specialized treatment programs: Community Cancer Center; ICU/CCU; Cardiac Health Center including cardiac cath, chest pain and stroke programs; Renal Care Center; Transitional Care Unit; Scanning and Treatment Center.
Physical rehab services: Occupational Health Program-Work Recovery, ERGOS Work Simulator, Sports Recovery.
Outpatient health and wellness programs: CPR, first-aid, Lamaze and grandparenting classes; blood pressure and cholesterol screenings; stress management classes; multiple support groups.

Suburban General Hospital

2701 DeKalb Pike, Norristown; 610-278-2000. Doctors on active staff: 340 (75% board-certified). Number of beds: 118. RNs per bed: 1.15. Accreditation: AOA, CARF, AABB, ACR.

Ob/gyn programs: modern maternity suite with special birthing rooms; perinatal testing center; Suburban Ob/Gyn Center, which provides comprehensive diagnostic and medical services, including a full range of gynecologic and obstetric care, to women who are uninsured or are recipients of medical assistance, Medicare or Medicaid (some private insurances accepted).
Specialized treatment programs: pain management, cardiac rehab, Family Practice Clinic, Norristown Regional Cancer Center support groups (member of University of Pennsylvania Cancer Network), Suburban Geriatric Resource Center.
Physical rehab services: The Rehab Station.
Outpatient health and wellness programs: Suburban Seniors (free club for people age 50 and older, providing health education and special discounts); blood pressure, vision and cancer screenings; health fairs; support groups; CPR and first-aid classes; diabetes education; community health education program; Just for Women health resource center; Suburban Geriatric Research Center.

Atlantic County, N.J.

Atlantic City Medical Center

Two divisions: CITY DIVISION, 1925 Pacific Ave., Atlantic City, N.J., 609-345-4000; MAINLAND DIVISION, Jimmie Leeds Road, Pomona, N.J., 609-652-1000. Accreditation: JCAHO.

Special surgical units: Kligerman Digestive Disease Service, endoscopy, cardiac catheterization laboratory, same-day surgery, on-site trauma operating room, neurological surgery, Level II Regional Trauma Center, orthopedic surgery, plastic and reconstructive surgery, thoracic surgery, otolaryngology, ophthalmology.

Ob/gyn programs: neonatal intensive care unit, abnormal Pap smears and cervical disease, high-risk pregnancy, genetic testing and counseling, ultrasound, perinatal services, amniocentesis, childbirth classes, sibling classes, gynecologic oncology.

Specialized treatment programs: RNS Regional Cancer Center, Kligerman Digestive Disease Center, The Heart Center, hospice, Regional Children's Center specializing in respiratory illness, acute and chronic hemodialysis, Infectious Disease Service, HIV Care Consortium, geriatric services, mobile intensive care units.

Outpatient health and wellness programs: Kligerman Digestive Disease Center, Community Health Services, Back on Track, teenage pregnancy prevention, Stay in School programs, Teens Offering Support, Medical Explorer Teen Program, female gang intervention, Healthy Cities Project, Success by 6, free screening programs, outpatient mental health, stereotactic mammotest, RNS Mobile Mammography Unit, cancer support groups, dialysis, MRI, Expresscare, geriatric services, Junior Volunteers, infectious disease service, two child care centers, CPR classes, Lifeline Emergency Response System, faculty practice, family practice, community health education, Male Health Clinic, Ambulatory Care Centers, Family Planning and Women's Health Center.

Kessler Memorial Hospital

600 SOUTH WHITE HORSE PIKE, HAMMONTON, N.J.; 609-561-6700, 1-800-925-6478. DOCTORS ON ACTIVE STAFF: 150. NUMBER OF BEDS: 130. ACCREDITATION: JCAHO.

Special surgical units: same-day surgery.

Specialized treatment programs: pain management; Podiatry Clinic; Lyme Disease Service; Occupational Health Service; Wound Care Center.

Outpatient health and wellness programs: home health service, including infusion therapy.

Shore Memorial Hospital

1 EAST NEW YORK AVE. AND SHORE ROAD, SOMERS POINT, N.J.; 609-653-3500, 1-800-449-4SMH (*SMH Healthline Service and Physician Finder*). DOCTORS ON ACTIVE STAFF: 279 (*75% board-certified*). NUMBER OF BEDS: 373. ACCREDITATION: JCAHO. MEMBER AHA, NJHA, VHA.

Specialized programs: Cancer Care Center, Cardiac Care Center, Critical Care Unit, Emergency Department, Regional Dialysis Center, Metabolic and Diabetes Care Center, Neurological Care Center, Obstetrical Care Unit, Orthopedic Care

Unit, Pediatric Care Center, Substance Abuse Care, Urological and Renal Care Unit, Vascular Care Center, Health and Conference Center, Women's Center, Wellness Center.

Surgical services: Arthroscopic Surgical Center, Laminar Flow Operating Suite, Laparoscopic Surgery, Ophthalmology Laser Suite, Pediatric Surgical Program, same-day surgery.

Diagnostic services: Doppler imaging, CT, osteoporosis testing, angiography, MRI, mammography suite, nuclear medicine/SPECT gamma camera, special procedure suite, ultrasound, X-ray.

Treatment, testing and therapy services: cardiopulmonary lab, endoscopy unit, intravenous therapy, transfusion and outpatient Care Unit, noninvasive vascular lab, rehabilitation therapies, ShoreCare Home Health Care.

Outpatient health and wellness programs: bioethics services, community education programs, geriatric services, Prime Time Plus program for older adults, stroke prevention program, health care careers counseling, *Health Today* television show, humor therapy program, lactation consultant, language translation service, Medical Explorer program, medical and nursing lecture series, mental health service, radiology school, scholarships and fellowship programs, speakers bureau, walkers club, wellness program, weight loss and fitness program, Women's Center, wound and ostomy therapy, support groups (cancer, diabetes, loss of a child, etc.), auxiliary and volunteer programs.

Burlington County, N.J.

Memorial Hospital of Burlington County

175 MADISON AVE., MOUNT HOLLY, N.J.; 609-267-0700. DOCTORS ON ACTIVE STAFF: 220 (*99% board-certified*). NUMBER OF BEDS: 369. ACCREDITATION: JCAHO, ACR, ACS.

Sample charges for surgical services: vaginal delivery, $1,539; standard local anesthesia, $137.24; hourly operating room charge, $1,516.

Base cost for ER visit: $134.50 (Level 1).

Special ER services: Chest Pain Clinic, Fast Track (quick service for minor problems).

Ob/gyn programs: a full range of neonatal, perinatal, parenting and midlife wellness services through Women's Health Network (609-261-7482).

Specialized treatment programs: dialysis, psychiatry, pediatrics, Speech and Hearing Center, same-day surgery center, geriatric assessment, incontinence program.

Physical rehab services: physical and occupational therapy (inpatient and outpatient).

Outpatient health and wellness programs: Senior Health-Link (a wellness program for those over 55; 609-265-7900).

Graduate Health System
Rancocas Hospital

218A Sunset Road, Willingboro, N.J.; 609-835-2900, 1-800-GRAD-LINE (*physician referral*). Doctors on active staff: 302 (*88% board-certified*). Number of beds: 318. RNs per bed: 1.4. Semiprivate room cost: $1,195. Private room cost: $1,245. Accreditation: JCAHO, FDA, ACR, AABB, CAP, licensed by NJDH.

Special surgical units: general operating suites, eye surgery center, same-day surgery.
Base cost for ER visit: $112.
Ob/gyn programs: Woman's Center, mammography and ultrasound testing, complete childbirth services, neonatology, antenatal testing, genetic counseling, six LDRs (labor and delivery suites), ob/gyn residency program.
Specialized treatment programs: Sleep Laboratory; comprehensive cancer program accredited by the American College of Surgeons' Commission on Cancer; mental health; Eye Surgery Center.
Physical rehab services: speech, physical and occupational therapy.
Outpatient health and wellness programs: 55 Plus or older adults when they're well and when they're sick, state-certified diabetes education, lectures and screening.

Camden County, N.J.

The Cooper Health System

One Cooper Plaza, Camden, N.J.; 609-342-2000. Doctors on active staff: 540 (*91% board-certified*). Number of beds: 552. RNs per bed: 1.45. Semiprivate room cost: $902. Private room cost: $1,018. Accreditation: AABB, ACS, AHA, CAP, JCAHO, MSNJ.

Cooper Hospital/University Medical Center
Special surgical units: endoscopic and laser surgery, cardiothoracic, bone marrow transplantation, pediatrics surgery, neurosurgery, gynecologic oncology, colorectal, orthopedics, otolaryngology, plastic and reconstructive, cleft palate program, urology, ophthalmology, traumatology and emergency. Cooper is a Level I Regional Trauma Center.
Ob/gyn programs: antenatal testing, comprehensive breast care center, maternal/fetal medicine, perinatal center, gynecologic oncology, reproductive endocrinology, in-vitro fertilization, genetic counseling, maternal advanced care.
Specialized treatment programs: Comprehensive Cancer Center,

Cardiovascular Center, Sleep Disorders Laboratory, Geriatric Assessment Program, Diabetes Care Center, epilepsy program, radiation therapy, high-risk pregnancy program, Colorectal Care Center, Perinatal Center, Special Care Nursery, Children's Epilepsy Center, Young Adult Care Center, maternal advanced and intermediate care, Comprehensive Breast Care Center, Institute for Systemic Radiation Therapy.

Physical rehab services: physical and occupational therapy, psychiatric evaluations, prosthetics and orthotics, speech pathology, comprehensive oncology rehab, swallowing evaluations, electromyography and nerve conduction studies, audiology, chronic pain, comprehensive lymphedema treatment, balance disorders, gait dysfunction, movement disorder therapy.

Outpatient health and wellness programs: Community Health Affairs Department, Understanding Menopause, breast surgery, Pregnancy After 35, Stress Management, Diabetes Management, Childhood Nutrition, Cancer Prevention Through Nutrition, breast cancer screening.

The Children's Regional Hospital at Cooper

Specialized programs: Child Development Center, birth defects and genetic disorders, pediatric hematology/oncology, pediatric and neonatal intensive care, sickle-cell anemia, Diabetes Center, speech pathology, spina bifida, SIDS and infant apnea evaluation, young adult care, play therapy program.

Kennedy Health System

500 MARLBORO AVENUE, CHERRY HILL, N.J.; 1-800-321-4KMH. KENNEDY-CHERRY HILL, 2201 WEST CHAPEL AVE.; 609-488-6500. KENNEDY-STRATFORD, 18 EAST LAUREL RD.; 609-346-6000. KENNEDY-WASHINGTON TOWNSHIP, 435 HURFFVILLE-CROSS KEYS RD., TURNERSVILLE, 609-582-2500. DOCTORS ON ACTIVE STAFF: 792 (*81% board-certified*). NUMBER OF BEDS: 607. RNS PER BED: 1.1. ACCREDITATION: NJDH, AOA, JCAHO (PENDING), ACR (MAMMOGRAPHY), CAP (LAB).

Special surgical units: three hospital-based same-day surgery units; Kennedy Surgical Center in Sewell, a free-standing ambulatory surgical center to open in September 1996.

Ob/gyn programs: Women and Children's Services include perinatal testing unit, neonatal intensive care nurseries, genetic counseling, mammography, childbirth classes, dads-on-call beepers, sibling classes, breast-feeding classes, Motherwell maternity and fitness program, Women's Resource Center, infertility treatment, breast pump rental, parenting education.

Cardiology: affiliated with Our Lady of Lourdes Medical Center, Camden, as part of The New Jersey Heart Institute, providing cardiac catheterization.

Behavioral health: The Access Center provides comprehensive inpatient and outpatient mental health and substance abuse treatment for children, adolescents and adults.

Specialized treatment programs: Gerontology Center includes ElderMed senior membership program and case management services; Dialysis Center; crisis intervention in affiliation with Steininger Center; Family Health Centers providing primary care for the underserved; Early Intervention Program providing treatment for HIV/AIDS patients; home health services; Access Center providing comprehensive inpatient and outpatient mental health and substance abuse treatment for children, adolescents and adults; Kennedy Teen Center at Echelon; Diabetes Control Center (to open in the fall of 1996).
Physical rehab services: comprehensive physical therapy and sports medicine.
Outpatient health and wellness programs: comprehensive health education programs for businesses and community, CPR training, babysitter certification programs.
Long-term care: Health Care Center at Washington Township.

Our Lady of Lourdes Medical Center

1600 HADDON AVE., CAMDEN, N.J.; 609-757-3500. DOCTORS ON ACTIVE STAFF: 312 (*81% board-certified*). NUMBER OF BEDS: 375. RNS PER BED 1.4. SEMIPRIVATE ROOM COST: $690. PRIVATE ROOM COST: $840. ACCREDITATION: JCAHO, CARF.

Sample charges for surgical services: coronary bypass without cardiac cath, $23,315; vaginal delivery, $3,807; standard local anesthesia, $55; hourly operating room charge, $550 (minor surgery), $850 (major surgery).
Special surgical units: kidney and pancreas transplantation programs, open-heart surgery.
Base cost for ER visit: $175.
Special ER services: psychiatric emergency service.
Ob/gyn programs: Level III Regional Perinatal Center, NICU, maternal and neonatal transport services, Osborn Family Health Center, newborn nursery and transitional nursery, LDR rooms.
Specialized treatment programs: pediatric, mental health, geropsychiatry, in- and outpatient dialysis units; home of The New Jersey Heart Institute at Lourdes.
Physical rehab services: 50-bed Lourdes Regional Rehabilitation Center; physical, occupational, speech and recreational therapy; electromyography; hand rehab; prosthetic-orthotic evaluation; videofluoroscopic swallowing studies.
Outpatient health and wellness programs: prenatal classes; infant, child and adult CPR; asthma workshops; massage; weight loss program; stress reduction courses; Christian yoga; meditation; foot reflexology; dance instruction; nutritional counseling; blood pressure, cholesterol, vision and cancer screenings; variety of support groups; parish nurse program.

West Jersey Health System

🖋️ 🏥 ⚖️ 🚫 E

CORPORATE OFFICES: 1000 ATLANTIC AVE, CAMDEN, N.J.; 609-342-4488. HOSPITALS LOCATED IN CAMDEN (609-342-4000), BERLIN (609-768-6000), VOORHEES (609-772-5000) AND MARLTON (609-596-3500). TOTAL DOCTORS ON ACTIVE STAFF: 889 (*85% board-certified*). TOTAL NUMBER OF BEDS: 763. ACCREDITATION: JCAHO, CAP, AABB, AHA, ABP.

Emergency services: regional services including on-ground teams and South star helicopter rescue team.

Ob/gyn programs: Women and Children's Center (5,000 babies born every year, highest among all South Jersey hospitals), NICU.

Specialized treatment programs: Children's Sleep and Breathing Center, after-hours children's urgent care, diabetes center, Alcove drug and alcohol treatment center, Good Life Center for older adults, cancer center, arthritis center, hip replacement and orthopedic surgery, cardiac rehab and education, geriatric units.

Physical rehab services: comprehensive regional occupational health services.

Outpatient health and wellness programs: Tatum Brown Family Practice Center, ambulatory care center, women's health lecture series, health education and prevention programs.

Cape May County, N.J.

Burdette Tomlin Memorial Hospital

🖋️ 🏥 ⚖️ 🚫 E

2 STONE HARBOR BLVD., CAPE MAY COURT HOUSE, N.J.; 609-463-2000, 1-800-362-4123 (PHYSICIAN REFERRAL SERVICE). DOCTORS ON ACTIVE STAFF: 100. NUMBER OF BEDS: 242. ACCREDITATION: JCAHO, CAP.

Special surgical units: General surgery; same-day surgery unit; Dramis Arthroscopy Center.

ER services: board-certified ER physicians on duty 24 hours a day, 7 days a week; diagnostic imaging with MRI and CT scanning; state-of-the-art customer-focused laboratory.

Ob/gyn programs: Labor, delivery, recovery and postpartum all in the same homelike room (LDRP); Healthstart maternity clinic; ultrasound; childbirth preparation classes.

Physical rehab services: Cardiopulmonary rehabilitation program; physical, occupational and speech therapy.

Outpatient health and wellness programs: Diabetes teaching and counseling; smoking cessation program; Vision Aerobics; bereavement; Growing Through Loss; Adult Care for the Caregiver; Exercise Is for Everyone; 55 Alive mature driving; Safe

Sitters; Beyond Dieting; individual and group counseling for personal growth and wellness, marriage/family, crisis and addiction; CPR and EMS training; speakers bureau; support groups for people with specific health problems; outreach programs to improve the health of the community.

Cumberland County, N.J.

Newcomb Medical Center

65 South State St., Vineland, N.J.; 609-691-9000. Doctors on active staff: 140 (*75% board-certified*). Number of beds: 235. Accreditation: JCAHO.

Special surgical units: same-day surgery; noninvasive cardiovascular lab; laparoscopy services; ob/gyn and general surgery; laser surgery; orthopedics.
Ob/gyn programs: surgery; midwifery; antenatal diagnostic center; community perinatal center (intermediate); women's primary care center; maternity patient education channel; maternity telephone helpline.
Pediatric services: dedicated inpatient pediatric center; children's primary care center; neonatal ICU.
Specialized treatment programs: chest pain center; outpatient substance abuse; child development center; early intervention program; acute dialysis; diabetes management; dedicated endoscopy suite.
Physical rehab services: physical, occupational, speech and sports therapy; cardiopulmonary rehab; audiology.
Outpatient health and wellness programs: comprehensive community health programs, screenings and lectures; Women's Health Network; Hospital with Heart; support groups for congestive heart failure, cancer, panic disorder, gambling and alcoholism; industrial health; adult primary-care center; oncology and dedicated chemotherapy suite; foot and ankle surgery; stress testing; echocardiography.

South Jersey Hospital

Corporate offices: 333 Irving Ave., Bridgeton, N.J.; 609-451-8700, ext. 2201. Hospitals located in Bridgeton (609-451-6600), Millville (609-825-3500), and Elmer (609-358-2341). 1-800-770-7547 (physician referral). Doctors on active staff: 400. Total number of beds: 424. Accreditation: JCAHO, American College of Surgeons Commission on Cancer.

Cancer care: The South Jersey Regional Cancer Center (in affiliation with Fox Chase Cancer Center) provides comprehensive inpatient and outpatient cancer

care, including medical oncology, radiation oncology, specialized surgery and clinical trials.
Ob/gyn programs: Family-centered maternity unit with three labor and delivery suites; ultrasound and mammography; free breast and cervical cancer screenings.
Mental health services: inpatient and partial care services for children, adolescents and adults; region's only children's crisis intervention service.
Specialized treatment programs: cosmetic/reconstructive surgery; occupational therapy; physical therapy; occupational/industrial medicine; cardiac rehab; pulmonary rehab; dialysis.
Outpatient health and wellness programs: diabetes management classes, cancer support groups, weight management/healthy lifestyle programs, senior citizens groups, free health screenings.

Gloucester County, N.J.

Underwood-Memorial Hospital

509 NORTH BROAD ST., WOODBURY, N.J.; 609-845-0100, 609-384-8884 (*physician referral*). DOCTORS ON ACTIVE STAFF: 323 (*80% board-certified*). NUMBER OF BEDS: 310. RNS PER BED: .25. SEMIPRIVATE ROOM COST: $672. PRIVATE ROOM COST: $747. SUITE COST: $821. ACCREDITATION: JCAHO, CAP.

Sample charges for surgical services: cataract eye surgery with interocular lens replacement, $2,000; laparoscopic cholecystectomy (removal of gallbladder), $3,200; arthroscopic knee surgery, $2,100; vaginal delivery with two-day stay, $4,300; operating-room charge, $400 per half-hour.
Special surgical units: cryosurgery for prostate cancer.
Base cost for ER visit: $54-$177.
Ob/gyn programs: obstetrics clinic; prenatal education; infant CPR classes; prenatal refresher course; fetal loss support group; grandparent, breast-feeding and sibling classes.
Physical rehab services: inpatient and outpatient physical medicine, occupational and speech therapy.

Mercer County, N.J.

The Medical Center at Princeton

253 WITHERSPOON ST., PRINCETON, N.J.; 609-497-4000, 609-497-4197 (PHYSICIAN REFERRAL). DOCTORS ON ACTIVE STAFF: 450. NUMBER OF BEDS: 410. ACCREDITATION: JCAHO.

Special surgical units: Same-day surgery.

Ob/gyn programs: single-room maternity care unit, family-centered maternity program that offers educational classes, exercise classes, Lamaze instruction, genetic counseling, a complete and intensive neonatal program with a special care nursery for sick babies and an infant apnea center.

Specialized treatment programs: Princeton House, a 70-bed psychiatric and addictions treatment unit providing inpatient and outpatient care for psychiatric patients and their families; Senior Link, a partial hospital day treatment program for older adults that offers intermediate psychiatric care.

Physical rehab services: Merwick, a 93-bed long-term care and rehabilitation unit providing services in residential and skilled nursing care, physical medicine and rehab as well as outpatient services in rehab, speech and audiology; Monroe Unit, offering complete outpatient rehab services including pulmonary and cardiac rehab and physical therapy.

Outpatient health and wellness programs: health education programs; home care, including intravenous and antibiotic therapy, hospice, Lifeline Emergency Response System and private-duty services; outpatient counseling services specializing in geriatric issues; bereavement, psychiatric and addictions counseling.

Mercer Medical Center

446 BELLEVUE AVE., TRENTON, N.J.; 609-394-4000, 1-800-255-3440 (PHYSICIAN REFERRAL). DOCTORS ON ACTIVE STAFF: 250 (*88% board-certified*). NUMBER OF BEDS: 318. ACCREDITATION: JCAHO.

Special surgical units: Ambulatory care unit; nine general operating rooms including orthopedic operating suite for joint replacement; minor surgical suite for outpatient procedures not requiring general anesthesia; cystoscopy suite; cataract surgical suite; otorhinolaryngology, gynecology, vascular and thoracic surgery.

Special ER services: two critical-care rooms; X-ray room; isolation room.

Ob/gyn programs: Designated by N.J. Dept. of Health as a Regional Perinatal Center. Offers comprehensive high-risk obstetrical and neonatal services with 24-hour in-house obstetrical, perinatal, neonatal and anesthesiology coverage; maternal/infant transport; high-risk pregnancy management; high-risk prenatal clinic and neonatal intensive care nursery. Also, reproductive endocrinology/fertility, ultrasound, genetic testing and counseling, and classes to prepare for baby's arrival. Maternity unit includes 48 private suites equipped for every aspect of birth.

Specialized treatment programs: Cancer care: designated Community Hospital Comprehensive Care Program by the Commission on Cancer of the American College of Surgeons. Also member of the University of Pennsylvania Cancer Network. Services include radiation oncology, chemotherapy, brachytherapy, surgery, 28-bed inpatient unit, psychosocial counseling, cancer prevention programs and screenings, Women's Breast Center and, with grant support, free mammography and cervical cancer screenings for minority and socioeconomically disadvantaged women. Heart and lung care: Mercer's Regional Heart and Lung Center includes acute coronary care facilities with monitoring equipment, pulmonary intensive care unit and neonatal intensive care unit; pacemaker insertion and follow-up; advanced diagnostic facility; pediatric cardiology; asthma program; noninvasive vascular lab; risk assessment and prevention programs; patient education and support groups.

Other specialties: Mercer Medical Wound Care Center for the treatment of chronic nonhealing wounds; Sleep Disorders Center accredited by the American Sleep Disorders Association.

Outpatient health and wellness programs: Adult Day Care Center; Mall Walkers clubs; blood pressure checks; Senior Advantage membership program; support groups for breast and prostate cancer, sarcoidosis, chronic pulmonary disease, smoking, caregiving, sleep apnea; health risk assessment; corporate wellness programs; HEARTCHECK healthy dining program; cholesterol and body composition screening; men's and women's health programs; pregnancy planning; sibling preparation; genetic counseling and testing; reproductive endocrinology; sleep studies; asthma workshops for adults and families; ambulatory surgery; cardiac disease; nonivasive diagnostics including TEE, echocardiography, stress testing, cardiovascular fitness and mammography.

St. Francis Medical Center

601 Hamilton Avenue, Trenton, N.J.; 609-599-5000. Doctors on active staff: 235. Number of beds: 436. Accreditation: JCAHO.

Nuclear and radiological diagnostic and therapeutic complex; same-day surgery; eight-room operating suite; state-of-the-art maternity center; Fox Chase Cancer Program; 24-hour emergency department; The Heart Institute at St. Francis, featuring the regional cardiac catheterization laboratory, comprehensible cardiac diagnostics and on-site Cardiac Rehabilitation Program; regional chest pain emergency center; Regional Neuromuscular Program, the only hospital-based program in Central New Jersey providing a comprehensive range of services to children and adults with a neuromuscular disorder; senior programs, such as the Sister Hyacinths Program for the homebound and Senior Choice, a free membership program for individuals 60 years and older; sleep disorders program; social services and home care planning.

Salem County, N.J.

The Memorial Hospital of Salem County

310 WOODSTOWN ROAD, SALEM, N.J.; 609-935-1000. DOCTORS ON ACTIVE STAFF: 140. NUMBER OF BEDS: 150. ACCREDITATION: JCAHO. AFFILIATED WITH BECKETT HEALTH PARK, CHILDREN'S HEALTHCARE CENTERS, COOPER HEALTH SYSTEM, MEDICAL CENTER OF DELAWARE AND PREMIER ALLIANCE.

Specialized surgical units: same-day surgery, Southern New Jersey Oncology Center.
Special ER services: Radiation Treatment Program, helicopter access.
Ob/gyn programs: Family Birth Center, early pregnancy program, childbirth education, Motherwell exercise classes, infant safety, SafeSitter classes, sibling classes.
Specialized treatment programs: Breast Evaluation Center, Diagnostic Imaging Center and CT scanner, outpatient dialysis in conjunction with Cooper, Healthy Start program, Home Health Care and Hospice, ICU and telemetry units.
Physical rehab services: inpatient services; outpatient services provided by South Jersey Physical Therapy and Back Rehabilitation Center; Cardiac Rehabilitation Program.
Outpatient health and wellness programs: blood pressure and cholesterol screenings, Community Walking Program, CPR classes, diabetes information group for adults, Medical Explorers, label reading tours, Lose and Win weight loss program, smoking cessation and Weight Loss Through Hypnosis, "Understanding Diabetes" series, various support groups.

Delaware State

Alfred I. duPont Institute

1600 ROCKLAND ROAD, WILMINGTON, DEL.; 302-651-4000. DOCTORS ON ACTIVE STAFF: 253 (*95% board-certified*). NUMBER OF BEDS: 128. RNS PER BED: 1.56. PRIVATE, SEMIPRIVATE AND SUITE COST: $535. ACCREDITATION: JCAHO, CARF.

Special surgical units: neurosurgery, urology, ophthalmology, orthopedic, otolaryngology, plastic surgery, kidney transplantation.
Base cost for ER visit: $36.
Special ER services: 24-hour staffing by pediatric emergency medicine specialists, in-house surgical capabilities, pediatric transport team.
Specialized treatment programs: traumatic brain and spinal cord injury and comprehensive outpatient rehab, end-stage renal disease program, critical care,

NICU, audiology, child and adolescent psychiatry and psychology, gastroenterology, neurology, orthopedics, sports medicine, genetics, rheumatology, infectious diseases, endocrinology, growth disorders.
Physical rehab services: 20-bed inpatient rehab unit; comprehensive outpatient rehab program; physical, occupational and speech therapy; academic and child life therapy; assistive technology and psychological services.

Beebe Medical Center

424 SAVANNAH ROAD, LEWES, DEL.; 302-645-3300. DOCTORS ON ACTIVE STAFF: 100. NUMBER OF BEDS: 119. ACCREDITATION: JCAHO.

An acute care hospital offering a broad range of inpatient and outpatient medical, surgical and psychiatric services. The hospital's not-for-profit mission of providing comprehensive care also includes a commitment to meeting the psychosocial needs of the patient with mental health services as needed, pastoral services as desired and case management as appropriate.
Specialized treatment programs: Three freestanding diagnostic imaging and laboratory specimen collection facilities in Georgetown, Millville and Millsboro; a high-quality, cost-efficient ambulatory surgical facility in Millsboro dedicated to ophthalmologic procedures; a licensed emergency facility in Millville that operates during the summer months.
Outpatient health and wellness programs: five primary-care centers staffed by employed primary-care physicians in the communities of Rehoboth, Milton, Georgetown, Millville and Millsboro; a pediatric practice with an employed board-certified pulmonologist/geriatrician, oncologist/hematologist and, in the near future, an infectious disease specialist to expand the level of service to HIV/AIDS patients at the Medical Center and Lewes Convalescent Center with intermediate care and skilled nursing care beds; a home health agency; a geriatric day care facility in Rehoboth.

St. Francis Hospital

7TH AND CLAYTON STS., P.O. BOX 2500, WILMINGTON, DEL.; 302-421-4100, 302-652-LIFE (PHYSICIAN REFERRAL AND INFORMATION HOTLINE). DOCTORS ON ACTIVE STAFF: 570. NUMBER OF BEDS: 295. ACCREDITATION: JCAHO. MEMBER OF CATHOLIC HEALTH INITIATIVE.

Special surgical units: patient-focused inpatient and outpatient surgical services including cardiac catheterization lab and cardiovascular, cosmetic/plastic, general, gynecologic, laser, neurologic, ophthalmology, oral/maxillofacial, orthopedic, otologic, outpatient, retinal, thoracic and urologic surgical services.
Ob/gyn programs: modern maternity department and family birth center; Level II

neonatal intensive care with on-site neonatologists; labor/delivery/recovery suites; nurse-midwifery; maternal/child home care; childbirth, breast-feeding/lactation and sibling education classes; mammography; ultrasound; and gynecological surgical services; West End Neighborhood—prenatal care for low-income women (Tiny Steps program).

Specialized treatment programs: home care services (including maternal/child and IV infusion); cardiovascular services (including inpatient and outpatient catheterization, rehabilitation, electrophysiology, echocardiography, electrodiagnostics and stress testing); radiology services (including CT scanner, diagnostic radioisotope, digital radiography, angiography, mammography, SPECT camera, vascular laboratory, nuclear medicine, ultrasound and affiliate MRI services); psychiatric services (inpatient and outpatient); critical care services (including intensive care, intermediate care and neonatal intensive care); pulmonary services; 24-hour emergency department staffed with board-certified emergency physicians and nurse practitioners and Fast Track minor emergency care; pain management center; family, pediatric and ob/gyn and midwifery physician practices; Family Practice Residency Program affiliated with Temple University.

Physical rehab services: cardiac rehabilitation; occupational therapy; inpatient and outpatient rehabilitation services; physical therapy; recreational therapy; respiratory therapy; speech therapy; and work conditioning.

Outpatient health and wellness programs: childbirth, sibling preparation and breast-feeding/lactation education classes; breast cancer support group; diabetes education program; caregivers support group; physician referral; community health newsletter; employee wellness programs; pastoral care; pediatric day care for sick children; emergency care education program for children; Ministry of Caring—primary care for area uninsured, low-/no-income and homeless (St. Clare Medical Outreach); West End Neighborhood—prenatal care program for low-income women (Tiny Steps); community health education and screening programs.

Specialty Hospitals

Children's Seashore House

3405 Civic Center Blvd., Philadelphia; 215-895-3600, 1-800-678-3773. Doctors on active staff: 19 (*100% board-certified*). Number of beds: 77. RNs per bed: 1. Semiprivate room cost: $1055. Accreditation: JCAHO.

Special treatment programs: biobehavioral; Center for Complex Medical Management; developmental disabilities; dysphagia and feeding management; musculoskeletal rehab; neurorehab and respiratory rehab; Attention Deficit/Hyperactivity Disorder; cerebral palsy clinic; child development; cochlear implant program (in affiliation with Children's Hospital of Philadelphia), Down's

syndrome.
Special services: Communication disorders (audiology and speech/language pathology), child life therapy, nutrition, occupational therapy, physical therapy, prosthetics and orthotics, psychology, psychiatry, rehab nursing, social work.

Deborah Heart and Lung Center

200 TRENTON ROAD, BROWNS MILLS, N.J.; 609-555-1990, 1-800-214-3452 (*physician referrals*). DOCTORS ON FULL-TIME STAFF: 64 (*more than 90% board-certified*); NUMBER OF BEDS: 161; NURSE-TO-PATIENT RATIO 1 TO 5 (*telemetry*), 1 TO 1 (*SICU*), 1 TO 1 OR 2 (*MICU*); ACCREDITATION: JCAHO, CAP, AABB, NJDH.

Specialized programs: adult, pediatric and neonatal cardiac medicine; fetal echocardiography; adult pulmonary medicine; Phase III clinical trial site for cardiomyoplasty; outpatient cardiac cath; minimally invasive coronary artery bypass; cardiac imaging; home-based pulmonary rehab; sleep apnea clinic; interventional catheterization program including angioplasty, coronary artery stenting, atherectomy and valvuloplasty; video-assisted thoracoscopy and bronchoscopy.
Outpatient health and wellness programs: full range of cardiac and pulmonary diagnostic testing, cardiac cath, bronchoscopy.

Fox Chase Cancer Center

7701 BURHOLME AVE., PHILADELPHIA; 215-728-6900, 1-800-FOX-CHASE. DOCTORS ON ACTIVE STAFF: 131 (*99% board-certified*). NUMBER OF BEDS: 100. RNS PER BED: 2.8. SEMIPRIVATE ROOM COST: $858. PRIVATE ROOM COST: $967. SUITE COST: $1,500. ACCREDITATION: PDH, JCAHO, ACS, ACR, AHA, CAP, ACCME, COTH, ACGME.

One of 27 institutions nationwide designated as Comprehensive Cancer Centers by the National Cancer Institute.

Special surgical units: intraoperative radiation therapy, pain management, endoscopy, cystoscopy, bronchoscopy.
Ob/gyn programs: gynecologic oncology.
Physical rehab services: physical, occupational and speech therapy.
Outpatient health and wellness programs: multidisciplinary evaluation and treatment programs for breast, ovarian, colorectal, lung, gastrointestinal, prostate, gynecological, head and neck cancers and sarcomas; genetic screening and family risk assessment; smoking cessation; mobile mammography; home health care, hospice; home infusion; community education programs.

Pennsylvania College of Optometry
The Eye Institute
🎓 E ✉

1200 West Godfrey Ave., Philadelphia; 215-276-6210. Outpatient only. Doctors on active staff: 37. Accreditation: AOA.

ER services: immediate eye care, 24-hour on-call ocular emergency service.
Specialized treatment programs: low vision, sports vision, corneal and specialty contact lens, neuro eye.
Physical rehab services: low-vision rehab.

Scheie Eye Institute
🛏 🍴 📺 💊 ⚖ 🚫 🎓 E

Department of Ophthalmology/University of Pennsylvania School of Medicine and Presbyterian Medical Center, Myrin Circle, 51 North 39th St., Philadelphia, 215-662-8119. Shares services with Presbyterian Medical Center and Hospital of the University of Pennsylvania. Doctors on active staff: 19 (*100% board-certified*); room and gourmet food costs: refer to Presbyterian Medical Center and UPMC; accreditation: JCAHO.

Sample surgical charges: hourly operating-room charge, $1,820 for the first hour; preadmission testing: lab work, $270; chest X-ray, $132; EKG, $142.
Special surgical units: cornea transplants, trauma, retina/vitreous, cataract and lens implants, glaucoma, oculoplastics, strabismus, radial keratotomy.
Base cost for ER visit: $40-$85. ER services run through Presbyterian Medical Center and UPMC.
Specialized treatment programs: primary and tertiary ophthalmological services, genetics, glaucoma, laser treatments for diabetic retinopathy and macular degeneration, oculoplastics, neuro-ophthalmology, pediatrics.
Outpatient health and wellness programs: contact lens service, low-vision service provides social service and rehab referrals for low-vision and legally blind patients.

Burn Centers

Crozer-Chester Medical Center
St. Agnes Medical Center
St. Christopher's Hospital for Children

Skilled Nursing Facilities

An SNF is a transitional stop for physician-directed care and rehabilitation. It falls somewhere between a hospital and a nursing home. It's for patients who no longer need the high-tech, acute, expensive care of a hospital, but are not yet ready for the next step. The cost of one night at Pennsylvania Hospital's Skilled Care Center is $505, as opposed to $1,125 for the same amount of time in a hospital room. The difference lies in the intensity of the services provided. Many hospitals have SNFs on their premises and simply transfer patients there until they are either recuperated enough to return home or able to move into the longer-term care of a nursing home. SNFs provide services such as wound care, tube feedings, colostomy care, insulin injection and IV therapy. The following institutions have skilled nursing facilities:

Albert Einstein Medical Center, Doylestown Hospital, Episcopal Hospital, Fitzgerald Mercy Hospital, Germantown Hospital and Medical Center, Grand View Hospital, Holy Redeemer Hospital and Medical Center, Presbyterian Medical Center, Riddle Memorial Hospital, Roxborough Memorial Hospital, St. Luke's Quakertown Hospital, Taylor Hospital

Trauma Centers

Trauma centers offer a more complete range of crisis services than ordinary emergency rooms. They are designated by the Pennsylvania Trauma Systems Foundation as either Level I or Level II. A Level I facility must be equipped to handle situations such as cardiac bypass, pediatric trauma, renal dialysis and reattachment of limbs. It must also have a general surgical residency, education programs and on-going research. A Level II facility may have many of the same capabilities but does not conduct research.

Level I Trauma: Albert Einstein Medical Center; Allegheny University Hospitals, Center City (formerly Hahnemann University Hospital); Allegheny University Hospitals, East Falls (formerly Medical College of Pennsylvania Hospital); Children's Hospital of Philadelphia; Cooper Hospital/University Medical Center; Temple University Hospital; Thomas Jefferson University Hospital; University of Pennsylvania Medical Center

Level II Trauma: Abington Memorial Hospital; Crozer-Chester Medical Center; Frankford Hospital, Torresdale Campus; Kennedy Memorial Hospital; St. Mary Medical Center

CHAPTER 9

Emergency!

The critical things to know when time is critical

Americans have come to rely on high-tech emergency rooms for dependable, quality health care. But emergency departments are actually designed to provide critical care "safety nets" for people with life-threatening illnesses and injuries. All too often, ERs become congested with people seeking help for minor conditions like sore throats, sprained ankles and upset stomachs. The results of this misuse have been well documented: inefficient care, escalating medical costs and wasted health care resources.

Because many ER patients fail to understand the way the system operates, it's not unusual for them to become disgruntled when they must wait for care, especially when they spot new arrivals being seen immediately, says Dr. Frederic H. Kauffman, director of the department of emergency medicine at Temple University Hospital. ERs aren't run on a first-come, first-served basis, he says, and with good reason. Instead, they are organized around the triage system, adapted from military methods of handling mass casualties in the field.

Here's Kauffman's description of how emergency departments work: When a patient comes in for care, a specially trained triage nurse records information about the person's chief complaint and measures his vital signs—temperature, pulse, respiration and blood pressure. These indicators reveal how well the patient is doing with his ABCs—that's ER-speak for airway, breathing and circulation, the vital functions that support life. The more worrisome the chief complaint, such as massive bleeding or an obstructed airway, and the more unstable the vital signs, the higher the priority assigned to that patient's case. Using this highly effective system, the patient who arrives with blunt trauma to the head following a motor vehicle accident will understandably be seen before one who is constipated.

Coverage counts

With the advent of managed care, it literally pays to learn about your insurance coverage before the need for emergency treatment arises. Although emergency patients have traditionally been brought to the closest hospital, some carriers now prefer that their insureds travel to the hospital they contract with, regardless of distance. In addition, some insurance companies may mandate the authorization of the patient's primary care physician before they will cover charges for ER care.

In many cases, you can avoid a trip to the emergency room altogether by simply contacting your primary care physician first. Since your doctor already knows you and your medical history, he or she is well prepared to do an over-the-phone assessment of your problem. The doctor can discuss your symptoms, advise you on how to manage them, phone in a prescription to your local pharmacy and arrange for prompt, in-office follow-up care, if necessary. Of course, if you are facing a truly life-threatening emergency and the delay of a phone call would jeopardize your health, a rapid trip to the emergency department is in order.

Help yourself to better ER care

Let's assume you've made it past your insurance company and the triage nurse with a truly emergent—or at least urgent—complaint. What can you do to ensure the best care possible? According to Kauffman, physicians base the vast majority of their diagnoses on medical history, which means you can expedite your visit by thinking through some pertinent facts about your past illnesses, chronic conditions and current complaint.

First, suggests Kauffman, it's important to have an up-to-date listing of all the prescription and over-the-counter medications you take, especially if your medication regimen is complex. Be sure to include all of your medication and food allergies on this list, too. For example, an allergy to seafood or to iodine is significant, because it places you at higher risk for an allergic reaction to the contrast dye used in many diagnostic imaging studies. If you do not have such a list, at least grab your medication containers before you leave the house; they can provide the doctor with important clues about your medical condition. If you have an old EKG or chest X-ray around the house, bring that along too.

Generally speaking, the more pertinent details you provide to the emergency medicine physician, the more rapid your diagnosis and treatment will be. The doctor will ask you to describe your complaint as fully as possible, says Kauffman. When did it begin? Is it a new problem or one you have experienced before? Does anything exacerbate or relieve your distress? If you are having pain, you will be asked to characterize the discomfort as dull, sharp or burning. Also be prepared to discuss your family medical history and personal history, including past hospitalizations and surgeries. In addition, if your problem is likely to require any kind of surgical procedure, the staff will want to know when you last ate or drank in order to be able to administer anesthetics safely.

While this list is far from all-inclusive, here are some conditions that do warrant emergency-level care, according to Dr. Paul G. Alexander, an attending physician formerly with the department of emergency medicine at the Medical Center of Delaware in Newark:

Pain: Sudden severe pain is a warning sign that should be heeded. Of particular significance, says Alexander, is abdominal pain accompanied by weakness and low blood pressure (signs of which include rapid heart beat, a sensation of sweatiness and nausea), which may indicate a ruptured abdominal aneurysm, or stomach distress with dark-colored or bloody stools, a sign of gastrointestinal bleeding, particularly if you have a history of ulcer.

Chest pain, pressure or tightness: Of particular concern is chest discomfort attended by shortness of breath, sweating, or neck, arm or jaw discomfort, which is usually associated with heart attack.

Fainting: This is especially worrisome in older adults, since it may indicate a cardiac problem. If you are younger and the event is associated with hot, crowded conditions or an intense emotional state, and is relieved with rest, you can probably forgo a visit to the ER.

Sudden weakness, dizziness or change in vision: These symptoms may indicate an impending stroke, especially when the visual change is similar to the sensation of a curtain being pulled down in front of the eyes. Visual changes are also associated with migraine headache.

Difficulty breathing or shortness of breath: This symptom should not be taken lightly, especially if you are an asthmatic with a history of severe attacks. If you do not have access to your usual inhalant medication, seek emergency care, particularly if your symptoms are worsening and are accompanied by nausea and increasing anxiety. Left untreated, asthma attacks can be fatal.

Blood loss: To avoid shock, significant bleeding should be controlled in an ER.

Trauma: Includes blunt trauma (for example, a blow to the chest or abdomen from a steering wheel, or falls from heights greater than 15 feet for adults and 6 feet for children) and penetrating trauma (knife wounds, gunshot wounds or wounds caused by being impaled on sharp objects). Note: Do not try to remove embedded objects—they act as stoppers to control blood loss. Instead, go to the emergency room, where the object can be removed surgically.

Violent encounters: These include elder, partner and child abuse and sexual assault (to aid collection of evidence, do not shower, bathe or change clothing before going to the ER).

Altered state of consciousness: This is evident when a person is difficult to awaken or cannot stay alert.

Exposure to extreme heat or cold: These conditions are of particular danger to the elderly and young children, says Alexander. Hyperthermia (increased body temperature) can be particularly life-threatening, since it may lead to cardiac arrhythmia and sudden death.

Pelvic pain: Any woman of childbearing age who has missed a period or two and who develops sudden, severe pelvic pain—possibly accompanied by dizziness, fainting and/or spotting—should seek emergency care without delay. These symptoms may indicate an ectopic (tubal) pregnancy, which can cause a potentially fatal hemorrhage.

Head trauma: Particularly dangerous if protective head gear was not in place.

Burns: Seek care for burns severe enough to result in blistering or charring of the soles of feet, hands, face, abdomen or genitalia.

Deep cuts or penetrating/puncture wounds: Even if the wound is not severe, consider seeing your family doctor for a tetanus booster. One is required every five years to be protected.

Accidental ingestions: Occupational or home-based. This can be particularly troublesome with toddlers if harmful household substances are not locked up or kept out of reach. Call Poison Control first for guidance (Philadelphia: 215-386-2100; New Jersey: 1-800-962-1253). Based on the substance, they will advise you whether to induce vomiting or whether it is safer to give milk to dilute the chemical. Be sure to have syrup of ipecac on hand at home at all times, says Alexander.

Psychiatric emergencies: Includes suicidal, homicidal or delusional behavior.

A foreign body in the eye that results in diminished or blurred vision.

Special circumstances

In addition, the very young, the very old and those with certain preexisting conditions may require an extra measure of vigilance and should seek prompt evaluation for symptoms that would not necessarily require emergency care in a healthy young or middle-aged adult:

Children

Fever: From birth to six months, fever could result in a hospital admission. Bring these young infants directly to the emergency room for evaluation. In older infants, toddlers and school-age children, fever is generally treated at home with acetaminophen and lukewarm (*not* ice cold or alcohol-based) sponge baths. (Don't give aspirin to kids up to age 14—it can lead to Reye's syndrome, which causes a serious brain inflammation.) Encourage fluids, and if the child is old enough, give cool foods like Jell-O and popsicles. If the fever remains high (above 102 degrees Fahrenheit orally or 103 degrees rectally) and does not break in 30 minutes using these measures, bring the child to the emergency department. In addition, if at any time the child appears extremely lethargic, displays any seizure activity (tremors, convulsions) or just doesn't "look right," proceed to the emergency department.

Difficulty breathing: Children, particularly those between the ages of two and seven years, who develop stridor (a musical, high-pitched sound when they inhale) should be rushed to the emergency room. They are prone to a condition called epiglottiditis, which can obstruct the airway, says Alexander.

Vomiting and diarrhea: Dehydration is a real threat for kids, and infants are at particularly high risk. Call your pediatrician for advice and keep in close contact with him or her if the condition persists.

Note: Although adult hospitals can and do provide good pediatric emergency care, it is generally best—time permitting—to bring children to a pediatric hospital ER. There, staff are equipped with child-sized tubes and lines, have top-of-the-mind familiarity with pediatric medication, enjoy ready access to appropriate pediatric specialists and can offer emotional support geared to your child's stage of development. Plus, if your child requires admission, you won't waste time waiting to be transferred to a pediatric hospital.

Older or chronically ill adults

Urinary tract infections: Although generally uncomplicated in younger patients, untreated urinary tract infections can lead to serious illness in the elderly, says Alexander. Be alert for fever, foul-smelling urine and chills, especially in a bedridden or diabetic older woman. If it will not be possible to see your family physician within 24 hours, seek emergency care.

Diabetes: Any person with diabetes who has unusual symptoms such as weakness, lethargy, rapid breathing, confusion or agitation due to abnormal blood sugar levels and who does not respond to self-care measures (such as drinking orange juice) should seek emergency care.

Pregnancy

For the vast majority of expectant mothers, pregnancy is a healthy event, albeit one fraught with minor discomforts such as indigestion, increased urinary frequency and leg cramps; however, the advent of certain signs and symptoms should be considered serious and are legitimate reasons for emergency care:

Vaginal bleeding: Always a concern, and considered a dire emergency during the second half of pregnancy.

Abdominal pain

Headache, blurred vision, swelling of the fingers

Trauma, such as falls and motor vehicle accidents.

Hospital discharges

Any person recently discharged from the hospital for any reason should be brought to the ER if his or her condition relapses or worsens. Again, rely on the expert advice of your doctor before making the trip.

—Joyce Brazino

Section

You Are What You Eat

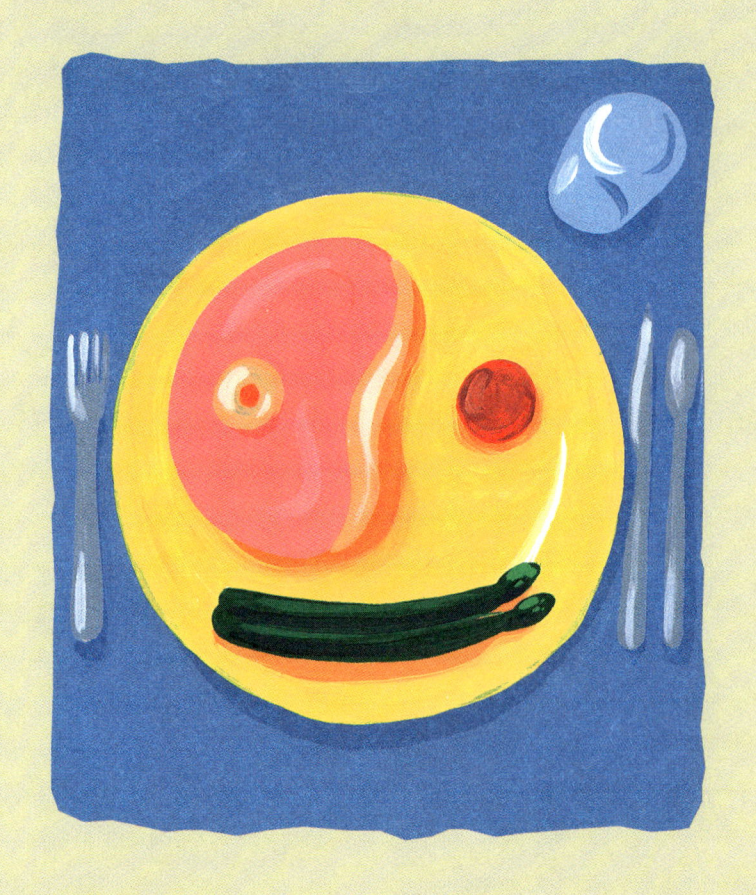

Four

Chapter 10
 A Carrot a Day
  Answers to 16 questions about eating right

Chapter 11
 Dining for Life
  How to eat healthy when you're eating out

CHAPTER 10

A Carrot a Day

Some of the area's top nutritionists answer 16 questions about how to eat right

It is a well-known fact that eating right and exercising not only make you feel good, but will help you live a longer, healthier life. It sounds easy enough—just eat a well-balanced diet and exercise a couple of times a week. No problem, right? Wrong. According to Linda Brugler, a registered dietitian at St. Francis Hospital in Wilmington, obesity is a growing problem among Americans. Although the market has been saturated with fat-free and sugar-free foods, most people have taken this as license to eat as much as they want. "The problem with this kind of thinking is that although these foods are fat-free and sugar-free, they still contain calories, and people tend to be making up for what they are saving in fat with a higher calorie count," says Brugler. "They don't realize that this is just as detrimental."

But if new chemicals and miracle foods aren't the answer, which way can we turn? We asked some of the area's top nutritionists to cut through the consumer hype and give us tips on getting our eating back under control. When it comes to daily nutrition, a little education goes a long way toward better health.

1. Why does fat make you fat?

Liz Emery, Registered Dietitian, Pennsylvania Hospital: Excess fat can mean a double whammy for your waistline. First, fat is high in calories. At 9 calories per gram, it has more than twice the calories of protein or carbohydrates. Secondly, dietary fat is quite readily converted to body fat. For every 100 excess fat calories you eat, your body will store 93 of them as body fat. For every 100 extra carbohydrate calories you eat, your body can store only about 76 of them as fat. The message is this: Not only is fat higher in calories than other nutrients, but those fat calories stick with you more easily than do other calories.

2. What types of food should you eat to increase your energy without increasing your fat and cholesterol?

Lisa Basel-Brown, M.S., R.D., Clinical Nutrition Manager, Marriott Management Services, The Graduate Hospital: Eating a variety of foods daily is the best way to get all the essential nutrients your body needs. Eating a balanced diet and exercising regularly may increase your energy level. Good choices that may boost your energy and are low in fat and cholesterol include foods that are high in complex carbohydrates, such as fruits and vegetables; whole-grain cereals, breads and rolls; and beans and legumes.

3. How many calories should you eat each day if you want to lose weight, and how many should you eat if you want to gain weight?

Lisa Basel-Brown, The Graduate Hospital: Calorie requirements are very individual, depending on your height, weight, age, sex and activity level. The Recommended Daily Allowance (RDA) for women is 2,200 calories per day (36 calories per kilogram of body weight). For men the RDA is 2,900 calories (37 calories/kg body weight). To determine energy needs for weight gain or loss it is important to know that one pound of fat is equal to 3,500 calories. To lose approximately one pound per week, decrease your calorie intake by 500 calories per day or increase the amount of calories you burn by 500 per day. To gain one pound per week, increase your calorie intake by 500 calories per day. Remember: You should never consume fewer than 1,000 calories a day, to be sure you take in all the vitamins, minerals and fiber needed for good health.

4. Is it better to eat three large meals or several smaller meals throughout the day?

Barbara Lohan, R.D., a wellness and therapeutic nutrition consultant based in Paoli: It is better to eat several small, well-balanced meals a day than three large ones because the body can burn the fewer calories throughout the day without having to store them as fat. The important point is not to consume more calories grazing than you would in your three meals.

5. Everybody always discusses the five food groups. How would they differ for a vegetarian?

Debra DeMille, R.D., Pennsylvania Hospital: The main difference for vegetarians is in the meat and milk or dairy groups. The primary nutrients available in the meat group are protein and iron. Legumes and soy products are wonderful sources of protein. Additional protein is also available through vegetables, grains, cereals and rices. For lacto-ovo vegetarians (who eat eggs and dairy products), protein is not an issue. For strict vegetarians, iron is available in beans (lima, kidney, lentils, etc.) and enriched cereals like Cream of Wheat or Total, peanuts, peanut butter and raisins. A vegetarian who does not eat dairy must consume alternative sources of calcium and vitamin B12. Some meat analogues (soy-based products such as tempeh) may also be fortified with vitamin B12.

6. When are vitamin supplements a good idea?

Lauren Swann, M.S., R.D., president of Concept Nutrition, Inc., in Bensalem: Food is the best way for your body to get vitamins and minerals, particularly because there are other substances in food—phytochemicals—that strengthen and reinforce the value of all nutrients. However, some experts do believe that individuals at risk for certain health conditions may benefit from nutrient supplements to prevent problems or limit their severity. Beta carotene may be valuable in fighting heart disease or cancer; vitamin C may help boost immune function; chromium may help with energy and metabolism. But it is important to remember that we can rely on our food supply for extra amounts of many nutrients. For example, one cup of sweet potato has 50,000 international units of beta-carotene—ten times the RDA; one large orange contains 100 percent of the RDA for vitamin C. One possible exception is vitamin E, as it is found primarily in oils, nuts and seeds, all high-fat foods.

7. Can certain vitamins become toxic if taken in megadoses?

Maureen Dube, R.D., South Jersey Hospital System, Bridgeton Division: Vitamins A, D, E and K tend to become toxic quickly because they are fat soluble. Water-soluble vitamins can be diluted and break up in the body quicker. The fat-solubles can be stored in the fat tissue for a long period of time and can become toxic when too much is consumed. You would have to take an exorbitant amount to be toxic, but this is happening more because of the megadoses that are being sold by some health food stores. Toxicity depends on a person's size and weight, but it is not recommended to take above the RDA unless you are advised to do so by a physician.

8. How can I satisfy a sweet tooth without diving into the cakes, cookies and candy?

Cheryl Marco, R.D., manager of outpatient nutrition at Thomas Jefferson University Hospital: Fruits are always a good avenue to choose when you crave something sweet. But allow yourself to eat a small amount of whatever you want to satisfy a craving. If you crave a candy bar and refuse to satisfy that craving, often times you will eat around the craving and eat a lot more.

9. How do you get a child with a finicky palate to eat something from all five food groups?

Lisa Basel-Brown, The Graduate Hospital: Children have an uncanny knowledge of how much and what kind of food their bodies need. Even if a child is going through a phase of eating only one type of food, he or she will almost always manage to take in the calories, protein, vitamins and minerals the body needs. But it is always a good idea to allow your child to try a variety of different foods. Kids should never be forced to eat something they don't want. If a child refuses a new food, try it again another time. If your child won't eat cooked vegetables, try raw ones cut into small pieces by themselves or with a yogurt dip. If veggies won't work, let the child eat fruit. Kids who don't like meat can try cheese, yogurt, tofu or beans as a protein source. Try to be flexible! One important note: Never restrict the fat intake of a child under two years of age. They need the fat for energy.

10. What foods help to lower cholesterol? What foods should you avoid?

Peggy Schiavo, R.D., Pennsylvania Hospital: Foods that help to lower your cholesterol are low in total fat, especially saturated fat, and have a special kind of fiber called soluble fiber. Good examples are beans, oatmeal and oat bran, fruits and vegetables and products made from soy. Avoid whole-fat dairy products, like cheese and ice cream, and most meats, like ground beef, marbleized steaks and ground turkey that contains the skin. Choose the leanest cut of meats, like pork tenderloin, beef round, white-meat chicken and turkey without the skin and, of course, fish. It is also helpful to keep your portions of these items small—about 3 ounces once or twice a day is plenty. Try some bean or soy vegetarian meals a few times a week, but skip the high-fat cheese types. Veggie burgers or vegetarian chili are a good place to start.

11. What are some healthful snacks?

Peggy Schiavo, Pennsylvania Hospital: Healthful snacks can be satisfying, but it depends on what you are craving. Watch out for muffins, excessive amounts of low-fat cookies and cakes, buttery crackers, chocolate candy bars and nuts. Some suggestions? Starchy: whole-grain toast with cottage cheese and/or apple butter, low-fat popcorn (air-popped or low-fat microwaveable), hot or cold cereal, baked potato. Sweet and juicy: popsicles (the frozen-juice type or make your own with Crystal Lite), applesauce, grapefruit, ½ cup low-fat frozen yogurt, grapes, hard candy, jelly beans. Crunchy: ½ cup Frosted Mini-Wheats or other sweet cereals, hard pretzels, celery with low-fat cream cheese, pickles. Creamy: diet puddings, 100-calorie yogurt and Cream of Wheat.

12. Is eating a lot of fruit healthy, or can the sugars be stored as fat?

Lauren Swann, Concept Nutrition, Inc.: Any extra calories in the body are broken down and then stored as fat if not used as energy. Some individuals find that too many carbohydrates (which fruits provide) all at once can actually intensify their hunger a short while later, a condition known as carbohydrate intolerance.

13. How can women control their weight while pregnant?

Christine Schwarz, R.D., Pennsylvania Hospital: A woman should gain, not lose, weight during pregnancy. In fact, most women should gain at least 25 pounds while pregnant. It is important to gain weight at a steady pace by eating healthful foods. In the first three months, most women gain three to six pounds, and then average one pound per week during the second and third trimesters.

About three to five servings of vegetables and two to four servings of fruits per day supply the necessary vitamins, particularly A and C. Recommended fruits include citrus, apples and bananas. Choose pure fruit juice over fruit drinks, which contain added sugar and provide little nutritional value. Fresh fruits and vegetables are best, but frozen or canned may be used. Among the grain products, whole-grain and whole-wheat are the best choices. About six to 11 servings per day are recommended. A serving is one slice of whole-grain bread, ¾ cup ready-to-eat enriched cereal, ½ cup oatmeal, ½ cup brown rice, or ½ cup pasta.

Calcium, for strong bones and teeth, is found in milk and milk products. Four servings a day of milk and milk products are suggested. These may include one cup milk, yogurt or cottage cheese, or two one-inch cubes of cheese. It may be best to choose low-fat products such as skim or one-percent milk to control weight gain.

An important nutrient during pregnancy is protein, which helps the growth of the baby's body tissues, placenta, the mother's increased blood volume and the amniotic fluid. About two to three servings a day (six to nine ounces per day) are recommended. Lean meats, eggs, beans and tofu are excellent sources of protein.

14. Are there certain foods that are good to eat while breast-feeding? Are there some that are harmful to the baby?

Christine Schwarz, Pennsylvania Hospital: As a breast-feeding mother, your body will change naturally to make you hungrier and thirstier, so you will eat enough to meet the extra needs required for milk production. As a general rule, if you are eating enough to feel full, your milk will have everything your baby needs for normal growth and development. Junk foods and fast food will not ruin your milk. But if you do not eat right, you will probably feel hungry or weak. Spicy foods do not usually cause problems.

You can always make some changes in your diet if your baby is one of the few who get gas or colic from certain foods. Some babies get very active and have trouble sleeping if their mothers drink lots of coffee, tea or colas that have caffeine in them. If this is the case, drink less, and wait until after you have nursed the baby. A better idea is to drink decaffeinated coffee or caffeine-free colas and other soft drinks. Also, the alcohol in beer, wine and liquor goes into your milk. Try to avoid it or cut down on how much you drink, and drink only after you have finished breast-feeding.

You should eat a balanced diet as often as possible as well as continue taking your prenatal vitamin daily. But if there are occasional times when you do not eat right, you will still make healthful milk, and your baby will still get the right nutrients.

15. What can I eat to prevent osteoporosis?

Sheh Chowdhry, R.D., Pennsylvania Hospital: In addition to a well-balanced diet, calcium and exercise play an important role in preventing osteoporosis. Foods rich in calcium include milk, yogurt, cheese, soy beans, spinach, broccoli and kale. Research shows that the absorption of calcium from most plants is poor. Therefore, two to three servings of milk or milk products are recommended daily. The following are examples of a serving size: 1 cup of milk, 1 cup of yogurt, 1½ ounces of cheese.

16. Do you think the consumption of reduced-fat items has increased? If so, how is this affecting the average diet?

Linda Brugler, R.D., St. Francis Hospital, Wilmington: The consumption of these items is definitely increasing. Consumers think that if it is low in fat it isn't bad for them. The fact is, these foods still have calories, and people should still pay attention to their total caloric intake. Many times people who eat fat-free items have no regard for the quantity they are eating and end up with their previous caloric intake. While lowering our fat intake in any way we can is a good idea, reduced-fat items should not be substitutes for a balanced diet. The basics still apply: Try to eat more fruits and vegetables, which are naturally fat free.

Nutrition Resources

The American Dietetic Association's National Center for Nutrition and Dietetics Consumer Nutrition Hotline: 1-800-366-1655

Philadelphia Dietetic Association: 215-646-7707

Dial-a-Dietitian (a service of the Philadelphia Dietetic Association): 215-322-7824

—*Nancy Houtz*

CHAPTER 11

Dining for Life

How to take a stand against bland when you're eating out

A bagel on the way to work, fast-food tacos for lunch and pasta primavera for dinner. Sound familiar?

You're not alone. The average American eats out at least four times a week. While safe at home, it's easy to eat fresh fruits and vegetables and read the nutrition facts labels decorating packaged foods. It's simple to monitor our intake of total fat, saturated fat, cholesterol and sodium, and ensure that we're partaking of all five necessary building blocks in the food pyramid.

But despite our current national crusade for healthful living, it's not always easy to keep a vigilant eye on selecting nutritious alternatives when we're dining out. We all have at least one health-conscious friend who interrogates the waiter with questions every time we go out: "Is the soup cream-based? Any green vegetables? Does the sauce have butter in it? No butter, please. And bring the sauce on the side." Yesterday's calorie-counters have turned their attention to fat grams.

The scoop on fats

Let's face it: We like fat. Fat enhances the taste and flavor of foods, from french fries to chocolate cake. Fat is also an essential part of our diet and a source of energy. But the body takes much longer to turn fat into energy than carbohydrates and protein. Fat is calorie-dense: One gram contains nine calories, whereas one gram of carbohydrate or protein contains less than half of that, roughly four calories.

Over the past few years, Americans have been waging war against fat. Check out any aisle in the grocery store to see how many bottles and boxes bear labels with the words "low fat," "fat free" and "cholesterol free."

Too much fat, especially saturated fat, can raise the risk of cardiovascular disease, cancer and other health problems. And saturated fat raises blood cholesterol more than anything else in the diet, according to Cheryl Marco, a registered dietitian at Thomas Jefferson University Hospital. Today's dietary guidelines recommend consuming no more than 30 percent of calories from fat, and no more than 10 percent of that as saturated fats.

The body makes enough of its own cholesterol. In fact, cholesterol is present in every cell membrane. Cholesterol is the precursor of bile acids, without which it would be almost impossible to digest fat, says Dr. David Kritchevsky, an internationally renowned researcher on fats, cholesterol and diet at Philadelphia's Wistar Institute. Cholesterol is also the precursor of adrenocortical steroids, such as cortisone, and even of sex hormones, without which ... well, none of us would be here.

The real trouble begins when there is too much cholesterol coursing through the bloodstream. Cholesterol needs special protein carriers called lipoproteins to travel around the body. This family of proteins differs in size and composition, but is categorized by density. The low-density lipoprotein (LDL) is called the "bad" cholesterol because of the way it can build up along the walls of the arteries, increasing the risk of heart disease. The high-density lipoprotein (HDL), called the "good" cholesterol, is produced by the liver and released into the bloodstream. Medical specialists believe that HDL helps carry cholesterol from the arteries back to the liver, slowing the growth of LDL along the arteries.

Some people metabolize cholesterol more efficiently than others, says Kritchevsky. Other factors, such as eating a high-fat diet, not exercising, being overweight, consuming caffeine and smoking, can elevate cholesterol levels. Recent research indicates that stress plays a role, too. One study at Mount Zion Hospital in San Francisco tracked the cholesterol levels of tax accountants before and after April 15th. During the pre-tax season, the cholesterol levels overall were quite elevated, says Kritchevsky. After April 15th, the cholesterol levels dropped significantly.

What does all this really mean? Today, more than 60 million Americans suffer from some kind of cardiovascular disease, ranging from high blood pressure to congenital heart defects. Coronary heart disease strikes men and women with the same vengeance, making it the number-one killer of both sexes, at about 1 million people annually. While many women worry about the odds of getting breast cancer, the risk of heart disease is far greater. According to the National Cancer Institute, nearly 50,000 women died of breast cancer last year. According to the American Heart Association, 500,000 women died from cardiovascular disease.

Enough is enough

About every five years, the Federal Drug Administration and the U.S. Department of Agriculture issue the latest round of dietary guidelines. "Each time these government agencies reissue the guidelines, the grammar gets better, but the suggestions remain basically the same," says Kritchevsky. As is commonly known, the guidelines suggest that we eat a variety of nutritious foods and eat a well-balanced diet, maintain a healthy weight and exercise.

While these guidelines may sound simple, they are not always easy to follow. On-the-go Americans grab food where and when they can find it, and lots of it.

Many restaurants are renowned for lavishly filling plates to the brim, often providing three or four times the daily protein allowances with an 18-ounce sirloin steak and triple the daily allowance of fat with a mound of french fries. Diners, in turn, try to finish every morsel because our parents cultivated a long-standing guilt that someone somewhere was starving.

But we can fight back. We can take our cue from the French, renowned for an abundance of rich foods, who keep their weight in check by keeping the food portions small. Instead of accepting the challenge of finishing an enormous entree, try ordering appetizers instead of a main course, or sharing an entree. And doggy bags are the perfect prescription for assuaging the vestiges of childhood guilt.

Low-fat options don't have to be tasteless and dull. For example, when your tastes turn south of the border, go for the salsas and fajitas and hold the guacamole, cheese and cream sauces. With Chinese food, go for the sizzling or stir-fried dishes with vegetables and tofu, that ever-versatile protein, and nix the monosodium glutamate (MSG). For Italian, go for pasta topped with a tomato-based sauce instead of creamy carbonara. And at the salad bar, stick to the greens and pass over the mayonnaise-rich pasta, tuna and chicken salads that pack in the calories. Likewise, creamy salad dressings can add 60 to 70 calories per tablespoon to those otherwise healthy greens.

What's on the menu

Philadelphia may get star billing for cheesesteaks, but we're also up to date with nutritious dining options. For almost a decade, health-conscious alternatives have been appearing on menus throughout the region. Among the pioneers were Thomas Jefferson's cardiology, nutrition and marketing departments, which consolidated their interests nine years ago to launch a heart-healthy program called Dining With Heart in Philadelphia-area restaurants. Their brainchild applied the science of nutrition to the art of cooking.

Teamed with the Philadelphia Association of Restaurant Purveyors and the Philadelphia-Delaware Valley Restaurant Association, Jefferson's Dining With Heart program now links about 40 area restaurants. The Dining With Heart symbol appears next to menu items that meet special low-fat and low-sodium requirements. Specifically, to qualify for the Dining With Heart seal of approval, appetizers and salads must weigh in at an average 8 grams of fat and 200 milligrams of sodium. A typical restaurant selection may contain 50 grams of fat and 400 milligrams or more of sodium. A Dining With Heart entree averages 15 grams of fat and 450 milligrams of sodium, compared to 100 grams of fat and 1,000 milligrams of sodium at a typical restaurant. Desserts average 3 grams of fat and 150 milligrams of sodium compared to 40 grams of fat and 600 milligrams or more of sodium. General Dining With Heart guidelines require no more than 30 percent of calories from fat, with fewer than a third of those calories from saturated fat.

Registered dietitians at Jefferson meet annually with chefs from participating restaurants to discuss heart-healthy ingredients and menus. Each chef can create his or her own signature Dining With Heart dishes. There are virtually no "unhealthy" ingredients—the key is moderation. A single slice of bacon can add flavor, just a teaspoon of butter can impart richness, and a tablespoon of cream can provide the feel of smoothness. Flavorful vinegars, fruit chutneys and puréed vegetables add contrast and interest to heart-healthy fish and pastas. "Color, texture and flavor are three crucial elements to any dish," says Paul Verica, chef at Carolina's in Center City Philadelphia. For Verica, spices and fresh herbs become nature's salt. Even his desserts can be savored without guilt—with fresh berries or his signature chocolate angel food cake.

Dietitian Cheryl Marco says Dining With Heart has dropped its cholesterol listing because of the relationship between cholesterol and saturated fat. Shrimp, for instance, is high in cholesterol but low in saturated fat. And limiting saturated fat is our main concern. Coconut oil, on the other hand, is cholesterol-free yet high in saturated fat, the real culprit in elevating blood cholesterol. So a few shrimp in a vegetable stir-fry is well within the guidelines.

Though most area chefs have no trouble preparing dishes for Dining With Heart, participating restaurants are continuously policed by a team of "secret agents" with discriminating palates. These undercover evaluators sample Dining With Heart selections at random in participating restaurants and bakeries. Their findings, ranging from how thoroughly questions were answered about the ingredients of the dish to its taste and nutritional composition, are reported to dietitians at Jefferson. The Dining With Heart "police," most of whom are cardiac patients and relatives, are specially trained food experts who can easily detect excess butter at a taste or an oversized portion of chicken by sight. One restaurant was reprimanded for serving a heart-healthy turkey burger with french fries. After the "police" reported the incident, the restaurant substituted a tossed salad. But the majority of chefs create dishes well below the listed fat and sodium limits.

Other area hospitals offer similar heart-healthy dining options. Winner's Choice, previously sponsored by Bryn Mawr and Lankenau hospitals, recently joined Dining With Heart in the MainLine Health Systems and Thomas Jefferson Health System merger. The Women's Board of Abington Memorial Hospital also offers its Eat Heart-y program in 38 restaurants in Northeast Philadelphia. In South Jersey, Memorial Hospital of Burlington County teams up with area restaurants for HeartCheck®. Other restaurants, such as the Swann Lounge and the Fountain at the Four Seasons Hotel in Center City, independently include low-fat, low-sodium alternatives on their menus for the health-conscious diner.

The American Heart Association has just started a national campaign to put its own symbol on healthful food items. The AHA's symbol—a red heart with a check mark through it—will decorate heart-healthy groceries and restaurant items that help consumers stay within the organization's daily guidelines: total fat less than 30 percent of calories consumed, consisting of no more than 10 percent each of saturated fats, polyunsaturated fats and monounsaturated fats; less than 300 milligrams of cholesterol; and less than 3,000 milligrams of sodium.

Here's to your health

Prehistoric man may have eaten a diet of mostly meat, but the lifespan back then, Kritchevsky points out, was about 21 years. People didn't live long enough to worry about the long-term effects of a carnivorous diet. Today, he says, "we can try to better our odds against heart disease and cancer" by following the basic guidelines to good health:

Eat a variety of nutritious foods, including vegetables, fruits and whole grains.

Select foods that are low in saturated fat.

Exercise.

Maintain a healthy weight.

Use sugar, salt and alcohol in moderation.

Don't smoke.

For more information on Dining With Heart, call 215-JEFF-NOW. For Eat Heart-y, call 215-576-2000. For HeartCheck®, call 609-267-7575.

—*Barbara Brynko*

Philadelphia MAGAZINE

Guide to Good Health

Yes, I would like information from the following advertisers:

1	2	3	4	5	6	7	8	9	10	11	12	13	14	15	16	17	18	19	20
21	22	23	24	25	26	27	28	29	30	31	32	33	34	35	36	37	38	39	40
41	42	43	44	45	46	47	48	49	50	51	52	53	54	55	56	57	58	59	60
61	62	63	64	65	66	67	68	69	70	71	72	73	74	75	76	77	78	79	80
81	82	83	84	85	86	87	88	89	90	91	92	93	94	95	96	97	98	99	100

Please type or print the following information. Please allow 6-8 weeks for processing. All requests fulfilled if received by July 1, 1997.

Name: _____

Address: _____

Telephone: _____ Age: _____ Male/Female: _____

If you have children, how many? _____

Requesting information for: ☐ Yourself ☐ Parent ☐ Other

Where did you purchase this guidebook? _____

Why did you purchase this guidebook? _____

_____

What different topics would you like covered in the next edition of PHILADELPHIA Magazine's Guide to Good Health?

_____
_____
_____
_____

I currently subscribe to PHILADELPHIA Magazine: ☐ Yes ☐ No

I would like information on becoming a subscriber to PHILADELPHIA Magazine: ☐ Yes ☐ No

NO POSTAGE
NECESSARY
IF MAILED
IN THE
UNITED STATES

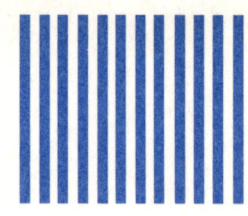

BUSINESS REPLY MAIL
FIRST CLASS MAIL PERMIT NO. 34137 PHILADELPHIA, PA

Philadelphia
MAGAZINE

1818 MARKET STREET
PHILADELPHIA, PA 19103-9467

Index of Advertisers

Advertiser	Page	Reader Service #
Alfred I. duPont Institute of the Nemours Foundation	198 & 231	1
Allegheny University of the Health Sciences	82 & 288	2
Cathedral Village	242	3
Chester Valley Obstetrics and Gynecology, Inc.	299	4
Children's Hospital of Philadelphia	204	5
Children's Regional Hospital at Cooper Hospital	309	6
Children's Seashore House	211	7
College of Podiatric Medicine	301	8
Community Rehab Center	303	9
Fox Chase Cancer Center	16	10
Frankford Hospital	178	11
Genesis Eldercare	264	12
Graduate Hospital Gastroenterology Associates	8	13
Harry Lawall & Son, Inc.	285	14
Hospital Home Care	295	15
Independence Blue Cross/PA Blue Shield/ AmeriHealth in New Jersey & Delaware	2 & 195	16
Jefferson Center for Women's Medical Specialties	164	17
Jenkintown Hearing Aid Center/Jacobson's Hearing Aid Center	294	18
Kremer Laser Eye Center	60	19
Montgomery Hospital	293	20
Philadelphia Fertility Institute	186	21
Philadelphia Health Associates	297	22
Howard Posner, M.D.	287	23
Procare Health Services	252	24
Reproductive & Medical Endocrine Associates	291	25
Riddle Memorial Hospital	307	26
The Rosenblum Center for Urologic Care	311	27
Mark P. Solomon, M.D., F.A.C.S.	289	28
Temple University Hospital	40	29
Thomas Jefferson University Hospital – Dept. of Surgery	46	30
University of Pennsylvania Health System – Cardiovascular Center	286	31
University of Pennsylvania Health System – Cancer Center	305	32
University of Pennsylvania Health System	94	33
University of Pennsylvania Health System – Penn Health Aware Line	25-37	34

Section

The Healthy Woman

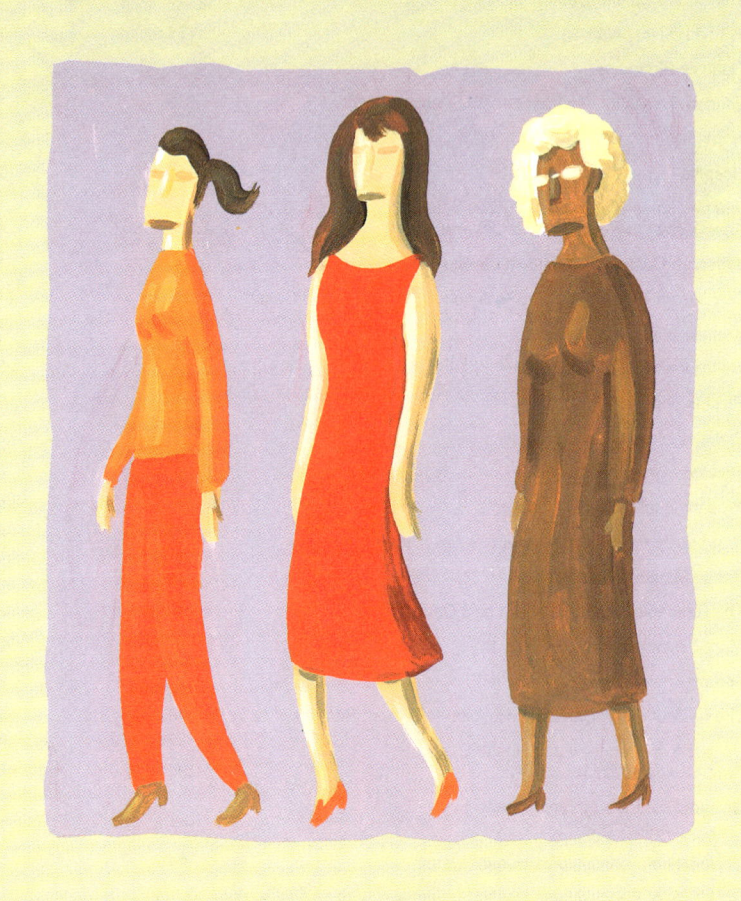

Five

Chapter 12
In Sickness and in Health
Straight talk about female problems

Chapter 13
A Change of Thought on Change of Life
A look at hormone replacement therapy

Chapter 14
Women's Services
Area centers, hotlines and support groups

JEFFERSON FACULTY FOUNDATION
DEPARTMENT OF OBSTETRICS AND GYNECOLOGY
Chairman: Richard Depp, M.D.

Jefferson Center for Women's Medical Specialties
Benjamin Franklin House, 834 Chestnut Street, Suite 300
Philadelphia, PA 19107   (215) 955-5000

GENERAL OBSTETRICS & GYNECOLOGY

Benjamin Franklin House
- **Thomas A. Klein, M.D.
- *Hee-Ok Park, M.D.
- *Howard L. Kent, M.D.
- *Cynthia G. Silber, M.D.
- *Joanne Armstrong, M.D.

Thomas Jefferson University Hospital
111 S. 11th Street, Ste. 8100
Philadelphia, PA 19107
(215)955-0400
- *Burton L. Wellenbach, M.D.
- *Carmen J. Sultana, M.D.
- Sonya S. Erickson, M.D.

GYNECOLOGIC ONCOLOGY
- **John A. Carlson, Jr., M.D. †
- **Charles Dunton, M.D. †
- **George C. Lewis, Jr., M.D.

HIGH-RISK OBSTETRICS
GENETICS/PRENATAL DIAGNOSIS
- **Ronald J. Wapner, M.D. †
- **Richard Depp, M.D.
- **Kathleen A. Kuhlman, M.D.
- **George H. Davis, D.O.
- **Neil S. Silverman, M.D. †
- **Arnold Cohen, M.D.
- ***Patrice M. L. Trauffer, M.D.
- **Amy B. Levine, M.D.
- Vincenzo Berghella, M.D.

ENDOCRINE & INFERTILITY
- **Craig A. Winkel, M.D. †
- *Alvin F. Goldfarb, M.D.
- *Michael I. Sobel, D.O.
- **Gregory T. Fossum, M.D.

IN-VITRO FERTILIZATION
- **Gregory T. Fossum, M.D.
- *Michael I. Sobel, D.O.

ULTRASOUND
- **Kathleen A. Kuhlman, M.D.

URINARY INCONTINENCE
- *Joseph M. Montella, M.D. †

Participate with most insurance plans
Complete Ob/Gyn Laboratory & Diagnostic Services
*Board Certified **Double Board Certified ***Triple Board Certified

†Noted in "Top Doctors" in Philadelphia Magazine, 1994, 1996

CHAPTER 12

In Sickness and in Health

Finally, women's diseases and conditions are getting the attention they deserve

For too long, women have gotten the shaft from the male-dominated medical establishment. Consider: Back in the '60s, epidemiological studies suggested that the hormone estrogen helped protect women from heart disease. So what did the government do? It spent millions on two huge studies investigating the effects of estrogen on the heart—in men!

This exasperating story is but one example of the way research dollars have favored men, giving scant attention to women's diseases and helping produce treatment models of questionable relevance to 51 percent of the population. But in recent years women have gotten smart and turned militant, demanding their fair share.

The result has been a mini-tidal wave of activity in Washington. In 1993, the government launched the Women's Health Initiative, which is spending $625 million over 15 years testing prevention and treatment strategies for three major diseases affecting older women: osteoporosis, heart disease and cancer. And in 1994, the Centers for Disease Control (CDC) in Atlanta established the Office of Women's Health, which will serve as a focal point for women's health issues throughout the CDC. That same year the FDA made its commitment to women's health more official by establishing its own Office of Women's Health, which will, among other things, sponsor projects that study the impact of medicines and other products on women. And in 1996 the Women's Health Initiative added an ancillary study to its research repertoire; in May the National Institutes of Health announced The Memory Study, which will test whether hormone replacement therapy (HRT) is effective in the prevention and treatment of Alzheimer's disease.

Things are also heating up in Philadelphia. In late 1995 the Medical College of Pennsylvania/Hahnemann University—now Allegheny University of the Health Sciences—established its own Institute for Women's Health. Under the charge of

Jean Hamilton, M.D., a nationally recognized authority on women's health, the Institute's aim is to help provide a higher quality of medical care to women. Among other things, the Institute is working on integrating women's health issues into the case studies used to teach medical students, incorporating women's health issues into students' clinical experiences, evaluating medical textbooks to highlight gender bias, running a model clinical program that provides comprehensive, integrated care to women in one convenient location, coordinating various research programs on women's health care, conducting community education programs for women and developing, training and supporting women who aspire to leadership positions in their fields. In sum, the Institute is one manifestation—right here in Philadelphia—of the big changes taking place in medicine with regard to women's health.

Despite these gains, women must be careful not to forget one primary lesson that still applies: Educate yourself. The best guarantee of good medicine is an informed patient.

To help you along, here is an overview of the diseases and conditions of particular concern to all those with birth certificates marked female.

Look for Lumps: Breast Cancer

When it comes to killers, cancer—all forms combined—is the second-leading cause of death among women. Included in that group is a cancer that's taken a powerful hold on the American psyche: breast cancer. Ask any woman you know and chances are she can rattle off the statistic: You have a one-in-eight chance of getting breast cancer.

But there's a lot of misunderstanding about just how much risk each woman faces. One in eight is your lifetime risk. That's not the risk you face at 25, 35 or even 45 years of age. At 25, the chance is 1 in 21,411. At 35, it's 1 in 622, and at 45, it's 1 in 96. The younger you are, the lower your risk.

The disease is on the rise. An estimated 186,000 new cases will be diagnosed in 1996, says Dr. Gordon Schwartz, professor of surgery at Thomas Jefferson Medical College. But the death rate from breast cancer is going down, says Schwartz. Recent statistics indicate that the death rate is 5 percent less than it was 5 to 10 years ago, he says.

There is no better way of surviving breast cancer than detecting the disease early. The five-year survival rate of women with breast cancer that is found early is 80 percent. Most breast lumps are found by women themselves, a strong argument for performing your monthly breast self-examination. Mammograms are also critical. The guidelines are in a state of flux, but, in general, a baseline study between 35 and 40 is advised, followed by biannual mammography from 40 to 50 and annual tests thereafter. On the horizon lies the prospect of using magnetic resonance imaging (MRI) to detect breast cancer. While the method is currently accepted and reimbursable by insurance companies in the case of leaky implants, it's still quasi-experimental for use in the detection of breast tumors. "It is still experimental because we do not know how benign and malignant tumors light up on MRI," says Schwartz. "The gold standard for the detection of a tumor that is too small to feel is a good mammogram."

A good mammogram is particularly vital in the case of carcinoma in situ, also known as inductal carcinoma or noninvasive carcinoma. This form of breast cancer cannot be detected through breast self-exam. Today doctors are seeing more of the disease. Twenty years ago carcinoma in situ made up 5 percent of all breast cancers; now it constitutes roughly 20 to 25 percent.

Risk factors

Heredity looks like a prime risk factor: 20 percent of breast cancers seem to be genetically linked. Women are at increased risk if one or more of their close relatives—mother, sisters or grandmothers—have had it. The history of the mother's side of the family appears to be more important than that of the father's side, and the younger the relatives were when the disease struck, the more likely it is that the cancer will be passed on.

Hormonal cycles, too, seem to have an impact. Early onset of menstruation (the average age for American girls is 12) and the late onset of menopause (the average age is 50) are associated with increased risk, while breast-feeding is associated with reduced risk. Obese women and those who have never had a full-term pregnancy are probably also at increased risk, as are women who have used birth-control pills for more than six years and before childbirth. Hormone replacement therapy is thought by some to increase the incidence of breast cancer in certain women (see Chapter 13, "A Change of Thought on Change of Life"). The effects of alcohol and dietary fat have yet to be determined, although preliminary evidence points to some connection between breast cancer and a high intake of either one. Studies are currently under way examining the link between breast cancer and pesticides, as well as other environmental factors.

The incidence of breast cancer rises with age, and women who have had it once are more likely to get it again. Benign lumps are not predictive of cancer, but they can complicate its detection.

The preventive value of the drug Tamoxifen is being studied and is still uncertain, says Schwartz. The good news is that for women treated with Tamoxifen for breast cancer, the treatment span is now shorter. While women used to be told they would need to take the drug forever, they are now told they can take it for five years, says Schwartz.

Recent discoveries include the identification of two genetic markers for breast cancer—BRCA1 and BRCA2. These markers seem to be present in women whose families have a strong history of breast or ovarian cancer, and their presence indicates a higher than average risk for breast cancer, says Schwartz. The problem is that finding a marker doesn't predict that you will definitely get breast cancer, and the absence of a marker does not guarantee that you will avoid the disease.

Until research comes up with more definitive answers, screening, self-exams and awareness are as good as it gets.

No Prevention or Cure: Ovarian Cancer

The statistics are worse than grim: One in 70 women in the United States will develop ovarian cancer; 21,000 new cases were diagnosed last year, and 13,000 women died from it—61 percent of them within five years of diagnosis. Ovarian cancer usually strikes after menopause, with incidence peaking in the early 60s and then subsiding. Women who have never been pregnant and women who enter early menopause also appear to be at increased risk. Studies have implicated high-fat diets and the use of talcum powder on sanitary pads or genitals, but those results are not universally accepted. Use of birth-control pills appears to provide a measure of protection.

Ovarian cancer is almost never found early, in part because its symptoms—indigestion, fullness and pain in the lower abdomen—occur late. At least 75 percent of its victims are already in the third of four stages of the cancer when it is discovered, which means the tumors have spread. In 1989, after comedian Gilda Radner died of ovarian cancer at the age of 42, her husband, Gene Wilder, launched a television advertising campaign to persuade more women to seek a trio of tests that can help screen for the disease. One of them is for CA-125, a tumor byproduct secreted into the bloodstream. It was developed to help manage patients with known ovarian cancer, which is its only FDA-approved use. The CA-125 test has an enormously high rate of false positives and is not a reliable screening tool.

There are three types of ovarian cancer, but 85 percent are of the epithelial variety, affecting the surface of the ovary where the egg breaks free once a month, creating opportunities for abnormal cell transformations. A 1990 Italian study suggested that about 5.8 percent of ovarian cancers occur in women whose family members have a predisposition to the disease, and tends to strike them in their 30s or 40s.

Women attempting to assess their risk should determine whether at least two first-degree relatives—mother or sisters—had ovarian cancer. But it is not at all clear what the next step should be. Little is known about the risk. Some high-risk women opt to have their ovaries removed, but there are cases of ovarian cancer occurring in the peritoneal cavity even in the absence of ovaries. For most women in 1996, medical science offers virtually no effective screening method and no preventive measures.

The Reason for Pap Smears: Cervical Cancer

After years of stressing that cancer is not contagious, scientists now suspect that one kind—cervical cancer—can be transmitted after all. It's not actually the cancer itself that's transmitted but a viral villain that can trigger its development. Since the 19th century, doctors have pondered the question of why prostitutes often get cervical cancer but nuns rarely do. Research published in 1980 convinced most doctors that the human papilloma virus—or HPV—is the culprit behind the cancer. HPV has more than 60 subtypes, including one that causes the common finger wart. Four other strains are associated with cervical cancer. (In other words, not everyone who gets HPV—about 40 million Americans are estimated to have it—is destined to get cervical cancer.) Scientists can neither culture HPV nor cure it, so once you are infected with this sexually transmitted disease (STD), you are infected for life. Certain strains of the virus can cause cauliflower-like warts to develop, while other strains trigger no visible symptoms. Sometimes the virus causes dysplasia, an area of abnormal cell growth on the cervix that is always treated when discovered, because it can lead to cancer.

About 13,500 new cases of cervical cancer were diagnosed in the United States last year, and 4,400 women died from it. The women most likely to be stricken fall between the ages of 20 and 40, have been sexually active since the age of 17 and have had many sex partners. Even intercourse with just one partner—male or female—can mean a high risk of exposure to HPV if that partner has had multiple sexual contacts. Women who smoke more than four cigarettes a day and those whose immune systems are suppressed by AIDS or other medical conditions are also at increased risk.

Preventive measures, as for any other sexually transmitted diseases, are pretty standard: Limit your number of sex partners and use a condom (even if you are using another method for birth control). Better yet, ask any new partners to be tested for STDs before you have sex. Be advised, though, that when it comes to HPV, "safe" sex is not completely safe, because the virus can be transmitted through contact between the genitals, not just through semen. To prevent the development of full-blown cervical cancer, the best step by far is to have a yearly Pap smear starting at age 18 or when you become sexually active. This inexpensive test, while sometimes inaccurate, helps doctors identify cell abnormalities before they become cancerous and has contributed to a high overall five-year survival rate of 66 percent.

Sex and STDs

While HPV is the only sexually transmitted disease associated with cancer, there are a host of other STDs that threaten women's health. While about the same number of women as men—about six million members of each gender—are infected each year, women are more susceptible to certain STDs than men. In particular, women are twice as likely to contract gonorrhea and chlamydia, and half again as likely to get syphilis.

That's a matter of anatomy: Most STDs are transmitted in semen—which pools inside the vagina, whose thin mucosal lining is highly susceptible to infection. STDs can result in the upper genital tract infection known as pelvic inflammatory disease, infertility, ectopic or tubal pregnancy, stillbirths, spontaneous abortions and premature and low-birthweight babies.

At present the best protection against STDs is to know whom you are sleeping with; find out your partner's sexual history and ask him or her to be tested before you sleep together (not all STDs produce symptoms, so a verbal assurance that your partner is free of infection is no guarantee). Next in line is using protection, in the form of either latex condoms or the polyurethane female condom. Finally, be sure to get screened yourself: Just because you're symptom-free doesn't mean you're in the clear. Early detection and treatment may help you prevent a minor infection from becoming a more major, harmful one.

While the condom is the most effective protection method currently available, researchers are working on new methods known as microbicides—jellies and creams with anti-STD powers that can be used without interfering with contraception.

If you've contracted a viral STD such as herpes or HPV, you're not alone. For support you can turn to Philadelphia Help, a support group for individuals infected with herpes. Or call the American Social Health Association in Research Triangle Park (919-361-8400).

Dem Bones, Dem Bones: Osteoporosis

Osteoporosis, the scourge of the elderly, is in a sense a childhood disease, because the scene is set early in life for trouble later on, when osteoporosis causes thin, weak bones to fracture, sometimes spontaneously, crippling bodies and curbing independence. Building strong bones between the ages of 11 and 24 is essential so that a woman has a full deck when she reaches her peak bone density, in her early to mid-30s. From then on, according to current medical research, she only discards bone mass and can never build more naturally.

Some 25 million Americans suffer from osteoporosis, and that number is expected to swell to epidemic proportions as the population lives longer and baby boomers age. The disease disproportionately affects women; four-fifths of that 25 million are women. Aside from demographics, data shows that between 1955 and 1983, for unknown reasons, bone fracture rates increased. Osteoporosis affects more than half of all women over 65. In their 50s, six women suffer from osteoporosis for every man; by their 80s the proportion is two to one.

Scientists believe estrogen protects women from bone loss until after menopause, which ushers in a five-year period of rapid decline (as much as 20 percent of bone mass) followed by continuing loss of 1 to 3 percent per year until death. Although osteoporosis is not in itself deadly, geriatric hip fractures often force women into nursing homes, and complications are fatal 20 percent of the time.

Risky business

Gender and advancing age are the main risk factors for osteoporosis. Caucasians and Asians are more likely victims than blacks. Thin women with small frames are at a disadvantage, although height itself is not a predictor. Poor nutrition, a sedentary lifestyle, smoking, excessive caffeine and boozing—especially in youth—are all associated with osteoporosis. Excessive exercise and abnormal menstruation—as is common among anorexics—can permanently disrupt the formation of bone mass, as can some drugs, including corticosteroids, anticonvulsants and thyroid hormones that suppress the pituitary gland. Family history appears to be relevant as well.

It's important to note, says Dr. Ann Honeybrink, co-director of Allegheny University's Center for Women's Health, that studies show that people without risk factors for osteoporosis can also get the disease. It's such a common problem that there are actually more people with no risk factors who get the disease than people with risk factors.

The calcium connection

Calcium builds strong bones, just as your mother told you, and after age 55 it actually helps to retard bone loss. Premenopausal women should ingest between 1,000 and 1,200 milligrams per day. After menopause, when the ability to absorb calcium diminishes, 1,500 milligrams is preferred for women on HRT, says Honeybrink. For women not taking hormone therapy, the recommendation is higher—about 1,800 milligrams, she says. Foods that are rich in calcium include milk (an eight-ounce glass provides about 300 milligrams) and some other dairy products; green leafy vegetables like broccoli, collard greens and spinach; oysters; salmon; sardines; and tofu. Vitamin D helps the body absorb calcium. It's available, along with calcium, in tablet form; the antacid Tums is a good source. One note on calcium supplements like Tums and Mylanta: The milligram amount specified as "elemental calcium" is the amount your body will actually absorb.

The estrogen connection

Doctors are increasingly prescribing estrogen, along with progesterone, for menopausal women at high risk of osteoporosis. The hormone retards bone loss and reduces the risk of both fractures and heart disease by 50 percent. The doctors interviewed for this chapter were against routine prescription of hormone replacement therapy for all women, but believed it to be beneficial for many. One indicator would be a measurement of bone density. The test—which varies in cost from medical center to medical center—is not cost-effective for all premenopausal women but is worth considering for those in high-risk categories.

Currently under investigation and on the horizon is a new urine test that can measure the excretion of the components of bone breakdown, says Honeybrink. It's not yet clear what the clinical implications of the test are, she says, but it may enable doctors to monitor the effect of HRT on bone on a more ongoing basis, instead of having to wait several months or years to assess the effect of treatment.

The guaranteed, no-risk prevention for osteoporosis is weight-bearing exercise—important for bone health throughout life, but crucial for the elderly.

For those women already suffering with osteoporosis, there is some good news. Two new drugs on the market—Calcitonin and Foximax—have recently been approved for the use in strengthening bones, says Honeybrink. That means doctors now have the capability to treat osteoporosis after it has developed, she says; however, the drugs aren't really recommended for people with milder forms of the disease. So if you are a perimenopausal or menopausal woman deciding about hormone replacement therapy, don't let the fact that there are treatments available for osteoporosis dissuade you from taking it. Prevention is still your best bet.

For additional information, contact the National Osteoporosis Foundation in Washington at 202-223-2226.

Hysterectomy

Name the second-most-frequent major surgery in the United States. Did you guess gallbladder? Nope. Mastectomy? Heart bypass? Laminectomy? All wrong. The correct response: hysterectomy, a far-too-frequently performed operation that removes a woman's uterus and perhaps her ovaries too. (Cesarean sections are in first place.) An estimated 650,000 hysterectomies are performed annually in the United States, five times the rate in Europe. Typically the surgery occurs around age 43, and by age 60 more than a third of American women have bid their reproductive organs goodbye.

The uterus is one of the few organs that gets taken out even when it's not diseased. The criteria for recommending a hysterectomy have been about as flexible as a Slinky. At least two of them—cancer prevention and birth control—are not valid. And with increased information that the uterus plays a lifelong role in certain hormonal activity, it can no longer be viewed as being nothing more than a fetal residence. The question a woman facing a hysterectomy ought to be asking isn't whether she needs her uterus, but whether she needs to undergo a major surgery after which 25 to 50 percent of patients experience some complications, albeit usually minor.

What's behind the American love affair with the hysterectomy? There are a variety of reasons ranging from economics (it's a great income producer for doctors) to acceptance (because doctors do so many, they've become relatively safe) to attitude (many still consider the uterus a useless organ after childbearing) to lack of viable alternatives. But all these traditional arguments for hysterectomy have begun leaking like a torpedoed water tower. More and more gynecologists, joined by the voices of women's health consumer groups, are railing against using hysterectomy as a routine answer to the common female problem of benign tumors and excessive bleeding.

When is it necessary?

Thomas Jefferson University Hospital gynecologist Dr. Marty Weisberg says there are only a handful of legitimate grounds for performing a hysterectomy. From a doctor's point of view they are cancer (the kind that can be cured by taking out the uterus), fibroid tumors that are so large they are threatening other organs, anemia from excessive bleeding, massive infections that don't respond to antibiotics and a prolapsed uterus (one that has lost its support and is protruding through the vagina). That's it. From a patient's perspective, the surgery may be valid if the woman has intolerably heavy periods that turn her into a menstrual cripple, unusually painful menstrual cramps that aren't amenable to any other treatment or very large fibroid tumors that make it impossible for her to button her skirts. "For a doctor, the decision usually relates to life-threatening issues," says Weisberg. "For the patient it may be more to improve the quality of life than to save it."

At the very least, no woman should agree to a hysterectomy without getting a second opinion. "Well over 90 percent of instances [of hysterectomy] are performed electively to improve the quality of a woman's life. It is rarely performed as a lifesaving procedure, so that's why a second opinion is essential," says Dr. Francis Hutchins, a gynecological surgeon at The Graduate Hospital. There are more and more alternatives to hysterectomy, so it is becoming less and less the only option one has, he says. "In the majority of circumstances, it is not the only option."

Keep in mind that doctors like to operate. As Hutchins puts it, "If your only tool is a hammer, every problem looks like a nail." Questions you want to raise include: Do I have a disease? Is it serious? What are the consequences of doing nothing? What are my treatment options?

Ask about myomectomy

A woman with fibroid tumors, a benign condition responsible for about one-third of all hysterectomies, may consider an operation called a myomectomy if she's of childbearing age and/or doesn't want to lose her uterus. This operation, often performed by fertility specialists, cuts out the tumors but leaves the uterus functional. Depending on the size or placement of the tumor, a myomectomy can be done by opening the abdomen, with a minimal incision using a laparoscope or through the vagina using a hysteroscope. "Myomectomy is best used in selected cases with few tumors of moderate size," Hutchins says. "Though once considered more complicated than just removing the uterus itself, today we have improved techniques with drugs and certain instruments that can reduce the blood loss, and that's key to reducing complications." Myomectomies, which are popular in Europe, require a high level of technical skill—more than a standard hysterectomy—so choose your surgeon carefully and ask how often he or she does the procedure.

On the other hand, a woman approaching menopause who has fibroid tumors that aren't causing pain or a bulging belly may want to try to sweat it out until she's through menopause; at menopause, fibroids shrink by 40 to 60 percent. The growth of these tumors depends on estrogen, so as that hormone level drops, the tumors start to shrivel.

Help for heavy bleeders

As for excessive bleeding, the other common cause of a hysterectomy, it can be handled by birth control pills, a variety of hormones that turn off the ovaries temporarily, or surgically. The surgical alternative to hysterectomy is a procedure called endometrial ablation, where the lining of the uterus is destroyed but the uterus itself remains intact. There are various techniques for performing endometrial ablation, says Hutchins. The original method used a laser to zap the lining; later methods employed electrosurgery, in which an electrical device was used to cauterize the lining. Now several devices are being tested that deliver either extreme heat or extreme cold to the uterine lining, he says. One group in Philadelphia is using hot water, while another is using a freezing probe to basically induce frostbite in the uterine lining. "All of these methods are being hotly pursued right now," says Hutchins.

Endometrial ablation should be done only by someone who does it often and very well. "It's not easy," says Weisberg, "until you learn how to do it." It's one of a number of procedures done through the increasingly popular hysteroscope, which is inserted into the vagina. When equipped with lights and lenses, this is a terrific diagnostic tool, especially to examine the uterus, perhaps take a biopsy and determine the cause of pain or bleeding.

Another new technique under investigation for women with fibroids causing bleeding is something called uterine artery embolization, says Hutchins. In this technique a material is injected into the arteries feeding the uterus; the blood supply is basically cut off, tumors shrink and bleeding abates.

Old vs. new

Speaking of gadgets, your surgeon may offer a new way of doing hysterectomies through the vagina using a laparoscope instead of a big incision in the abdomen. In the right hands and under the right circumstances, this can be a very good operation that leaves only a tiny scar and substantially reduces recovery time. But proceed cautiously before accepting this operation because it is being heavily marketed by the companies who make the equipment and used as a marketing tool by doctors who don't have enough experience in its usage.

On Again, Off Again: PMS

The old jokes about women getting out of whack when their monthlies come along are no longer considered funny now that premenstrual syndrome has been recognized as a very real and chronic problem for as many as half of all women in their reproductive years. The symptoms encompass a broad range of emotional and physical responses that occur between ovulation and menstruation. This cyclical pattern and timing is critical in diagnosing the problem, because the varied symptoms—things like mood swings, food cravings, angry outbursts, breast tenderness, fluid retention, migraines, anxiety, backaches and tension—mimic other disorders.

The causes are unknown but thought to be related to hormonal changes. Sometimes diet helps, but when PMS begins to interfere with work and relationships, a more aggressive medical approach may be in order. The Women's Health Connection, an organization devoted to holistic education and research in women's health, reports significant success in treating PMS with natural micronized progesterone. This is a substance derived from plants that is reportedly an exact chemical duplicate of what the ovaries produce, as opposed to synthetic progesterone, which is similar but not identical. The vast majority of the medical literature doesn't support the improved effects of natural progesterone, but it seems to help many women and may be worth examining.

More promising is the discovery that the antidepressant drug Prozac effectively relieves the anxiety, depression and food cravings associated with PMS. It has become a frontline treatment for the problem. Hormonal treatments are also used as a last resort, as are oral contraceptives.

PMS is a debilitating syndrome and should not simply be endured as a curse of being female. While finding the right treatment make take some trial and error, looking is worth the trouble.

For additional information

The University of Pennsylvania Medical Center operates the respected PMS Clinic under the direction of Dr. Steven Sondheimer (215-662-3329). Other hospitals that maintain women's health centers, such as Allegheny and Graduate, can also be helpful.

PMS Access (1-800-222-4PMS) is a national information hotline for education as well as referral to support groups and physicians who specialize in PMS treatment.

Women's International Pharmacy (1-800-279-5708) is affiliated with the Women's Health Connection. They will answer questions about natural progesterone and PMS, as well as other holistic medicines for treating menopause, infertility, postpartum depression and thyroid and adrenal disorders. They also send detailed information packets free of charge.

—*C.S. and Elisabeth Torg*

CHAPTER 13

A Change of Thought on Change of Life

For years menopausal women worried about the risks of hormone therapy. Now they're talking about the benefits

"Is it warm in here or is it me?" asked one of the four women at the table, fanning herself furiously with the menu. Her three companions, all successful career women closing in on their 50th birthdays, nodded sympathetically at the classic symptom of a hot flash.

"Aren't you taking hormones?" one of them asked.

"No, I've read too much about the risks of breast cancer and I'm afraid," she replied. "I'm trying to tough it out, but I don't think I can last. I haven't had a full night's sleep in months. I wake up two or three times; my nightgown's soaked. And talk about moody. I'm up and down like a yo-yo."

"Well, I think you're nuts," her friend said. "I've been on hormones for four years. It took a while to get the dosage adjusted and I'm not thrilled with getting my period every month, but I must say I feel terrific. It's kind of like slowing down the aging process." She grinned. "And that includes getting my sex drive back."

The third woman listened intently. "I need to be convinced that hormones are safe," she said. "My sister's doctor swears by hormones, but my doctor has some reservations. How do you know who to believe?"

To take hormones—or not to take them. That is the question plaguing millions of middle-aged women entering menopause, the change-of-life event that happens to all women who manage to reach their 50s. As the baby-boom generation ages, some 40 to 50 million women will enter menopause in the next two decades. And with that change comes the big decision of whether to take hormone replacement therapy (HRT), the treatment regimen aimed at lowering a woman's risk for heart disease and osteoporosis, as well as mitigating the uncomfortable and annoying symptoms of hot flashes, vaginal dryness, lowered sex drive, skin changes and more.

Prompt Treatment & Support

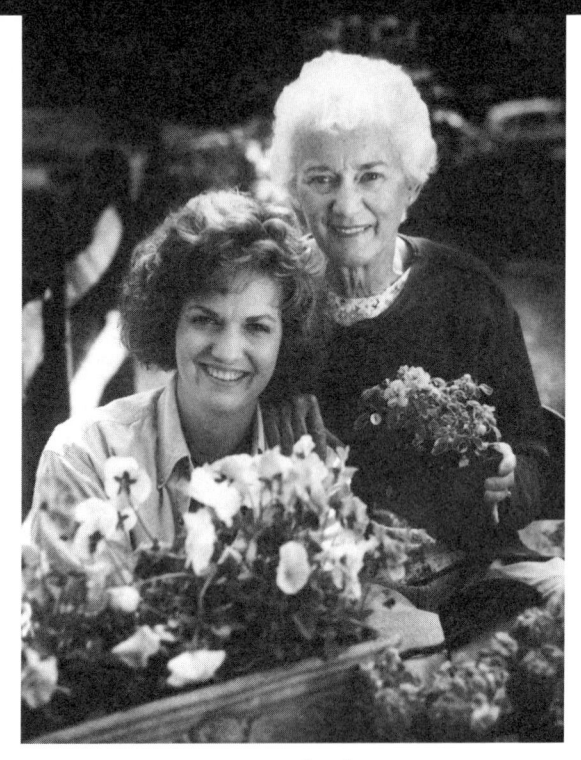

Breast Health Program

Frankford Hospital's Breast Health Program provides immediate diagnosis and prompt treatment for women experiencing breast problems. Unlike the traditional approach that requires scheduling numerous appointments, our Program takes only one call. By coordinating necessary tests and physician specialist consultations into a single appointment, our innovative approach drastically reduces delays and alleviates patient anxiety.

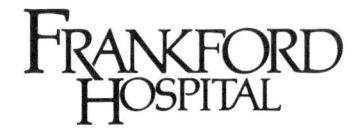

Frankford Hospital

For more information or to schedule an appointment, please call 215•612•4999.

Having reached that transition stage once quaintly labeled "the change of life," women want assurance that it's safe to take replacement hormones to augment the body's declining production of estrogen and progesterone. What they're getting however, is a very mixed message. One day the media hype the risk of hormones; the next they tout the benefits. Studies seem to conflict in their findings. Medical professionals are either enthusiastic or cautious. Some hormone users rave about the results; others rail against the side effects. Instead of helping women make a decision, the abundance of information is just making them more confused.

In the view of most experts, the benefits of HRT outnumber what most people call "the risks"—but what Dr. Marie Savard, an internist and women's health expert in Philadelphia, prefers to call "the uncertainties." Two of them are significant. One is the issue of breast cancer, which has jumped from a striking 1 in 22 lifetime risk in 1977 to one in eight lifetime risk today. Estrogen has been established as a growth factor in breast tumors, but not as a cause. More about that later.

The other cloudy area—until fairly recently—has been the role of progesterone in HRT. Until February 1995, when the preliminary results of a major study known as the PEPI trial were released, experts weren't sure if progesterone would interfere with estrogen's protective effect on the heart. They also weren't clear how synthetic progesterone would respond compared to natural (or micronized) progesterone. The study, however, revealed that estrogen can still exert a positive effect on our heart health, even in the presence of progesterone. Read on for more details.

What is menopause?

The term menopause refers to a woman's last menstrual period. The several years during which she cycles from erratic periods to none at all are called perimenopause; the time after her periods cease is called postmenopause. Approximately one-third of all premenopausal women in America are surgically thrust into instant menopause by hysterectomies. The rest gradually begin the hormonal descent sometime in their 40s, when the ovaries start putting out less and less estrogen and progesterone. The uneven spiking of hormone levels causes the symptoms of perimenopause—the hot flashes, mood swings, irregular bleeding, night sweats and vaginal dryness—that send women to their gynecologists in search of relief. At this point, many doctors will commence HRT based strictly on a woman's symptoms, or on the results of a simple blood test that measures an increase in her follicle-stimulating hormone level. The rise of that pituitary hormone signals the beginning of the end of menstrual cycles and fertile life as the woman once knew it.

The case for HRT

Today some 43 million American women are candidates for hormone replacement therapy, an option that was not available to most of their mothers. A Gallup poll conducted for the North American Menopause Society found that fewer than half the women eligible for HRT have ever tried it. Many complained that they hadn't gotten sufficient information from their physicians.

In the view of some HRT opponents, the mere fact that women now live far beyond menopause is not reason to mess with Mother Nature. Nora Coffee, director of HERS (Hysterectomy Education and Resource Services), says, "You can't improve on what nature gave you. The idea that women need hormone substitutes suggests we are somehow deficient and should have been born with an estrogen pump." Jerome Check, a reproductive endocrinologist, counters with the more popular position: "Just because women are living longer doesn't mean deterioration is appropriate."

In-depth research into hormones dates back only to the 1940s. By the mid-'60s, doctors were actively writing estrogen prescriptions at five times the dosages used today. The first sign of trouble came with the release in 1975 of a major study that reported a fourfold increase in endometrial cancer among women taking estrogen by itself. Estrogen causes changes in the lining of the uterus that can lead to cancer. It has since been proven—and reconfirmed in the 1995 PEPI results—that adding progesterone to the hormone package causes a monthly sloughing of this lining and completely eliminates the danger. Nevertheless, the widely reported 1975 study planted fear of hormones in women and gave rise to persistent misunderstandings of the links between hormones and cancer.

"Endometrial cancer is the only cancer ever unequivocally validated at a cellular level to be related to *unopposed* estrogen," says Dr. Winnifred Cutler, president of the Athena Institute for Women's Health and author of several books on women's health and sexual function. An advocate of combined hormone therapy, Cutler has examined 3,500 studies on women's health and hormones and published 30 papers of her own. She says, "Those who suggest hormones may cause any other cancer are not in the labs studying cells, where to date there has been no cause and effect established."

The bottom line on HRT when it comes to endometrial cancer is this: The results of the PEPI trial showed that women who took estrogen alone had a 30 percent increased risk of significant endometrial hyperplasia, says Savard. The findings told us convincingly that a woman shouldn't take unopposed estrogen if she has a uterus, and if she takes it, it's at her own risk and she runs a one-in-three chance of developing cancer, she says. Some women choose to take unopposed estrogen anyway, she says, and these women must undergo yearly monitoring of the endometrium.

How to interpret the research

The whole area of hormone therapy research does a disservice to women. At present there is an appalling absence of solid, double-blind scientific studies comparing hormone takers with matched control groups. One long-term study recently launched by the National Institutes of Health—the HERS study—should provide this much-needed information, but not for several years. A second long-term study out of NIH—the PEPI trial—has revealed some astounding preliminary findings about the effect of HRT on heart disease risk factors. But the long-term results from

PEPI on the effect of HRT on the incidence of heart attacks and angina are yet to come. In the vacuum, organizations like the Washington-based National Women's Health Network remain cautiously critical of HRT and supportive of only short-term (one- to three-year) hormone replacement for menopausal complaints.

What's not well understood by the general public is that the bulk of research data about hormones comes from epidemiological studies. These are statistical compilations, not standard clinical tests. The results measure only the rate at which a disease occurs in a particular group.

Of 36 epidemiological studies performed over the past decade examining the link between HRT and breast cancer, 32 showed no effect; the other four found minimal increased risk. Not long ago, the Centers for Disease Control and Prevention lumped together a slew of major studies in a trendy new procedure called meta-analysis and arrived at an overall 1.3 percent increase in breast cancer among women taking estrogen for 15 years or longer, but no increase in risk among five-year users.

What do these figures amount to? Not much more than a minor warning in the jargon of epidemiologists and even less than that according to Dr. Lila Nachtigall, a respected New York reproductive endocrinologist who has been working in the field of hormone replacement therapy for 22 years. She says, "So long as the figures for estrogen and breast cancer hover at 1.1 to 1.3 percent, that's too low for the likelihood of a carcinogen. For an obvious cancer link, the incidence would be three, four or five times greater, like it was with endometrial cancer."

Recently released results of a huge observational study—known as the Nurses Study—revealed a similar figure in terms of breast cancer risk. The study's ten-year results said women on HRT have a relative risk of 1.3 percent for breast cancer. Yet the study was contradicted by another study released a month later. So when it comes to the few clinical studies on HRT and breast cancer that have been conducted, there appears to be no clear-cut conclusion. "There is tremendous debate about whether HRT increases or decreases the risk of breast cancer," says Cutler. "The issue is not resolved in a way that is at all clear."

Estrogen and cancer growth

While nobody has any proof that hormones trigger cancer, it has been definitely found that estrogen does speed up the growth of some breast tumors. This is the reason hormones are not generally prescribed for women with a family history of breast cancer. Among the important questions yet to be answered: Does estrogen precipitate tumors, or does it only accelerate the growth of certain already present lesions? What is the effect of progesterone? And if hormones make small cancers grow to the point where they can be detected and treated, is that all bad?

For a cancer specialist like Presbyterian Medical Center's Dr. Donna Glover, the "growth factor" alone is enough to give pause. "I wouldn't tell all women not to take hormones," she says. "I'd tell them to weigh the risks, since estrogen is definitely known to be a growth accelerator with ovarian, endometrial and breast cancer." She advises women on HRT to be extremely conscientious about monthly breast self-examination, and to have yearly mammograms. She says, "If you discover a breast lump and it doesn't disappear after you get your period, get a mammogram. Then get an excisional biopsy that cuts out a piece of the lump for a pathologist to examine. Conversely, if the mammogram indicates the lump is benign, don't go home and forget about it. Verify the diagnosis with either an ultrasound or a needle aspiration to see if the lump is a cyst or a solid mass that should be removed."

At this point, the worry about hormones and breast cancer stems more from what we don't know than what we do. For now, bear in mind that the cancer risks, on paper, are relatively small. That certainly doesn't mean hormone replacement is for everyone. In addition to personal or family history of breast cancer, there are other contraindications. Dr. Bernard Eskin, professor of obstetrics and gynecology in reproductive endocrinology at Allegheny University of the Health Sciences, would not give hormones to anyone with liver disease, a history of phlebitis or thrombosis, cardiac disease of unknown origin or uterine bleeding problems. A sliding scale of personal risk factors, including fibrocystic disease or cancer in a sibling or parent, should be discussed with your doctor.

Health benefits of HRT

In the view of many doctors the compelling case for the important health benefits of HRT far outweigh the hue and cry against it. Dr. Mona Shangold, director of The Center for Sports Gynecology and Women's Health, an affiliate of Pennsylvania Hospital in Center City Philadelphia, and author of *The Complete Sports Medicine Book for Women*, is often asked by her patients if it is safe to take hormones. "I tell them it is safer to take them than not to take them," she says. At least 25 studies, including the recent Nurses Study (which looked at more than 48,000 nurses over a ten-year period), have shown that women who take estrogen can expect a 50 percent reduction in heart disease, which kills more than twice as many women as all forms of cancer combined. And the preliminary results of PEPI released in February 1995 revealed that estrogen still exerts a protective effect, even in the presence of progesterone, says Savard. All of the cardiac risk factors that were looked at—including levels of HDL (the "good" cholesterol) and LDL (the "bad" cholesterol)—moved in a direction indicating protection, she says. The study compared the effect of estrogen alone on HDL and LDL to the effects of estrogen combined with micronized (natural) progesterone and estrogen combined with synthetic progesterone; the estrogen with the micronized progesterone had the second highest rise in HDL levels, indicating that natural progesterone is effective in warding off endometrial cancer while not interfering with estrogen's positive effect on heart disease risk factors.

The problem to date with micronized progesterone, says Savard, is that there is no standardized formula available for doctors to prescribe to women. The product is available through drugstores, but there's no assurance that you will always be getting the same dose, she says.

The next big benefit of HRT is the protection it offers against osteoporosis, a major problem for older women. The disease thins the bones substantially, to the point where they are so weak that many women never recover from falls or fractures. Although calcium and exercise can reduce the bone loss that accompanies menopause, neither is as effective as estrogen. (You can get a bone density test that will determine if you're at risk for fractures.) Estrogen and progesterone combined have been found to reduce the risk of fractures by 50 percent. There are new drugs on the market that have recently been approved for strengthening weakened bones, but that fact doesn't mean you should avoid HRT, says Dr. Ann Honeybrink, co-director of Allegheny University's Center for Women's Health (formerly MCP's Center for Women's Health). If you decide not to take hormones for protection against heart disease or osteoporosis, be sure to discuss the alternatives with your doctor.

In addition to its protection against heart disease and osteoporosis, HRT combats psychological and intellectual problems of menopause. The midlife woman can be a walking complaint department. Where has her sex drive gone? Why is she so irritable and moody? What the hell is wrong with her memory? All these changes are related to estrogen, which regulates sexual desire, enhances mood and even affects brain chemistry. For many women, HRT restores lost balance and provides a sense of well-being associated with feeling young and vigorous. The potential benefit of HRT to the powers of the mind is such that the Women's Health Initiative study has just added on an ancillary study—called the Memory Study—that will assess the effect of HRT on the development of Alzheimer's disease.

Will I gain weight?

In some women, taking hormones creates its own set of problems: breast tenderness, nausea, bloating, fluid retention, headaches. Often these can be eradicated by changing pills, dosages or regimens. Most doctors recommend taking a combination of estrogen and progesterone, because that mimics the natural production of the menstrual cycle. Don't be alarmed if your doctor has to juggle the formula for several months before finding what works for you. Because our bodies produce highly individual levels of hormones, there is no single right way to take replacements. Some women never adjust to the pills and quit. Others put up with several months of mild weight gain and then stay on hormones without trouble for years.

Of the myriad estrogen preparations on the market, the three most popular oral pills in the United States are Premarin (.625 dose), Ogun and Estrace. Some women prefer the estrogen patch—called Estraderm—which provides continuous-release estrogen through the skin. Be aware that the patch may not be as effective as oral pills; estrogen from pills goes through the digestive tract and liver and thereby exerts a positive effect on cholesterol levels, while estrogen from the patch goes directly into the bloodstream and can't affect cholesterol in the same way.

Provera is the most commonly used synthetic progesterone. Some women find the synthetic progestins make them irritable and headachey. As an alternative, the Women's International Pharmacy (1-800-279-5708) markets a natural micronized progesterone made from plants like yams and soybeans in both pill and cream form. They claim this natural product eliminates the aggravating symptoms of the synthetic form. And as we've said, these micronized progesterones have been studied for the first time in the PEPI trial, with very positive preliminary results. Now all we need is a pharmaceutical company to start producing it in a form our doctors feel comfortable prescribing.

The latest development with regard to progesterone is the start of a new trial—PRISM II—that will investigate a new method of administering the hormone. Studies are currently under way investigating the use of a natural progesterone-coated IUD for releasing progesterone directly to the lining of the uterus. The hope is that this method of administration will provide the progesterone needed to protect the endometrium from cancer while relieving women of one of the side effects of progesterone—the PMS-like irritability—they experience with synthetic, orally administered forms of the hormone. The study compares treatment with estrogen and orally administered progesterone to treatment with estrogen and the progesterone-coated IUD. About 700 women will be studied at 50 different sites throughout the country, one of them right here in Philadelphia at The Philadelphia Menopause Group. While some doctors are optimistic about the method, others, like Savard, feel the technique is too invasive.

Another hot trend in hormone packaging is estrogen combined with androgen, which is normally produced by the ovaries. However, its levels drop as much as 50 percent after menopause. There's research indicating that androgens have a positive effect on mood, memory, concentration and sex drive.

Beginning HRT: Is there a right time?

When it comes to the question of when should you start HRT, the answer is that it varies from woman to woman. If a woman is taking HRT to decrease her risk of osteoporosis and heart disease, she should start at the time of menopause, says Shangold. If a woman starts having symptoms like hot flashes before menopause—she's approaching 50 but is still having periods—then she may begin HRT at that time, she says. When it comes to the issue of estrogen forever "there is no evidence at present that taking it forever is harmful," Shangold says. Those in the more conservative school would set a five-year limit.

"It all depends on why you are taking it," says Savard. If you are taking it only to relieve the symptoms of menopause, then it should be for as short as possible, say three to five years, she says. But if you are taking it for the prevention of osteoporosis and heart disease, then that means taking it forever, she says. "Because once you stop, you immediately lose protection."

You may prefer to treat the symptoms of menopause with natural remedies. Among those tried but unproven are such things as acupuncture, biofeedback, large doses of vitamin E, herbs, garlic and ginseng, a Chinese medical plant that may contain estrogen-like compounds. Herbal supplements taken in moderation won't be harmful, but in excess they can cause damage. Talk to your doctor.

The hormone debate is likely to rage for years to come. Obviously no drug is risk-free—even aspirin can be dangerous. But until the gray areas of HRT are cleared up, women may have to rely on something besides research data to decide whether HRT is right for them. "Women know how they feel with hormones and without them," says Savard. "It's a quality-of-life issue, and nobody talks enough about that."

—*C.S. and Elisabeth Torg*

We proudly announce the formation of the

FERTILITY NETWORK OF GREATER PHILADELPHIA, INC.

MAIN LINE FERTILITY
610 649-0500 *Lankenau*
610 993-8200 *Paoli*

William Pfeffer, M.D.
Michael Glassner, M.D.

LOUIS MANARA, D.O.
609 783-2802 *Voorhees*

NORTHERN FERTILITY & REPRODUCTIVE ASSOCIATES
215 572-1515 *Abington*
215 938-1515 *Meadowbrook*

Martin Freedman, M.D.
Maria Platia, M.D.
Arthur Castelbaum, M.D.

PHILADELPHIA FERTILITY INSTITUTE
215 922-2206 *Philadelphia*
610 834-1230 *Plymouth Meeting*
215 757-4440 *Langhorne*

Stephen L. Corson, M.D.
Frances R. Batzer, M.D.
Benjamin Gocial, M.D.
Maureen Kelly, M.D.
Jacqueline N. Gutmann, M.D.

CHAPTER 14

Women's Services

A rundown of centers, hotlines and support groups

Women's health used to be completely synonymous with obstetrics and gynecology—you know, Pap smears, annual exams and all that below-the-belly-button stuff. Today, however, experts are recognizing that women's health encompasses much more. Medical doctors and researchers are finding that certain diseases affect women more frequently than men, and that certain diseases manifest themselves differently and even require different medications. Other problems are on the rise in women.

Consider the following:

Of individuals with the eating disorders anorexia and bulimia, 90 to 95 percent are women.

One-fifth to one-third of all American women will be assaulted or abused by a current or former partner in their lifetimes. Two million women are assaulted each year.

The health consequences of drinking are substantial in women: Chronic drinking can contribute to early menopause, osteoporosis, breast cancer, infertility, miscarriage, stillbirth and birth defects. Alcoholism can shorten a woman's life by 15 years and is the third-leading cause of death among women ages 35 to 55.

Women are twice as likely as men to be depressed.

Women are more readily infected with certain sexually transmitted diseases—namely gonorrhea and chlamydia—than men. And the consequences of STDs for women—infertility, tubal pregnancies, cervical cancer and chronic pelvic pain—can be devastating.

Women are the fastest-growing group infected with HIV, the virus that causes AIDS. Sixty percent of the heterosexually transmitted cases of HIV are among women. AIDS is currently one of the top-ten causes of death among women of reproductive age, and in several American cities it is the leading cause of death in this group.

Four-fifths of the individuals with osteoporosis are women.

Ninety percent of individuals with lupus are women of childbearing age. The disease strikes an estimated 1 in 400 Caucasian women and 1 in 250 African-American women.

Women tend to get headaches more frequently than men and often experience more pain. Migraines affect some 16 percent of women, compared to some 8 percent of men.

So today women's health encompasses more than reproductive health issues. With that in mind we have compiled the following list of health services for you to use as a resource list in looking for the help you need.

Abuse/Assault/Rape

WOAR—Women Organized Against Rape
1233 LOCUST STREET, SUITE 202, PHILADELPHIA;
215-985-3333 (HOTLINE)

Counseling and support services for children and adults, education groups and schools; 24-hour hotline. Court accompaniment available.

Domestic Abuse Project of Delaware County
MEDIA; 610-565-4590 (HOTLINE)

Counseling, case management, support groups, employment services, safe house, 24-hour crisis hotline.

Domestic Violence Program
215-739-9999 (ENGLISH)
215-235-9992 (SPANISH)

Free counseling, legal referrals, G.E.D. classes, employment counseling/training, teen-parent program.

Lutheran Settlement House
215-426-8610

Up to 30-day residency for victims of domestic violence; affiliated with Domestic Violence Program. Bilingual hotline: 215-739-9999.

Women Against Abuse
215-386-7777

Shelter for battered women and children, legal center, transitional housing.

Women in Transition
215-751-1111

Composed of four interrelated services: 24-hour hotline, counseling and advocacy, peer support groups, prevention education/community outreach.

Domestic Violence Hotline
WOMEN'S CENTER OF MONTGOMERY COUNTY;
215-885-5020, 1-800-773-2424

Provides a 24-hour, toll-free domestic violence hotline. Additional services include legal advocacy and court accompaniment, domestic violence support groups for women and a Korean Women's Support Committee. Also offers support groups in bereavement, divorce, separation. Individual counseling available. Offices in Norristown, Pottstown and Jenkintown.

Abused Women's Shelter
LAUREL HOUSE, MONTGOMERY COUNTY; 215-643-3150

A safe home for battered women that has been in service for 15 years. Offers support groups and continuing support services for women. Confidential location.

A Woman's Place
BUCKS COUNTY; 1-800-220-8116

A domestic violence program with 24-hour hotline for information and options. Legal advocacy, support groups and counseling for women in domestic abuse situations. Education programs around dating violence. Also has a shelter for women seeking safety.

Chester County Women's Center
610-431-1430

Domestic violence hotline and shelter.

Eliza Shirley House
PHILADELPHIA; 215-568-5111

Shelter in Center City for abused women and their children.

La Linea Directa
215-235-9992

Spanish-speaking hotline for domestic violence.

Casa Esperenza
PHILADELPHIA; 215-739-9999

24-hour domestic violence hotline.

Congreso de Latinos Unidos Inc.
PHILADELPHIA; 215-763-8870

Breast Cancer Resources and Services

The following organizations provide a range of help to breast-cancer patients and their families:

Breast Health Institute
1015 Chestnut Street, Philadelphia; 215-627-4447

A nonprofit center dedicated to raising money for breast-cancer research. Provides advocacy, educational seminars and research grants. Gives vouchers to uninsured, low-income women for mammography services at Allegheny University Hospitals, Center City. Sponsors the Race for the Cure, a well-attended fund-raising event for research money held annually on Mother's Day at the Philadelphia Art Museum.

Linda Creed Foundation
118 South 11th Street, Philadelphia; 215-955-4354

Dedicated to the early detection and treatment of breast cancer, this is a nonprofit organization sponsored by Jefferson University Hospital, offering seminars, advocacy and referrals. Operates free mammography services and free breast-cancer screenings at Jefferson Park Hospital, Methodist Hospital and Jefferson University Hospital. Provides educational programs through businesses and high schools on breast self-examination, risk factors and disease protection. Also runs a 12-week support workshop for breast-cancer patients.

Living Beyond Breast Cancer
P.O. Box 92; Narberth, PA 19072; 610-668-1320

Nonprofit organization established by radiation oncologist Marisa Weiss. In collaboration with various hospitals, it sponsors periodic educational conferences for survivors as well as physicians, featuring noted authorities as speakers. Call to be put on mailing list.

The Joan A. Karnell Women's Cancer Center
Ayer Building, 800 Spruce Street, Philadelphia; 215-829-7584

The center provides group and individual therapy for women and their families, cosmetology services and patient educational programs. Also specializes in cancer of the reproductive organs. A resource library is open, free of charge, weekdays from 9 to 4:30.

HIV/AIDS

CHOICE AIDS Hotline
215-985-AIDS; 1-800-985-AIDS-6

WATS—Women's Anonymous Test Site
ALLEGHENY UNIVERSITY OF THE HEALTH SCIENCES (FORMERLY HAHNEMANN UNIVERSITY), 1302 RACE STREET, 1ST FLOOR, PHILADELPHIA; 215-246-5210

Anonymous, free HIV testing and counseling.

Spectrum Health Services
HADDINGTON HEALTH CENTER, 5619-23 VINE STREET, PHILADELPHIA; 215-471-2750

A nonprofit community health agency. Identifies prenatal patients at high risk for HIV infection and offers HIV testing, pre- and post-test counseling and follow-up services.

ActionAIDS
1216 ARCH STREET, 4TH FLOOR, PHILADELPHIA; 215-981-0088

Women-only support group, case management services for women, infection prevention education program for women. The Family Program (215-981-0088) provides services to family members infected with AIDS.

Craig Foundation
1233 LOCUST STREET, SUITE 401, PHILADELPHIA; 215-546-6112

HIV/AIDS support group for women called Women Helping Women, case-management services.

Southwest Philadelphia Community Facts Center
5021-23 BALTIMORE AVENUE, PHILADELPHIA; 215-476-9790

An extended HIV/AIDs program for men, women and children.

Philadelphia Community Health Alternatives (PCHA)
1642 PINE STREET, PHILADELPHIA; 215-545-8686

Offers the Women's Health Series, monthly seminars on a variety of topics related to women and HIV. Meets the last Wednesday of every month. Also offers free, anonymous HIV testing.

ChesPenn Health Services
CROZER-CHESTER MEDICAL CENTER COMMUNITY DIVISION, 2600 WEST 9TH STREET, CHESTER; 610-874-6231

A community health center that provides health care for the entire family. All adult services except for ob/gyn exams, breast exams, routine physicals, STD testing and treatment, HIV testing and treatment. Also provides well-baby clinic, immunization services, dental care, family therapy, and drug and alcohol treatment. Self-esteem workshops for women and group therapy focus on body image for women. Nonprofit organization serving all of Delaware County but primarily the medically underserved in Chester. Sliding-fee scale available.

Chester AIDS Coalition
P.O. Box 253, Chester, PA; 610-874-4727

Home health parties for women to provide education and prevention information. Community outreach and early-intervention specialists. Provides food on an emergency basis. Assistance with financial payments.

Delaware County AIDS Network
Sharon Hill; 610-522-0549

Prevention and risk education; direct client services including HIV testing, buddy program, food bank, client-run drop-in center, educational resource library, educational programs for women.

Family and Community Service
Front and Olive streets, Media; 610-566-7540

Counseling and support groups for women with HIV/AIDS. Case-management services available.

Childbirth, Pregnancy and Prenatal Services

Childbirth Education Association of Greater Philadelphia
215-828-0131

La Leche League
215-666-0359

An international organization offering breast-feeding information and support for mothers. Call for information about meeting times and locations.

Pregnancy Hotline
215-829-5437

Hotline at Pennsylvania Hospital that provides information on the effects of medication and chemical exposure on pregnancy. Receives calls from all Pennsylvania residents. Hours: Monday through Thursday, 10 a.m. to 3 p.m.

Lamaze Educators of Southeastern Pennsylvania, Inc.
1-800-368-4404

Covenant House
215-844-1020

Health clinic for infants and adults. Prenatal care, payment on sliding scale.

Step-Ahead Walk-in Pregnancy Testing Centers

The following centers offer walk-in, confidential pregnancy testing:

>WOMEN'S CARE CENTER, ALLEGHENY UNIVERSITY HOSPITALS, CENTER CITY (FORMERLY HAHNEMANN); 215-762-7824
>COVENANT HOUSE HEALTH SERVICES, GERMANTOWN; 215-844-0181
>BROAD STREET HEALTH CENTER, NORTH PHILADELPHIA; 215-235-7944
>ADOLESCENT CLINIC, ST. CHRISTOPHER'S HOSPITAL, NORTH PHILADELPHIA; 215-427-3802
>DISTRICT HEALTH CENTER #10, NORTHEAST PHILADELPHIA; 215-685-0639
>DISTRICT HEALTH CENTER #2, SOUTH PHILADELPHIA; 215-685-1803
>JEFFERSON TEENAGERS IN TOUCH, CENTER CITY; 215-546-TEEN
>HADDINGTON HEALTH CENTER, WEST PHILADELPHIA; 215-471-2761
>UNIVERSITY OF PENNSYLVANIA MEDICAL CENTER, WEST PHILADELPHIA; 215-662-3118

Eating Disorders

The Renfrew Center
>75 SPRING LANE, PHILADELPHIA; 1-800-RENFREW, 215-334-8415

The country's first residential center exclusively for the treatment of women with eating disorders. Programs last seven to nine weeks, and there is an emphasis on the active participation of women in their own treatment. A new intensive outpatient program is based on the same philosophy, structured around 12 hours of group therapy each week along with designated meal times.

Women's Recovery Center
>110 NORTH ESSEX AVENUE, NARBERTH; 610-664-5858

Intensive outpatient programs for women with eating disorders, including anorexia, bulimia, binge eating, compulsive overeating and eating disorders that occur in conjunction with a drug or alcohol problem or as a result of a post-traumatic stress due to sexual, physical or emotional abuse. Also available: an evening intensive outpatient program as well as individual, group, family and nutrition counseling. Educational programs, individual and intensive therapy, day treatment and residential programs are available for survivors of abuse and women struggling with dissociative disorders, depression and anxiety.

Anorexia/Bulimia Association of Philadelphia
215-221-1864

Groups for individuals, family and friends.

Hysterectomy

HERS Foundation
215-387-6700

Hysterectomy education resources and services that focus on alternatives as well as consequences of surgery.

Infant Mortality

The Philadelphia Black Women's Health Project
5021-23 BALTIMORE AVENUE, PHILADELPHIA; 215-474-3066

Counseling and parental classes.

Lupus

Lupus Foundation of Philadelphia
215-743-7171

Lupus Foundation of the Delaware Valley
610-649-7171

Referral Services

Montgomery County Women and Families Commission
507 MONTGOMERY PLAZA, NORRISTOWN; 610-292-5000

Provides referrals to women's services.

Friends of the Delaware Valley Women's Commission
339 WEST STATE STREET, MEDIA; 610-565-3590

CHOICE Hotline
215-985-3300 (ENGLISH)
215-985-3350 (SPANISH)

Professional counselors provide information, short-term counseling and detailed referrals on birth control, pregnancy testing, prenatal care, abortion, adoption, sexually transmitted diseases, HIV/AIDS issues and other reproductive health concerns.

—*C.S. and Elisabeth Torg*

Guess Who Leans On The Blues®

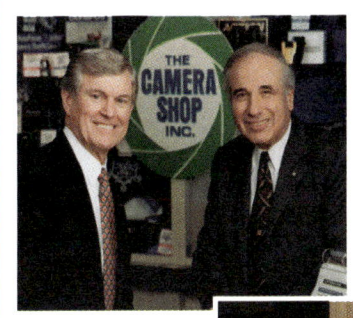

*Dick Vermeil with
John Bogosian,
President,
Camera Shop, Inc.*

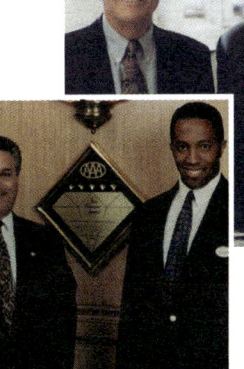

*Dick Vermeil with
Alan Hoffmann,
President,
Vitetta Group*

*David G. Benton, Vice President & General Manager,
The Rittenhouse Condominium Residences and Hotel
(Pictured here, center, with employees
Dan Wills, left & Steve Jones, right)*

The Camera Shop and its sister company, Visual Sound, the *Five Diamond*
Rittenhouse Condominium Residences and Hotel and the nationally recognized
architectural and engineering company Vitetta Group have joined countless
other prestigious Delaware Valley businesses who have gone All Blue
by offering their employees health plans from
Independence Blue Cross and Pennsylvania Blue Shield.

For information on how your business can
Lean On The Blues, call: **(215) 241-3400.**

Personal
CHOICE™

Keystone
HEALTH PLAN EAST

**Independence Blue Cross
Pennsylvania Blue Shield**

Independence Blue Cross, Pennsylvania Blue Shield and Keystone Health Plan East are independent licensees of the Blue Cross and Blue Shield Association.
® Registered marks of the Blue Cross and Blue Shield Association, an Association of Independent Blue Cross and Blue Shield Plans.

Section

The Healthy Child

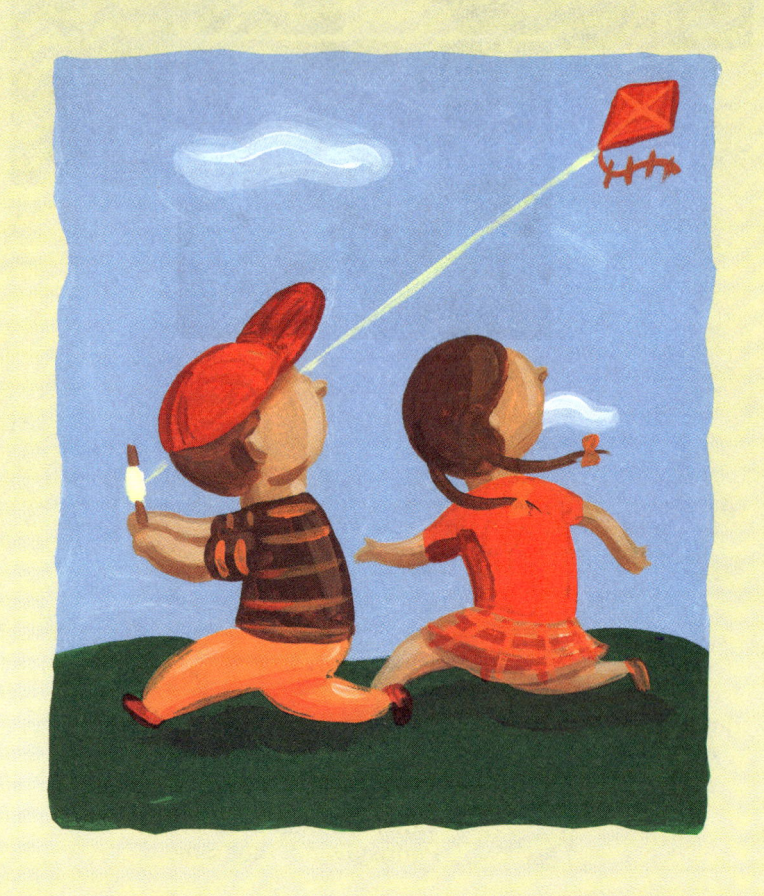

Six

Chapter 15
   Accidents Will Happen …
   Tips for handling emergencies with children

Chapter 16
   Your Attention, Please
   Advice and support for the child with ADHD

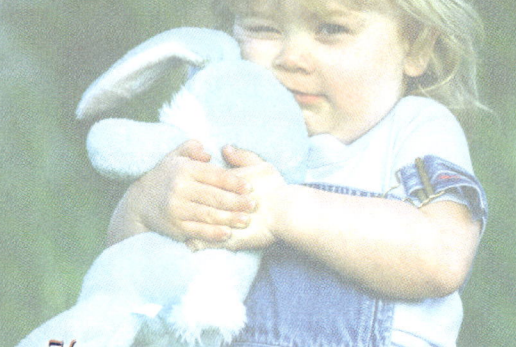

Something So Precious Deserves Only The Best.
Alfred I. duPont Children's Hospital

Known as one of the country's best children's hospitals, the Alfred I. duPont Children's Hospital has over 220 specialists providing care for children from birth through age seventeen.

Areas of specialty include:

- Adolescent Medicine
- Allergy/Immunology
- Anesthesiology
- Apnea Program
- Arthrogryposis Program
- Asthma Rehabilitation
- Audiology
- Augmentative Communication
- Cardiology
- Cerebral Palsy Program
- Critical Care Medicine
- Cystic Fibrosis Program
- Day Medicine
- Dentistry
- Dermatology
- Developmental Pediatrics
- Early Childhood Programs
- Emergency Medicine
- Endocrinology
- Enuresis Program

- External Program
- Gait Lab
- Gastroenterology and Nutrition
- General Pediatrics
- General Surgery
- Genetics
- Headache Program
- Hematology/Oncology
- Infectious Disease
- Lyme Disease Program
- Lymphedema Program
- Medical Imaging
- Muscle Disorders Program
- Musculoskeletal Tumor Program
- Neonatal Intensive Care
- Nephrology
- Neurology
- Neurosurgery
- Occupational Therapy
- Ophthalmology

- Orthopedic Surgery
- Otolaryngology
- Pathology Laboratories
- Physical Therapy
- Plastic Surgery
- POPS (Pediatric Outpatient Surgery)
- Prosthetics Program
- Psychiatry
- Psychology
- Pulmonary Function Lab
- Pulmonary Medicine
- Rehabilitation
- Rehabilitation Engineering
- Rheumatology
- Speech Pathology
- Spinal Dysfunction Program
- Sports Medicine
- Urology
- Weight Management Program

The Alfred I. duPont Children's Hospital knows how to care for your child. Something so precious deserves only the best --a hospital only for children.

Visit our web site for Kids Health information
http://KidsHealth.org

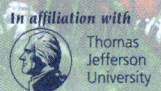

In affiliation with Thomas Jefferson University

Alfred I. duPont Institute
OF THE NEMOURS FOUNDATION
A CHILDREN'S HOSPITAL

P.O. Box 269 • 1600 Rockland Rd. • Wilmington, DE 19899 • (302) 651-4000

CHAPTER 15

Accidents Will Happen ...

... and when they do, knowing the basics of first aid for children can make the difference

Every parent's nightmare: A screaming eight-year-old runs through the kitchen, crying, bleeding from a scrape on his arm. The solution: a little tender, loving care, a Band-Aid and maybe a chocolate-chip cookie and milk. But what if the child had been severely cut, or if he was choking on a piece of fruit? Any number of accidents could turn a sunny day into tragedy.

Parents need to know what to do. First of all, children aren't adults. Kids obviously differ in size, temperament and intellectual skills, for starters. That means they experience different kinds of emergencies in different ways and must be treated differently. Kids may be more likely to choke, drown or suffocate than adults, whereas chest pain in a child is more likely to be muscle pain than a heart attack.

Parents can take certain precautions to protect their kids from injury. Start with the basics: Make sure your children wear seat belts, always wear protective gear when riding a bike or skating, childproof your home to prevent falls, fires, choking and poisoning, learn where and how to contact the local emergency service and learn basic life support skills, such as CPR.

Parents should be prepared for potential emergencies before they happen, says Dr. Stephen Ludwig, associate chairman of the department of pediatrics at Children's Hospital of Philadelphia and professor of pediatrics at the University of Pennsylvania Medical Center. "More and more I see parents coming to the ER prepared," he says. "First, we recommend parents have some basic CPR training from the Red Cross or some local organization. The training would include how to define an emergency and steps to take to deal with a situation."

Ludwig suggests that families have an emergency manual on hand to provide easy-to-follow instructions for calling emergency numbers, including local hospitals, ambulances, 911 and poison centers. Parents should also have information on where to go if they need emergency care for their child. They should talk to their primary-care physician or pediatrician beforehand, Ludwig says.

He's frustrated by parents who ignore safety measures such as seat belts, particularly when he sees injured children after accidents. He notes that gun injuries fall into that category, especially in the city, where parents often buy guns for protection.

Though there is greater emphasis now on children using protective gear in skating or biking, not everyone is heeding the advice. The safety-conscious are still in the minority, Ludwig says.

Dr. Mark D. Joffe, director of emergency medicine at St. Christopher's Hospital for Children, notes that the number-one cause of death from birth to age 40 is accidents. He advises that the best way to treat an emergency is to prevent it, noting that emergencies are often predictable. Different injuries are often age-dependent, and parents need to think one step ahead of their child's possible injury. If you leave a one-month-old alone on a changing table, he can't roll over. But if you get into that bad habit, a couple of months later he'll be able to roll right off that table.

The first step in dealing with emergencies, Joffe says, is being able to tell when a situation is something a parent can handle at home and when the injury needs immediate attention from a physician or local hospital emergency room. This isn't always easy.

Choking or uncontrolled bleeding usually warrants immediate attention, says Dr. Brent King, associate professor of emergency medicine and pediatrics at Allegheny University of the Health Sciences. Most earaches, however, can usually be treated at home.

Childhood medical emergencies often include many types of respiratory problems, such as asthma, which is one of the most common reasons for a visit to the emergency room. Some premature children develop respiratory illnesses that are routine in most normal-sized healthy kids but become more dangerous in those with underlying health problems.

"Parents may be more protective and smarter today about preventing emergencies before they happen, but there's a lot of room for improvement," says Joffe.

Here are a few common emergencies and how to deal with them:

Ticks: Kids may meet ticks in the backyard as well as at camp. If a child may have been exposed, parents should examine him or her carefully. Large ticks are seldom a problem, but small deer ticks can cause Lyme disease, which may involve neurological complications. If parents notice a large ring-like rash around or near the bite site, they should talk to a doctor, advises Joffe. If your child develops seizures or shock, call 911 or the local emergency number.

Insect stings: Parents can take precautions to ward off stings before they occur. If a child is allergic to bee stings, however, keep a supply of the chemical epinephrine and syringes available, according to your physician's instructions. Allergic reactions aren't usually fatal, but parents have arrived at the ER with children whose windpipes had swollen shut. For typical stings, apply some ice to keep the swelling down.

Sunburns: Though sunburns are almost always handled home, Joffe says sunscreen and proper clothing should ensure that children—especially infants—never get sunburned. Burns can result in skin problems later in life, even leading to skin cancer. King suggests using a soothing lotion containing aloe vera on the sunburned area.

Fevers: A fever can be a symptom of either a serious or a minor illness. A baby under six months with a fever of 101 degrees should be seen in an emergency room, says King. A parent may only need to call and talk to the doctor if an older child has a high fever but looks okay or is sitting and playing normally.

Call the local emergency number or 911 if your child has symptoms of shock or impending respiratory failure. While waiting for the ambulance, check the child's airway, breathing and circulation and give CPR if the child stops breathing. Keep the child as calm as possible.

For children over six months, call the doctor if the child has an oral temperature of more than 102 degrees or a rectal temperature of more than 103 degrees. If any temperature is accompanied by seizures, labored breathing, extreme lethargy, pallor, severe headache or a stiff neck, go to the emergency room. Meningitis, though rare, is always a concern, cautions King.

If the temperature is less than 102, treat the child at home with acetaminophen and lukewarm sponge baths. Be sure to dress the child in lightweight clothing, such as light pajamas or underwear. Extra fluids always help. Call the doctor if a fever lasts longer than three days.

Sprains: For most sprains, the RICE formula works well: rest, ice, compression and elevation.

Poison: Call the Poison Control Center. If you know what your child has ingested, the center may tell you to induce vomiting by giving the child syrup of ipecac plus water. If you don't know what the child swallowed, tell the Poison Control Center what you do know.

King cautions against inducing vomiting unless the Poison Control Center tells you to do so. Ipecac may cause vomiting and empty the stomach, but it may actually get in the way of more effective treatments if the stomach fails to empty completely. Call 911 if the Poison Control Center advises.

Ear infections: If the child has symptoms of an ear infection, including ear pain, irritability and vomiting, see your doctor, give acetaminophen for pain and fever over 101 degrees and provide plenty of fluids. Most ear infections usually occur in the first year of life. King observes that doctors may overprescribe antibiotics—the traditional mainstay of treatment—which may not always be needed.

Nosebleeds: To stop a nosebleed, have the child sit and tilt his or her head slightly forward. Pinch the nostrils shut just below the bony part of the nose and apply pressure for five to ten minutes. Apply cold compresses over the nose. If the bleeding continues, place gauze into the nostrils. Apply petroleum jelly to the nostrils after the bleeding has stopped.

Call 911 if the nosebleed is associated with a blow to the head. Call your doctor if you can't stop the bleeding, if there's facial swelling or if bruising or the child has frequent nosebleeds.

For more information

For further reading, call or write to the Children's Hospital of Philadelphia for the booklet "What to Do for Childhood Emergencies and Illnesses." CHOP has also published *A Parent's Guide to Childhood Emergencies* by Lisa J. Bain, available at bookstores and libraries.

—*Steven Benowitz*

CHAPTER 16

Your Attention, Please

Helping the child with attention deficit/hyperactivity disorder

Soon after he could no longer blame the "terrible twos" for his son's behavior, John began sensing that something was wrong with Tim. (Names have been changed to protect privacy.) "From about age two to five, we noticed that he wasn't responding to normal directions or discipline. We'd correct him for something and a second later he would do it again, without any regard to consequences," says John. But this was nine years ago, long before attention deficit/hyperactivity disorder (ADHD) was a household name, and it would take several frustrating years before Tim was accurately diagnosed.

Today, ADHD is thought to affect roughly 5 percent of all school-age children. And while some argue that the pendulum has swung too far toward overdiagnosis, parents whose children have been helped by ADHD treatment are unconvinced.

Many experts agree. Greater awareness, says Dr. Anthony L. Rostain, associate professor of psychiatry and pediatrics at the University of Pennsylvania, leads to earlier diagnosis and earlier intervention, two of the most important factors in the long-term outcome for the child with ADHD.

Symptoms

The American Psychiatric Association lists 14 symptoms of ADHD in its *Diagnostic and Statistical Manual of Mental Disorders*. For a diagnosis to be made, a child must exhibit eight of these criteria over a six-month period, with onset occurring before the age of seven.

___
Is excessively fidgety, squirms in seat
___
Has difficulty remaining seated when required to do so
___
Is easily distracted by extraneous stimuli

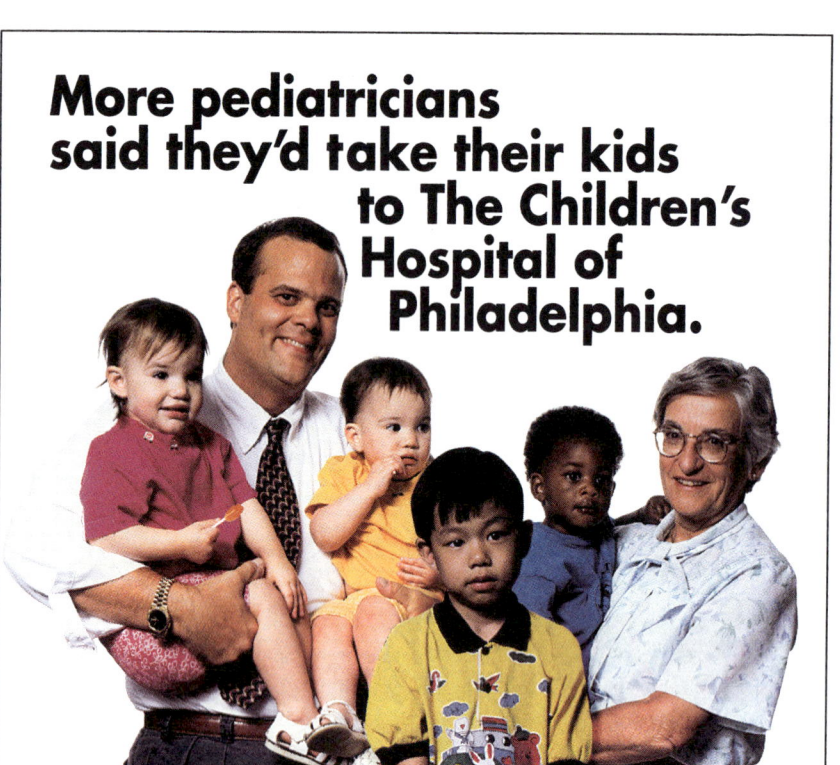

More pediatricians said they'd take their kids to The Children's Hospital of Philadelphia.

In a *Philadelphia Magazine** survey of 1,000 area pediatricians, more said they would take their kids to specialists at Children's Hospital than to any other area hospital.

Maybe it's because they know we're one of the leading pediatric centers in the world.

Maybe it's because we were named as one of the top two children's hospitals in the country by a *U.S. News and World Report*** survey of the nation's leading pediatricians.

And maybe, like you, they simply want the very best care available for their children.

Call today for more information about pediatric specialty services at
The Children's Hospital of Philadelphia,
34th Street and Civic Center Boulevard
Philadelphia, PA 19104

1-800-TRY-CHOP
1-800-879-2467

Philadelphia Magazine,* June 1992;
U.S. News and World Report,** July 13, 1995

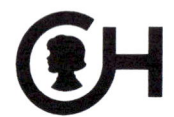

Solving Big Problems for Little People

_____ Has difficulty awaiting turn during games

_____ Blurts out answers to questions

_____ Has difficulty following instructions

_____ Has difficulty sustaining attention

_____ Shifts from one uncompleted activity to another

_____ Has difficulty playing quietly

_____ Often talks excessively

_____ Often interrupts

_____ Often does not listen to what is said

_____ Often loses things necessary for a task at home or school

_____ Often engages in dangerous activities without considering consequences

Once the disorder is actually diagnosed, the severity of ADHD is broken into three categories:

Mild: Few, if any, symptoms in excess of those required to make the diagnosis and only minimal or no impairment in school or social functioning.

Moderate: Symptoms or functional impairment intermediate between mild and severe.

Severe: Many symptoms in excess of those required to make the diagnosis, and significant and pervasive impairment in functioning at home and school and with peers.

Diagnosis: Will the real symptoms come forward?

Given that many children who don't have ADHD can exhibit these exact characteristics at times, how can you tell the difference between a child with ADHD and a child who is simply poorly behaved? Unfortunately, the answer is not so clear.

Much like Alzheimer's disease, there is no single test to definitively indicate ADHD. If a child falls within the parameters outlined above, doctors first try to rule out other possible causes. Allergies, brain tumors and seizure disorders can often elicit symptoms similar to ADHD, as can learning disabilities and emotional problems, such as those caused by abuse.

The key is to get multiple assessments of a child over a long period of time. "One teacher or one parent is not enough to diagnose a child with ADHD," says Rostain. "You need the assessment of a number of adults, particularly those who know the child well and have an understanding of the child's behavior in a variety of settings."

The ideal scenario is to have a "case" approach, where a team consisting of neurologists, child psychiatrists, developmental pediatricians, social workers, the child's parents and teachers observes and tests the child over a long period of time.

In the Delaware Valley, Children's Seashore House, the Philadelphia Child Guidance Center and The Children's Hospital of Philadelphia are well-known for their work with ADHD and for following the case approach.

Getting to the root of the problem

The idea that parents or a bad home life are to blame for ADHD has been flatly refuted by a number of research studies. Most memorable is a December 1990 report in the *New England Journal of Medicine* that found that adults with ADHD use glucose—the brain's main energy source—at a lesser rate than adults without ADHD. This reduced brain metabolism rate was most evident in the portion of the brain that is important for attention, handwriting, motor control and inhibition of responses, leading researchers to classify ADHD as a neurobiological disorder.

Interestingly, of the 5 percent of American children affected by ADHD, the ratio of boys to girls is 4 to 1. Rostain offers several possibilities: "First, boys' brains are slower to develop compared to girls'. Second, it appears that testosterone has some influence over the development of motor and impulse control, along with the development of frontal lobe functioning, which regulates attention skills."

Finding the help you need

The best course of treatment, says Rostain, is a multimodal approach that combines medicine and extensive behavior management, family therapy and work within the school setting.

This approach may actually be contrary to what most people think. "In most people's minds, ADHD means Ritalin [a commonly prescribed ADHD medication], and that's unfair," says Rostain. The idea that doctors are drugging up bad kids, he says, is truly misguided.

In fact, medication is far from a magic bullet. It is simply a starting point from which to launch the "real" work: behavior management for the child, modifying parenting skills, creating a more structured home environment and family therapy, to name just a few.

Medication

When medications are used, the stimulant methylphenidate (Ritalin) is generally the first line of attack. In a seemingly anomalous process, Ritalin and other stimulants actually provide increased mental alertness for children with ADHD, helping them to better focus and concentrate.

"We saw an immediate difference," says John, commenting on his son's experience with Ritalin. Once incredibly impulsive and highly aggressive, Tim became "more compliant, focused and less disruptive at school and at home."

But there are downsides to medication, as well. Side effects may include appetite suppression, headaches, insomnia, stomachaches, increased blood pressure and feeling "jittery." Antihypertensive drugs (such as Catapres) are used when stimulants produce too many side effects.

In addition, newer antidepressants are becoming available to replace tricyclic antidepressants (TCAs), which used to be prescribed when stimulants didn't work. TCAs have fallen out of favor in the past few years due to concern over side effects, which include increased heart rate and rhythm abnormalities.

Behavior management

ADHD children generally work with psychiatrists, psychologists, social workers and/or school counselors to learn how to adapt to their disorder. But the kids are not the only ones who have to change. Parents need to create a structure at home that takes into account the ADHD child's needs, teachers must understand how ADHD affects the learning process, and siblings must learn to cope with the inequities that can occur in the home.

For example, parents often develop different sets of reward and punishment scenarios—one for the child with ADHD and the other for his siblings. "Tim would be rewarded for not disrupting dinner, while his brothers and sisters were simply expected to behave," says John. Counseling for the entire family helped ease the frustrations brought on by these issues.

One father, whose son was diagnosed at age three, posted these parenting strategies on his ADHD World Wide Web site:

Transitioning

ADHD children have a difficult time adjusting to change. Providing forewarning (for example, telling the child "We're going to the supermarket in ten minutes" and then repeating it again in five minutes) can help ease the stress of a perceived sudden disruption.

Rules/Rewards

For children who can't focus, it's not enough to make subtle references to house rules, or worse yet, to have "unwritten rules." Parents need to regularly outline rules, detailing rewards and punishments for good and bad behavior.

Timeouts

This popular method of behavior modification works well with ADHD children because it takes them out of a situation, giving them time to reflect on their behavior.

Deflection/Redirection

Much like timeout, this form of behavior modification removes the child from a situation and helps to refocus energy on a more appropriate activity or behavior.

Structure/Consistency

To children with ADHD, the world and their own behavior seem out of control. Providing your child with consistency and structure can help.

Advocacy

Often misunderstood by other kids and labeled a "troublemaker" at school, the ADHD child often feels a sense of isolation and frustration. Parents can help by advocating for their children, educating friends, family and teachers about the disorder and the reasons for particular behaviors.

The importance of finding support

Another important aspect of living with ADHD is the support of others in the same situation. Support groups and national ADHD membership organizations serve as important social and educational resources, often advocating for the educational rights of children with ADHD.

John and his wife attended local support meetings for many years. "You immediately connect with these people," says John, whose son, Tim, now 14, is doing very well socially and academically.

Prognosis: What the future holds

According to Rostain, 50 percent of children with ADHD will have symptoms into adulthood. Of those, 50 percent will need continued treatment for ADHD. Again, the key is early detection.

"The longer the disorder goes undetected, the harder it is to treat," says Rostain. The potential long-term consequences for those who do not get help include school failure and dropout, depression, conduct disorders, failed relationships and even substance abuse.

Those who are diagnosed and treated early on can do quite well at adapting to their disability. Some, like Tim—now a standout sports star, thanks in large part to his impulsive, fearless personality—can even turn their disability into an advantage.

Local Resources

Here are a few organizations that specialize in ADHD:

Children's Seashore House
ATTENTION DEFICIT/HYPERACTIVITY DISORDER PROGRAM, 3405 CIVIC CENTER BOULEVARD, PHILADELPHIA; 215-895-3849

This program, coming up on its tenth year in operation, evaluates and treats children ages 3 to 14. In addition to full evaluation services, Children's Seashore House helps with the social side of ADHD through child and family therapy, school consultation and advocacy and group counseling in homework and behavior-change strategies.

Philadelphia Child Guidance Center
ATTENTION DEFICIT/HYPERACTIVITY DISORDER PROGRAM, 34TH STREET AND CIVIC CENTER BOULEVARD, PHILADELPHIA; 215-243-2700

This practice specializes in evaluating and treating ADHD in preschoolers, children and adolescents. Services include comprehensive individual and family evaluation, individual and family group therapy, psychological assessment, psychiatric consultation and medication management. The group also works with the schools, updating school case workers on children's progress.

Children's Hospital of Philadelphia
34TH STREET AND CIVIC CENTER BOULEVARD, PHILADELPHIA; 215-590-1719

CHOP's program includes nine doctors, all neurologists, who diagnose and treat ADHD. In 1991, the hospital published *A Parent's Guide to Attention Deficit Disorders* by Lisa J. Bain, a book that often is listed as a "must read" for parents of children with ADHD. This 200-page easy read addresses a broad spectrum of issues, including behavior management, medications and therapy. It's available at local bookstores and in the hospital's Daisy Gift Shop.

Education Law Center
801 ARCH STREET, SUITE 610, PHILADELPHIA; 215-238-6970

This group provides free legal advice on how to obtain special education for your child and publishes an educational booklet, "Your Rights to Special Education."

National Resources

Children and Adults With Attention Deficit Disorder (CHADD)
499 NORTHWEST 70TH AVENUE, SUITE 101, PLANTATION, FL 33317; 1-800-233-4050, 305-587-3700; HTTP://WWW.CHADD.ORG

With 35,000 members and 600 chapters throughout the country, CHADD is the largest national organization focused on ADHD. CHADD provides a support network for parents and children and serves as an education and information clearinghouse. Members receive a quarterly magazine, *ATTENTION!*, with articles by leading ADHD researchers, educators and clinicians, as well as first-person stories by children with ADHD, their parents and teachers.

National Attention Deficit Disorder Association (NADDA)
1-800-487-2282

Much like CHADD, NADDA offers support groups for parents and children, serving as an educational and information resource. By calling 313-769-6729, you can connect with the group's fax-on-demand system and have information sent directly to your fax.

ADD Warehouse
1-800-233-9273

The free ADD Warehouse catalog offers a wide range of books, videos and games.

—Lynn Selhat

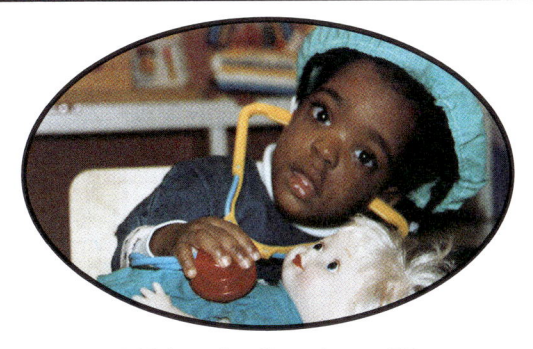

At Children's Seashore House, Our Specialized Care Begins With
LISTENING

With more than a century of ***listening*** to the special needs of our young patients and their families, Children's Seashore House leads the way in providing specialized care and rehabilitation to children with disabilities and chronic illnesses.

Our expanding outpatient specialty programs include:

Attention Deficit Hyperactivity Disorder
215-895-3849

• Audiology	215-895-3675
• Biobehavioral	215-895-3744
• Cerebral Palsy*	215-895-3835
• Child Development	215-895-3838
• Feeding Program*	215-895-3803
• Neurorehabilitation	215-895-3292
• Occupational Therapy	215-895-3790
• Physical Therapy	215-895-3780
• Psychology	215-895-3736
• Rheumatology	215-895-3845
• Social Work	215-895-3750
• Speech/Language	215-895-3680

*One of 50 "Centers of Excellence" featured in *Philadelphia Magazine*.

Children's Seashore House
A Regional Hospital for Specialized Care and Rehabilitation

3405 Civic Center Blvd. • Philadelphia, PA 19104 • 215-895-3600
35 S. Annapolis Ave. • Atlantic City, NJ 08401 • 609-347-6157

Section

Mind Over Matter

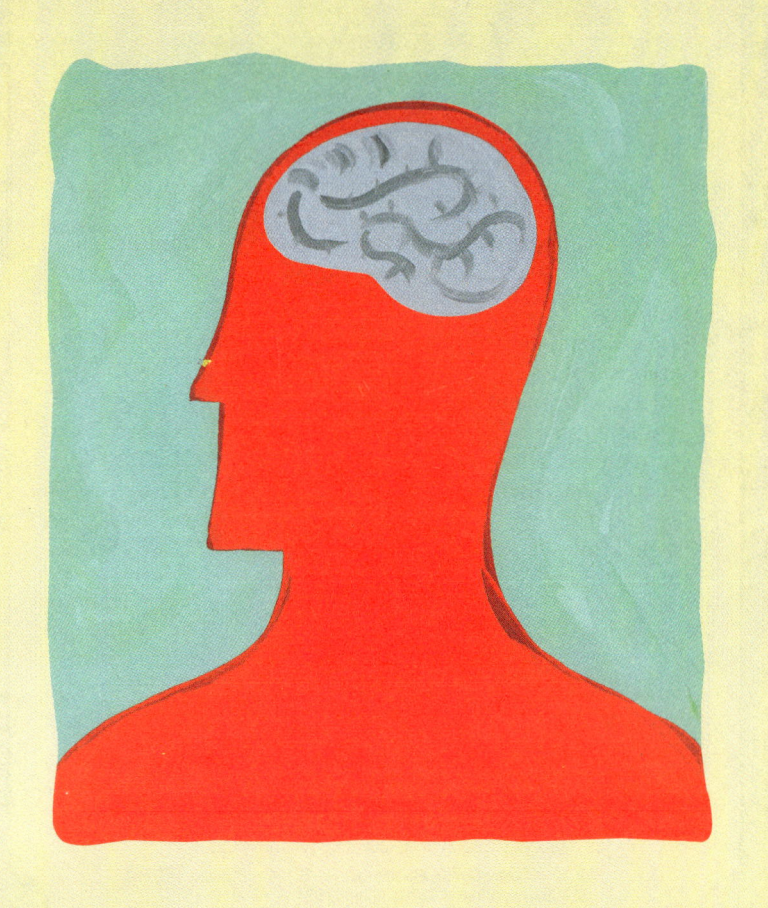

Seven

Chapter 17
The Drug Zone
Feeling sad? Hyper? Paranoid? Take a pill

Chapter 18
Where to Go for Help
Psychiatric treatment centers

CHAPTER 17

The Drug Zone

Move over, Dr. Freud. The prescription pad may be the answer to depression, anxiety and other problems once reserved for the shrink's couch

As cataclysmic as the ruminations of Sigmund Freud, a revolution is taking place in the field of psychiatry that has changed the way doctors view mental illness. One of every eight prescriptions written in the United States is for a drug to combat an emotional problem we used to take exclusively to a therapist's couch. That's still where many family and personal issues are best resolved. But Freud did not have the advantages of modern science, which has made astounding discoveries about the physiology of the brain, in particular the chemicals that affect mood and behavior. No longer is it generally accepted that, if you could only stop hating your mother or learn to love yourself even though you flunked out of college, you would cure your depression or reduce your anxiety. It's now understood that these and more serious mental disorders as diverse as panic attacks, bulimia and dissociative disorders can be treated by addressing a chemical imbalance in your brain.

Sophisticated technology has made it possible to see actual chemical changes taking place in the brain during a panic attack. And we now know the brain isn't really much like a computer; it's more like the hurly-burly floor of the stock exchange, with neurons shooting electrochemical messages to each other hither and yon. Scientists have established that psychotropic drugs work by affecting either the chemistry of these messages (the neurotransmitters) or the sites where the messages are received (the receptors).

The earliest psychotropic drugs arrived on the scene when very little was known about the brain; their discovery was as much accident as design. The first antidepressant, for example, was stumbled upon back in the '50s when doctors noticed that tuberculosis patients treated with the drug iproniazid became inexplicably cheerful. Someone shrewdly deduced that their exuberance might be drug-related, and that launched the use of one of the first mood elevators, the monoamine oxidase inhibitors.

These were followed by a larger group of antidepressants known as the tricyclates—drugs like Elavil and Tofranil—which, while effective in relieving depression, had a variety of unpleasant side effects ranging from dry mouth to constipation. The latest antidepressants, a group of drugs called SRIs (serotonin re-uptake inhibitors is the pharmacological jargon) are cousins to the tricyclates. They produce fewer side effects, however, because they act on fewer chemical systems. As many as 30 percent of the patients who did not respond to the older drugs—or wouldn't take them—seem to benefit from these second-generation antidepressants.

The warning signs of depression

How do you know whether you're a candidate for antidepressant medication? Ask yourself: Do I feel sad, blue, hopeless, down in the dumps or irritable, and am I getting less pleasure from the things I normally enjoy? If the answer is yes, then look at whether you have had any four of the following symptoms for at least two weeks:

1. Poor appetite and weight loss or increased appetite and weight gain.
2. Sleep disturbance, especially early-morning wakefulness.
3. Thoughts and actions slowed down or speeded up.
4. Loss of interest in normal activities and decreased sex drive.
5. Loss of energy; fatigue.
6. Diminished ability to think and concentrate; difficulty making decisions.
7. Feelings of worthlessness, self-reproach or inappropriate guilt.

These symptoms of biological or clinical depression often happen to people who have no reason to be depressed, yet they find they just aren't enjoying life like they once did and they are physically pooped. If this describes how you're feeling, you might want to visit one of the clinics listed in this chapter for an evaluation.

The warning signs of anxiety

There are three major categories of anxiety disorders. First are the phobias, such as fear of flying, fear of cats, fear of closed spaces, etc. Phobias do not respond particularly well to drugs. Second are panic disorders, the sudden onset of explosive, overwhelming feelings of terror, as if the body's alarm system is ringing for no apparent reason. The third and largest group is generalized anxiety. Someone with this condition can be treated with tranquilizers in concert with therapy; consider getting medical advice if three of the four following symptoms persist for at least one month:

Motor tension: shakiness, tension, aching muscles, inability to relax, jumpiness, fatigue.

Uncontrollable body sensations: sweating, heart pounding, clammy hands, dry mouth, dizziness, light-headedness, hot and cold flashes, upset stomach, lump in the throat, diarrhea, pallor or flushed face.

Apprehensive expectation: fear, worry, rumination, anticipation of misfortune to self or others.

Vigilance and scanning: constant hyperattention that makes it difficult to concentrate and leads to irritability, impatience, insomnia and always feeling on edge.

While not as easily treated as depression, anxiety disorders are significantly improved by drugs and/or psychotherapy 75 percent of the time. The Center for Psychotherapy Research (215-662-7993) at the University of Pennsylvania has low-cost programs with experienced therapists for people prone to worry.

If You Need Help

Memory Institute
1015 CHESTNUT STREET, ROOM 1303, PHILADELPHIA; 215-923-2583

Multisite research and treatment center that evaluates promising new medications for Alzheimer's disease. Free memory screenings and treatment programs are available to qualified individuals.

The University of Pennsylvania Mood and Anxiety Disorders Unit
UNIVERSITY SCIENCE CENTER, 3600 MARKET STREET, SUITE 872, PHILADELPHIA; 215-898-4301

This outpatient clinic provides free evaluation and treatment in a variety of research programs designed to help patients suffering from panic and other anxiety disorders, as well as depression and social phobia. Both standard and investigational medications, some not yet otherwise available in the United States, are used in treatment. The clinic also sponsors research programs designed to help persons who are physically dependent on tranquilizers such as Xanax, Ativan and Valium to stop using them.

Freedom From Depression
DEPRESSION RESEARCH UNIT, UNIVERSITY OF PENNSYLVANIA MEDICAL CENTER, 3600 MARKET STREET, 8TH FLOOR, PHILADELPHIA; 215-662-3462

This clinic is devoted to the treatment and investigation of biological depression. Each patient goes through a thorough psychiatric and medical evaluation, and those not considered appropriate are referred elsewhere. Treatment may combine antidepressant medication with supportive psychotherapy. If patients qualify for the research study, the evaluation is free.

Center for Cognitive Therapy
UNIVERSITY OF PENNSYLVANIA HEALTH SYSTEM,
3600 MARKET STREET, 7TH FLOOR, PHILADELPHIA;
215-898-4100

This program uses the behavioral concepts pioneered by Dr. Aaron Beck, which are based on the premise that anxiety and depression come from distorted ways of thinking. The therapy seldom uses drugs, relying instead on teaching how to recognize distorted thinking and change it. It has an excellent reputation and a high success rate. The sliding-scale fee is based on income.

Mood and Anxiety Disorders Program
ALLEGHENY UNIVERSITY HOSPITALS, EAST FALLS/EPPI,
3200 HENRY AVENUE, PHILADELPHIA; 215-842-4242

This program offers comprehensive clinical outpatient treatment programs for individuals having problems with depression, anxiety, anger, aggression and shyness. Treatment options include individual/group psychotherapy, cognitive/behavioral therapy and medication therapy. The sliding-scale fee is based on income. Treatment associated with participation in sponsored clinical research programs is provided at no cost to eligible individuals.

The Belmont Center for Comprehensive Treatment
4200 MONUMENT ROAD, PHILADELPHIA; 215-877-2000

Belmont provides outpatient and day-program treatment of depression and anxiety-based disorders, including panic disorder and obsessive-compulsive disorders. Special programs are available for women and the deaf. The anxiety and affective disorders inpatient unit provides intensive biological, psychological and social treatment of mood and anxiety disorders. Fees may be covered by insurance. The Belmont Center for Comprehensive Treatment is a member of the Albert Einstein Healthcare Network.

Mood Disorders Program
THE INSTITUTE OF PENNSYLVANIA HOSPITAL,
111 NORTH 49TH STREET, PHILADELPHIA; 215-471-2542

This program specializes in the treatment of mood disorders such as major depression, manic depressive or bipolar disorder, seasonal affective disorder, postpartum depression and chronic "blues." Institute clinicians specialize in working with patients who have not responded to medications, are experiencing recurrent depression or who have complex coexisting conditions, such as addiction and anxiety. A combination of therapies is used to help patients recover from painful symptoms and better cope with the challenges of daily living.

Child and Adolescent Anxiety Disorders Clinic
Temple University, Weiss Hall, 13th Street and Cecil B. Moore Avenue, Philadelphia; 215-204-7165

For children 9 to 13 whose anxiety interferes with daily functioning. Children acquire and practice behavioral skills in 16 to 20 individual sessions. Treatment is free.

Just What the Doctor Ordered

The following chart contains information about the most commonly prescribed psychotropic drugs. Before beginning any kind of drug therapy for a psychological problem, always discuss with your doctor your complete medical history, any other medication you're taking, risks if you're pregnant or nursing, and the interactive effects of alcohol with your prescription. A variety of side effects other than those noted may occur in vulnerable individuals, so you should carefully discuss your health profile with your psychiatrist.

Anxiety

Chemical Name: alprazolam
Brand Name: Xanax
Used For: Generalized anxiety disorder. Panic disorder.
Do Not Use If: You have a history of alcohol abuse or other misuse of addictive drugs. Be sure to tell your doctor if you have ever had any allergic reactions to medication, or if you have liver, kidney or lung disease or a history of seizures.
How Long Until It Works: Some relief within an hour. A week for patients with generalized anxiety disorder. Two to four weeks for patients with panic disorder.
Common Side Effects: Drowsiness. Gastrointestinal disorders. Heightens effect of alcohol. Bitter taste in mouth, dry mouth or excessive salivation. Headache. Nausea. Nervousness. Excessive sweating. Withdrawal symptoms, especially if stopped abruptly.

Chemical Name: buspirone
Brand Name: BuSpar
Used For: Generalized anxiety disorder.
Do Not Use If: You are taking a monoamine oxidase inhibitor (MAOI) or any other medication that would cause oversedation.
How Long Until It Works: About four weeks.
Common Side Effects: Nausea. Headache. Dizziness. Nervousness. Weakness.

Chemical Name: diazepam
Brand Name: Valium

Used For: Generalized anxiety disorder. Sometimes to treat muscle spasms.
Do Not Use If: You have a history of alcohol abuse or other misuse of addictive drugs. Be sure to tell your doctor if you have ever had any allergic reactions to medication, or if you have liver, kidney or lung disease or a history of seizures.
How Long Until It Works: 30 minutes to an hour. Substantial improvement within a week.
Common Side Effects: Drowsiness. Dizziness. Heightens the effect of alcohol. Gastrointestinal disorders. Withdrawal symptoms, especially if stopped abruptly.

Chemical Name: lorazepam
Brand Name: Ativan

Used For: Generalized anxiety disorder. Also, for calming agitated patients with mania or schizophrenia.
Do Not Use If: You have a history of alcohol abuse or other misuse of addictive drugs, or if you are taking any other medication that might cause oversedation.
How Long Until It Works: Some relief in about an hour. Much improvement within a week.
Common Side Effects: Bitter taste in mouth, dry mouth or excessive salivation. Drowsiness. Loss of appetite. Nausea, sweating or vomiting. Heightens the effects of alcohol. Withdrawal symptoms, especially if stopped abruptly.

Attention Deficit/Hyperactivity Disorder

Chemical Name: methylphenidate
Brand Name: Ritalin

Used For: Commonly used to treat children with attention deficit/hyperactivity disorder, it is increasingly being prescribed for adults as well.
Do Not Use If: You are taking an MAO inhibitor, hypertension medication, oral anticoagulants or anticonvulsants.
How Long Until It Works: Two to three weeks.
Common Side Effects: Restlessness. Mild dry mouth. Headache. Insomnia. This drug is related to amphetamines and may occasionally be habit-forming.

Bipolar Disorder (Manic Depression)

Chemical Name: lithium
Brand Names: Lithonate, Lithane, Eskalith

Used For: Acute and long-term treatment of bipolar affective disorder. Helps prevent extreme highs and lows.
Do Not Use If: You have kidney disease; you are taking diuretics for high blood pressure; you use anti-inflammatory drugs like Motrin.

How Long Until It Works: Hard to pinpoint. Usually the doctor observes the patient over a period of time for signs of lessened mood swings.
Common Side Effects: Gastrointestinal disorders. Metallic taste in mouth. Increased frequency of urination and increased thirst. Weakness. Drowsiness. Weight gain and bloating. Acne. Trembling of hands.

Chemical Name: valproate
Brand Names: Depakote

Used For: Acute and long-term treatment of bipolar disorder. Helps stabilize swings.
Do Not Use If: You have severe liver disease, history of problems with bone marrow, or history of allergy to valproate.
How Long Until It Works: Ten to 14 days in acute settings. May take months to determine if it helps to prevent or minimize recurrence of episodes of depression or mania.
Common Side Effects: Nausea. Sedation. Weight gain. Unsteadiness. Blurred vision. Low platelet count (rare). Liver damage (rare).

Depression

Chemical Name: amitriptyline
Brand Names: Elavil, Endep, others

Used For: Major depression.
Do Not Use If: You have a history of seizures, glaucoma, cardiovascular disorders, drug or alcohol abuse and/or are taking thyroid medication or an MAO inhibitor.
How Long Until It Works: Two to six weeks.
Common Side Effects: Dry mouth. Gastrointestinal disorders. Blurry vision. Difficulty urinating. Increased sensitivity to the sun. Dizziness when standing up quickly. Weight gain. Sleepiness. Increased sweating.

Chemical Name: doxepin
Brand Names: Adapin, Sinequan, others

Used For: Major depression.
Do Not Use If: You have a history of glaucoma, an enlarged prostate or cardiovascular disorders.
How Long Until It Works: Two to six weeks.
Common Side Effects: Dry mouth. Constipation. Blurry vision. Difficulty urinating. Increased sun sensitivity. Dizziness after standing quickly. Weight gain. Sleepiness. Increased sweating.

Chemical Name: fluoxetine
Brand Name: Prozac

Used For: Depression and several anxiety disorders, PMS.
Do Not Use If: You have severe insomnia or you are dangerously underweight.
How Long Until It Works: Two to four weeks.

Common Side Effects: Loss of appetite. Insomnia. Nausea, diarrhea or stomach cramps. Headaches. Nervousness. Sexual dysfunction.

Chemical Name: imipramine
Brand Names: Tofranil, Janimine, others
Used For: Major depression. Also, some anxiety disorders.
Do Not Use If: You have a history of glaucoma, an enlarged prostate or cardiovascular disorders.
How Long Until It Works: Two to six weeks.
Common Side Effects: Dry mouth. Constipation. Blurry vision. Difficulty urinating. Increased sensitivity to the sun. Dizziness after standing up quickly. Weight gain. Increased sweating. Drowsiness.

Chemical Name: nefazodone
Brand Names: Serzone
Used For: Major depression.
Do Not Use If: You are taking an MAO inhibitor, Seldane, Hismanol or concurrently with Xanax (alprazolam) or Halcion.
How Long Until It Works: Two to six weeks.
Common Side Effects: Sedation. Dizziness. Drop in blood pressure. Nausea. Headaches. Constipation.

Chemical Name: nortriptyline
Brand Names: Aventyl, Pamelor
Used For: Major depression.
Do Not Use If: You have narrow-angle glaucoma, an enlarged prostate or certain heart-rhythm irregularities.
How Long Until It Works: Two to six weeks.
Common Side Effects: Anxiety. Blurred vision. Dry mouth. Difficulty urinating. Gastrointestinal disorders. Sweating. Weakness. Weight gain or loss. Increased sensitivity to the sun.

Chemical Name: paroxetine
Brand Name: Paxil
Used For: Depression.
Do Not Use If: You have severe insomnia or you are dangerously underweight.
How Long Until It Works: Two to four weeks.
Common Side Effects: Weakness, sweating, nausea, decreased appetite, dizziness, insomnia, nervousness. Sexual dysfunction.

Chemical Name: sertraline
Brand Name: Zoloft
Used For: Depression.

Do Not Use If: You have severe insomnia or you are dangerously underweight.
How Long Until It Works: Two to four weeks.
Common Side Effects: Gastrointestinal disorders. Dizziness. Insomnia. Headache. Sweating. Dry mouth. Sexual dysfunction.

Chemical Name: venlafexine
Brand Name: Effexor

Used For: Depression.
Do Not Use If: You are taking an MAO inhibitor or other antidepressant; if you have a history of high blood pressure, discuss first with your doctor.
How Long Until It Works: Two to four weeks.
Common Side Effects: Increased blood pressure. Nausea. Headache. Insomnia.

Schizophrenia

Chemical Name: clozapine
Brand Name: Clozarile

Used For: Severely ill schizophrenic patients who fail to show an acceptable response to standard antipsychotic drugs.
Do Not Use If: You cannot comply with the need to have weekly blood counts.
How Long Until It Works: Two to four weeks.
Common Side Effects: Sedation. Increased salivation. Rapid heart rate. Dizziness caused by lowered blood pressure. Nausea and vomiting. Constipation. Dry mouth.

Chemical Name: fluphenazine
Brand Names: Permitil, Prolixin

Used For: Psychosis associated with schizophrenia, mania, severe behavioral problems.
Do Not Use If: Use carefully if you have a history of seizures.
How Long Until It Works: Two weeks.
Common Side Effects: Blurred vision. Dizziness. Fatigue. Gastrointestinal disorders. Dry mouth. Jitteriness. Weight gain.

Chemical Name: haloperidol
Brand Name: Haldol

Used For: Psychosis associated with schizophrenia, mania or depression.
Do Not Use If: You have a history of seizures.
How Long Until It Works: Two to four weeks.
Common Side Effects: Muscle stiffness. Tremors. Jumpiness. Weight gain.

Chemical Name: risperidone
Brand Name: Risperdal

Used For: Psychotic symptoms associated with schizophrenia, mania or depression.
Do Not Use If: You are hypersensitive to similar drugs.

How Long Until It Works: Two to three weeks.
Common Side Effects: Blurred vision. Muscle stiffness. Fatigue. Jitteriness. Sedation.

Chemical Name: thioridazine
Brand Name: Mellaril, Millazine, others

Used For: Psychosis associated with schizophrenia, mania and severe behavioral problems.
Do Not Use If: You are taking any other drugs that may cause oversedation.
How Long Until It Works: Two weeks.
Common Side Effects: Blurred vision. Gastrointestinal disorders. Dizziness. Drowsiness. Restlessness. Weight gain.

Chemical Name: trifluoperazine
Brand Name: Stelazine

Used For: Psychosis associated with schizophrenia, mania or depression.
Do Not Use If: You are taking any other drugs that may cause oversedation.
How Long Until It Works: The patient will probably become calmer and somewhat less violent after a few doses, but complete relief may take up to four weeks.
Common Side Effects: Sedation. Low blood pressure and dizziness. Dry mouth. Constipation. Difficulty urinating. Blurry vision. Muscle stiffness. Weight gain. Increased sensitivity to the sun.

CHAPTER 18

Where to Go for Help

Sometimes, the doctor's office isn't enough

When emotional problems require more attention than regular visits to a therapist's office, it may be necessary to head to a hospital for inpatient or daily outpatient care. As these listings show, there are treatment programs tailored to every kind of psychological disturbance, from stress to incest to obsessive-compulsive disorders to schizophrenia. Some psychiatric hospitals also treat mental retardation. In addition to the specialty facilities listed in this section, check Chapter 8 for those local hospitals that have psychiatric departments offering both in- and outpatient care.

Psychiatric Facilities

Belmont Center for Comprehensive Treatment

4200 MONUMENT ROAD, PHILADELPHIA; 215-877-2000, 215-456-8000 (*program information*), 215-581-3774 (*admission*), 1-800-220-HELP (*referrals*). DOCTORS ON ACTIVE STAFF: 209 (*82% board-certified*). NUMBER OF BEDS: 147. RNs PER BED: 2.3. ACCREDITATION: JCAHO, NATIONAL ASSOCIATION OF PSYCHIATRIC HEALTH SYSTEMS.

Emergency room services: access to psychiatric emergency at Albert Einstein Medical Center.
Special treatment units: inpatient, outpatient and partial hospitalization treatment programs for adolescents, adults and older adults for alcohol, chemical and gambling addictions; dual diagnosis for adolescents and adults; anxiety/affective disorders; adolescent treatment program; eating disorders program; step-down unit; Belmont House for Eating Disorders (residential facility); Woodside Hall Addictions

Treatment Program; CAREER Intensive Outpatient Addictions Program; Entry Point crisis intervention, triage and evaluation service.
Physical rehab services: physical medicine and rehab.

Belmont Center for Comprehensive Treatment, a core provider of Belmont Behavioral Health, is a private nonprofit psychiatric hospital and a part of Albert Einstein Healthcare Network.

The Charter Fairmount Institute

561 FAIRTHORNE AVENUE, PHILADELPHIA; 215-487-4000. STAFF COMPOSED OF MULTIDISCIPLINARY TEAM, INCLUDING PSYCHIATRISTS, PSYCHIATRIC NURSES, PSYCHOLOGISTS, ALLIED THERAPISTS AND SOCIAL WORKERS; NUMBER OF BEDS: 169; ACCREDITATION: JCAHO; LICENSED BY DPW AND ODAP; ACCEPTS MOST INSURANCE.

Specialized treatment programs: geriatric unit, child and adolescent programs (ages 5-18) including substance-abuse services and a school program, adult dual-diagnosis, adult special-care program (ages 18 and older) for those suffering from acute psychiatric disorders. Charter also specializes in the treatment of eating disorders and Tourette's syndrome.
Outpatient health and wellness: partial hospitalization day treatment.

Charter Fairmount, established in 1926, provides a variety of therapy programs, including recreational, music, art, family therapy and other ancillary services.

Eastern Pennsylvania Psychiatric Institute (EPPI)

3300 HENRY AVENUE, PHILADELPHIA; 215-842-4100. STAFF COMPOSED OF: 44 PSYCHIATRISTS (95% *board-certified*), 19 PSYCHOLOGISTS AND 15 SOCIAL WORKERS. NUMBER OF BEDS: 117. RNs PER BED: 2.29. ACCREDITATION: JCAHO.

Specialized psychiatry treatment programs: Behavioral Therapy Clinic; Center for the Treatment and Study of Anxiety, Child and Adolescent Depression Clinic; Child and Adolescent Psychiatry Outpatient Clinic and Inpatient Services; Crime Victims Program; Family/Couples Therapy Clinic; Family Coping Skills Workshop; Group Psychotherapy Clinic; Marital and Family Therapy Clinic; Mood, Anxiety and Personality Disorders Clinic; Preschool and School-Age Partial Hospitalization Program; a therapeutic nursery for preschoolers with neurodevelopmental delays; Psychiatric Consultation-Liaison Service; Psychotherapy Clinic; Schizophrenia Diagnostic Center; psychiatric emergency service for the clients of community mental-health centers throughout Northeast and Northwest Philadelphia. In addition, EPPI maintains general psychiatric units; an affective disorders unit, which treats patients with severe mood disturbances; psychiatric step-down units; a neuropsychiatric unit; a children's/adolescent unit; and a dual-diagnosis unit for treatment of mental health and substance abuse.

EPPI is the psychiatric arm of Allegheny University Hospitals. It houses several psychiatric units, the Sleep Disorders Center, the Mid-Atlantic Regional Epilepsy Center, the CIBA-Geigy Research Unit and the Pediatric Neurodevelopmental Program.

Friends Hospital

4641 ROOSEVELT BOULEVARD, PHILADELPHIA; 215-831-4600, 215-831-4870 (*for general information or referral, Monday to Friday 8:30-4:30*). STAFF COMPOSED OF 35 PSYCHIATRISTS (*90% board-certified*), 6 LICENSED PSYCHOLOGISTS, 15 REHABILITATIVE THERAPISTS AND 13 SOCIAL WORKERS. NUMBER OF BEDS: 192. RNS PER BED: .4. ACCREDITATION AND LICENSING: JCAHO, DPW, ODAP.

Specialized treatment programs: Young People's Unit (treating 13- to 21-year-olds with emotional, behavioral or psychiatric problems); Adolescent Dual-Diagnosis Program (treating young people with addiction and psychiatric diagnoses); The Sanctuary (an inpatient program for adult trauma survivors); The Eating Disorders Program (for male and female adolescents and adults); partial hospital programs (see outpatient); the Greystone Program (residential services); pain/stress management; Addictions Recovery Program; Geropsychiatry Service (for those with issues related to aging, loss or illnesses); horticultural, recreational, expressive, vocational and occupational therapy.

Outpatient programs: Partial hospital programs including the Day Program (for adults), The Garden (for older adults), Friends Recovery Center (intensive addictions recovery) and outpatient child and adolescent psychiatry. Additional outpatient treatment available in Abington, Philadelphia, Lower Bucks County and Bala Cynwyd.

Founded in 1813, Friends was the first private, not-for-profit psychiatric hospital in the country. Located on a beautifully landscaped 100-acre site, it offers a full range of in- and outpatient services for people of all ages. Friends Hospital is a Quaker hospital, with services available to all, regardless of race, religion or sexual preference.

Hampton Hospital

650 RANCOCAS ROAD, WESTAMPTON, N.J.; 609-267-7000, 1-800-345-7345 (*24-hour referral and assessment*). STAFF COMPOSED OF BOARD-CERTIFIED PSYCHIATRISTS AND CONSULTING PSYCHOLOGISTS. NUMBER OF BEDS: 100. RNs PER BED: 1.7. 1 SOCIAL WORKER FOR EVERY 8 PATIENTS. ACCEPTS MOST MAJOR INSURANCE, HMOs, MEDICARE AND MEDICAID. CHAMPUS APPROVED. ACCREDITATION: JCAHO.

A private psychiatric hospital offering a continuum of care. Patients may be admitted to the following inpatient programs: Adolescent, Adult, Dual-Diagnosis (for individuals with a primary psychiatric diagnosis and a substance-abuse problem), and Older Adult (which has both Affective Disorders and Dementia tracks). Outpatient services include day and evening sessions of intensive outpatient programs for adolescents and adults, partial hospitalization programs to adolescents and adults, short-term therapy and medication management. In addition, Hampton Academy, located in Mt. Holly, N.J., is a private day school for emotionally disturbed students and is accessible with a referral from a student's resident school district.

The Horsham Clinic

722 EAST BUTLER PIKE, AMBLER; 215-643-7800, 1-800-237-4447 (*24-hour assessment and referral center*). STAFF COMPOSED OF 24 PSYCHIATRISTS (*100% board-certified/board-eligible*), 11 PSYCHOLOGISTS, 23 SOCIAL WORKERS. NUMBER OF BEDS: 146. RNs PER BED: .55. ACCREDITATION: JCAHO; ACCEPTS MOST INSURANCE.

Specialized adult and older adult services: Short-Term Assessment Program (STAT)—adult intensive services that enable the patient to move down to the next level of care in as little as 23 hours; adult general psychiatric program, adult dual diagnosis program for patients with both a psychiatric illness and a substance abuse issue (includes medical detoxification for those who require such treatment); older adult inpatient program—a highly structured, comprehensive program designed to assist older adults in returning to a state of mental and physical well-being.
Specialized adolescent and children's services: Adolescent inpatient program for young adolescents (ages 11-13) and adolescents (ages 14-18) provides services that enable the teen to develop tools to manage issues that interfere with healthy functioning. Children's inpatient program (ages 4-10) assists children in acquiring skills, self-esteem and confidence to interact with peers, parents and school. Both programs are intensive-structured and include group and family therapy and daily academic tutorial services.
Partial hospital programs: Separate programs for various age groups are held daily as an alternative to inpatient treatment or as a transition from inpatient to

outpatient. Programs are held at various locations in Montgomery, Delaware and Philadelphia counties.

The Horsham Clinic is a private psychiatric hospital in a rural campus setting serving the greater Delaware Valley and New Jersey.

The Institute of Pennsylvania Hospital

111 NORTH 49TH ST., PHILADELPHIA, 215-471-2000. STAFF COMPOSED OF 260 LICENSED PSYCHIATRISTS, PLUS PSYCHOLOGISTS, PSYCHIATRIC NURSES, SOCIAL WORKERS AND ADDICTION COUNSELORS. NUMBER OF BEDS: 234. RNS PER STAFFED BED: .45. ROOM COST: $1,125. ACCREDITATION: JCAHO, ACGME, DPW, ODAP.

Emergency room service: access to psychiatric emergency at Pennsylvania Hospital.

Specialized treatment programs (in- and outpatient): substance-abuse treatment, including dual-diagnosis care; evaluation services; anxiety, eating, mood and dissociative disorders; adolescent, adult and geriatric psychiatry; Kirkbride Program (a supported-living program); Mill Creek School (a licensed high school for inpatients and day students); women's mental health program.

Outpatient health and wellness programs: speaker's bureau; outpatient clinic (child, adult and couples therapy offered on a sliding-fee scale); outpatient psychotherapy and pharmacotherapy; consultations; intensive partial hospitalization and day programs. The Hall-Mercer Community Mental Health and Mental Retardation Center provides community-based mental health services. The Counseling Program specializes in employee assistance programs and other services with managed care organizations. (See Pennsylvania Hospital listing, Chapter 8.)

The Institute of Pennsylvania Hospital was opened in 1841 to offer expanded, humane services to mentally ill patients of Pennsylvania Hospital, the nation's first hospital. Today, The Institute is a private, nonprofit facility serving adolescents and adults on a short- and long-term basis.

Malvern Institute

940 KING RD., MALVERN; 610-647-0330. NUMBER OF BEDS: 40. ACCREDITATION: JCAHO, PA DEPT. OF HEALTH, ODAP.

Malvern Institute is a comprehensive addiction treatment center that provides detoxification, rehabilitation and dual-diagnosis treatment to chemically dependent individuals in an inpatient or partial hospitalization setting; offers a drug and alcohol residential program and a residential program for adults with acute psychiatric disorders.

Mount Sinai Hospital

4TH AND REED STREETS., PHILADELPHIA; 215-339-3456. DOCTORS ON ACTIVE STAFF: 36 (*70% board-certified*). NUMBER OF BEDS: 220. ACCREDITATION: JCAHO, CAP.

Inpatient programs for adolescents, adults and older adults; partial hospital programs for adults and older adults; and subacute psychiatric program. Outpatient mental health services available. Also offers adult substance-abuse rehab program, detox unit, outpatient substance-abuse programs and services for the dual-diagnosed. Mt. Sinai is part of The Graduate Health System.

Northwestern Institute

450 BETHLEHEM PIKE, P.O. BOX 209, FORT WASHINGTON; 215-641-5300, 1-800-344-NWIP. OF PSYCHIATRISTS ON STAFF, 90% ARE BOARD-CERTIFIED. NUMBER OF BEDS: 146. ACCREDITATION: JCAHO.

Northwestern Institute is a private psychiatric hospital that provides acute inpatient treatment for children, adolescents, adults and older adults. Northwestern also offers specialty programs to treat women, dissociative disorders and dual diagnosis (mental health and addictions).

Philadelphia Child Guidance Center

34TH STREET AND CIVIC CENTER BOULEVARD., PHILADELPHIA; 215-243-2700 (*evening crisis hotline: 215-243-2888*). STAFF COMPOSED OF CHILD AND ADOLESCENT PSYCHIATRISTS, PSYCHOLOGISTS AND SOCIAL WORKERS. NUMBER OF BEDS: 38. RNs PER BED: .33. ACCREDITATION: JCAHO.

Specialized treatment programs: day treatment program on Main Campus and in Cherry Hill, N.J.; two residential apartment units for families undergoing intensive inpatient treatment.
Outpatient programs: assessment; individual, group and family therapy; medication clinic; intensive family/home-based program; therapeutic preschool program; drug and alcohol treatment; therapeutic foster homes.

The Philadelphia Child Guidance Center, a comprehensive mental health organization serving children and adolescents with emotional/behavioral problems and their families, is internationally known for expertise in family therapy, eating disorders and psychosomatic illness. It is a teaching hospital affiliated with the University of Pennsylvania School of Medicine and Children's Hospital of Philadelphia. Outpatient offices in Voorhees, N.J., and Doylestown, Pa. Evening and weekend appointments available.

Progressions Health Systems
Behavioral Health Centers

450 BETHLEHEM PIKE, P.O. BOX 209, FORT WASHINGTON; 1-800-344-NWIP.

Outpatient and partial hospital programs are offered throughout eastern Pennsylvania and New Jersey for acute psychiatric treatment at a less restrictive level of care than in an inpatient setting: Fort Washington and Pottstown in Montgomery County; Reading in Berks County; Allentown in Lehigh County; Media in Delaware County; Cherry Hill in Camden County, N.J.; and North Brunswick in Middlesex County, N.J. Specialty programs are offered for specific groups of people, such as Latinos, older adults and women.

The A. I. duPont Institute Children's Hospital

Jump on Board
KidsHealth.org
Get on track with your child's health.

If you're looking on-line for kids' health information, log on at http://KidsHealth.org. Put your kids on track toward better health.

At KidsHealth.org, kids can learn about their bodies, their feelings and more. For parents, the site offers valuable information on subjects from nutrition to immunizations to surgery. The award-winning site is written by leading pediatric health experts — use it as a resource you can trust.

Kids Vote
"[√] I Agree [√] I Disagree"

Nemours Guide to Children's Health Care Media
"Where can I find a great video on asthma?"

Win a Free T-Shirt!
Do you have a health tip you'd like to share? If so, be sure to click on the **Health Tip of the Day** page on our site. If you give us a tip we think people can use, we'll put it on-line where the whole world can see it. And we'll send you a brand new KidsHealth T-shirt—as our way of saying thanks!

http://KidsHealth.org
Where parents & kids go for reliable health information.

Alfred I. duPont Institute
of THE NEMOURS FOUNDATION
A CHILDREN'S HOSPITAL

The Nemours Foundation operates the Alfred I. duPont Institute Children's Hospital. A hospital only for children.
1600 Rockland Road, Wilmington, Delaware 19803

1-800-829-KIDS

Section

Making Sense for Seniors

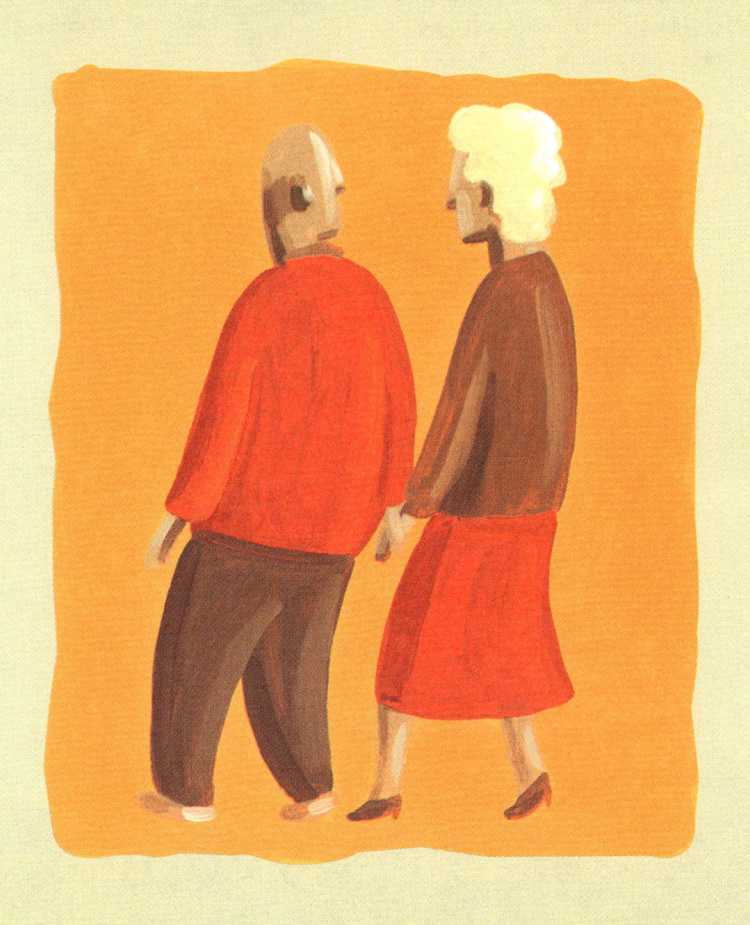

Eight

Chapter 19
   The Dosage Dilemma
   How to keep your medications straight

Chapter 20
   The Lowdown on Life-Care
   A guide to continuing care

CHAPTER 19

The Dosage Dilemma

For seniors, managing prescriptions can be a matter of life and death

We may not like to think about it, but with advancing age comes an increased chance of developing chronic illnesses like heart disease, arthritis, glaucoma, diabetes and cancer. So, as we grow older, it's a safe bet that the number of medicines we must take will begin to mount. Deal with a "simple" case of high blood pressure, and you might need to take one or two pills a day. Throw in a few more conditions and the volume of medicines can become truly staggering. It's not unusual for older adults to have to juggle more than 25 medications daily. Doing this is a formidable task—even for the young and healthy.

Medicines are potent chemicals. Using them properly isn't just a matter of getting effective medical therapy—make a mistake and your life could be in jeopardy. Experts say dangerous drug reactions, interactions and other problems associated with medication use result in hundreds of thousands of avoidable hospitalizations, including some deaths, each year. According to Dr. Lesley Carson, assistant professor of medicine in the division of geriatric medicine at Allegheny University of the Health Sciences, illnesses and deaths related to medications are probably underestimated since identification of a precise cause isn't always possible.

Some medication-related problems stem from the user. The patient may not comprehend how to use the medicine correctly or may be deliberately noncompliant due to concerns about cost or troublesome side effects. Add self-medication with a plethora of seemingly harmless over-the-counter drugs, and you've got the potential for a deadly chemical stew. In other cases, adverse drug interactions can occur when two or more physicians prescribe without knowing all the other drugs a patient is taking. And in still other instances, the problem is strictly physiological: As we age, our ability to effectively excrete these powerful medicines declines, leading to an increased risk of side effects and toxic reactions. Fortunately, physicians like Carson offer a number of suggestions to help us make sure we're getting optimal benefit from our medications and are using them safely.

Carson advises patients to make sure their prescriber knows their medication allergies, before he or she begins to write up a prescription. Also, she says, present the prescriber with an up-to-date list of every prescription and over-the-counter medication you take. (It's a good idea to keep a copy of this list with you at all times in the event of an emergency.) These two simple steps, says Carson, will help you work with your physician to prevent dangerous drug reactions and interactions.

The learning curve

There is much more we can do, however. When a new medication is prescribed, learn as much as you can about it from your physician or pharmacist. While you won't need to know any complex chemical formulas, it will help to have some basic information about the drug.

Make sure you understand what the drug is for; later, write this directly on the label: "for diabetes," "for blood pressure," and so on, says Dr. Christine Arenson, clinical assistant professor of family medicine at Jefferson Medical College of Thomas Jefferson University. This is perhaps the most important bit of knowledge you can have about your medications. During an emergency, you are more likely to recall that you are on diabetes medication than the actual name of that medication.

It is also helpful to have a fundamental understanding of how the medication works, says Arenson. For example, digoxin, also known as Lanoxin, increases the heart's ability to contract, giving each beat greater pumping efficiency. Be familiar with the amount of each dose—most often expressed in milligrams, micrograms, milliequivalents or units—and how often it should be taken: daily, every other day, or whatever. If the medication is to be taken four times a day, does that mean every six hours, or may it be taken on a more convenient schedule, such as with meals and at bedtime?

Arenson also advises patients to ask if the drug requires any special monitoring or follow-up. Some drugs, like Dilantin, a commonly prescribed anti-seizure medicine, and digoxin, for example, have narrow therapeutic ranges, and can easily reach toxic levels in the bloodstream. So, at least during the initial period of therapy, frequent blood studies should be ordered to help assess the correct dosage for each patient. Other drugs, such as anti-cancer drugs, can alter blood components, and require regular blood work throughout the course of therapy.

And, Arenson adds, if your new medication is an oral one, ask whether it should be taken on a full or empty stomach. Food intake may influence your ability to absorb the medication or tolerate therapy. For example, NSAIDs, a broad category of drugs commonly used to control the inflammation and pain of arthritis, can cause stomach upset and even gastrointestinal bleeding, especially if taken without the buffering effects of food.

Find out if this is a drug you will be taking "for life," as most medications to control chronic illnesses are, or if the therapy will be time-limited, as is usually the case with antibiotics. Some drugs, such as pain medications, are to be taken only on an "as-needed" basis.

While you're at it, recommends Arenson, find out if you'll need to avoid alcohol or any other drugs, what to do if you miss a dose, and if there are any dangerous side effects that should prompt an immediate call to your physician. Often, your doctor or pharmacist will be able to give you all of this general information in a concise patient education handout.

If your new medication is not in capsule or tablet form, you'll need to learn the correct way to apply topical ointments, measure liquids, use an inhaler or instill eye, ear or nose drops. Also, some heart and blood pressure medications are most safely used when the patient self-monitors his pulse or blood pressure. It may be possible for you or a helper to learn these relatively simple skills. Ask your doctor or nurse-practitioner if this would be beneficial for you.

Jeffrey A. Bourret, R.Ph., FASHP, director of pharmacy services at the University of Pennsylvania Medical Center, recommends that patients use one pharmacy for all their prescription needs. This way, you'll be putting your pharmacist to work for you, says Bourret. He or she can maintain one comprehensive record of all the medications you take and can act as the first line of defense against inappropriate prescriptions and potentially dangerous drug interactions.

Does all this seem like a lot of work? It is, but it's worth it. If you stop taking your antibiotics when you begin to feel better, you'll be inviting a relapse of your infection; skip a few doses of your high blood pressure medication and you risk a disabling stroke. Pop a Motrin for a headache while on Coumadin therapy (both are blood thinners) and you may wind up with dangerous internal bleeding.

But wait, your work isn't done quite yet. Once you get your new prescription home, take a good look at it to become familiar with its color and shape. And at some point, suggests Bourret, try to learn to identify your new medication by both of its names. Every drug has both a generic name and a trade name, which can lead to some confusion—even among health professionals. For example, Dilantin is also known as phenytoin—its generic name. Knowing both names will help you avoid double-dosing yourself by inadvertently filling two prescriptions. Bourret says this happens with alarming frequency, especially when multiple prescribers are treating the patient and are unaware of his or her current medications.

Finally, says Bourret, update that all-important medication list, because an out-of-date list is almost as useless as no list at all. Keep it in a prominent place in your home so that it can be found in an emergency, and be sure to review it regularly. When you go to the doctor or emergency department, remember to take your medication list with you.

Fill 'er up

If you are on long-term therapy, don't wait until the last minute to have your prescription refilled, suggests Bourret. When you see you are beginning to run low, check the label to determine how many refills are available. If there are no refills, and you are certain that your prescriber intended you to have ongoing therapy, call the office. Perhaps it is time for a routine office visit, or maybe your prescriber wanted to check your progress and ability to tolerate the drug before prescribing it again.

A complex interplay of skills

If you are the child of aging parents, or are concerned about older adults in your life, you may be wondering if they are up to the task of managing their medications successfully. According to Dr. Bruce Silver, chief of geriatrics at Lankenau Hospital, a seemingly simple thing like managing a medication regimen actually requires a moderately high degree of intellectual functioning, judgment and skill. "First, it is essential for the person to be able to understand the need for the medication," says Silver. "That's because this knowledge acts as an important, though not the only, factor in motivating the patient to comply with the medication schedule. Also critical is a good short-term memory. Without it, it's likely that double-dosing or skipped doses will become a problem."

Other assets Silver deems important to successful medication management are well-developed organizational skills and the physical stamina necessary to make and keep ongoing physician appointments, get prescriptions filled and have waning supplies replenished. Equally important, he says, are fine motor and sensory skills. Good manual dexterity is required for opening containers and for getting those minuscule pills out of the bottle without dropping them. And let's not forget the importance of visual acuity for reading labels.

Dispensing aids: Gadgets to keep you organized

Recognizing that sticking to a complex medication schedule is difficult, the pharmaceutical products industry has developed handy medication dispensing aids to help organize pills. Some are even alarm-equipped for audible reminders of when a dose is due. Although there is no perfect system, these containers can serve as a helpful aid to avoid skipped doses and provide evidence of doses already taken. For those who need assistance, some containers can be filled in advance by a helper. You have several varieties to choose from at your pharmacy. Here is a brief description of the various kinds:

The daily planner: A one-day container that separates doses with flip-top lids labeled "breakfast," "lunch," "dinner" and " bedtime." Small and easily portable, this container is helpful if you must take medication more than once a day.

The seven-day planner: This container is based on the same principle as the daily planner, but holds medications for an entire week in a larger, rectangular plastic box. This is especially useful if an assistant is available to help with medications only once a week. You can even work with several containers to provide coverage for longer periods of time. However, the person who sets up this system will need to do so with extreme care. Any mistake made repeatedly can result in a medication error for seven straight days, or more.

The prescription bottle minder: This special lid fits onto your prescription bottle to show in LCD numbers the last date and time the bottle was opened. Although it can be a helpful memory aid, initial programming can be tricky and requires a high degree of manual dexterity.

Alarm boxes: "Electronic" pill boxes can be programmed to beep when a dose is due. However, the audible signal may be too low for those with hearing difficulties. Note: An undivided container may work well for those taking one kind of medicine several times a day, but dumping several different kinds of pills into a pillbox of any kind is inviting medication errors.

If you are still skipping doses despite these organizers, try setting a wristwatch alarm or ask a friend or relative to remind you when your medication is due.

If your medication regimen seems truly complex and unwieldy, ask your pharmacist to review it. He or she may be able to make consolidation suggestions to the prescriber or other changes that will allow for an equal therapeutic effect with simpler scheduling requirements.

A place for everything

Unfortunately, the bathroom medicine cabinet is not the best place to store your medicines. Excessive heat and humidity generated by showering and bathing can alter the integrity of your medicines, causing them to lose their effectiveness. Instead, keep medications in a dry, cool environment. And for safety's sake, do a regular survey of all prescription and over-the-counter medications. Toss out:

Any that are outdated

Aspirins that have a vinegar-like smell

Tablets that are powdery or crumbly

Liquid medications that have formed a residue or become cloudy, crusted or crystallized

Any half-used medications prescribed for past illnesses.

In addition, it is best to store your medications in their original containers—except, of course, for those you may be moving to a dispenser box. And if there are any children in your house, even for occasional visits, have the pharmacist give you childproof caps, or be sure to store the medicines well out of their reach.

In the hospital

One of the benefits of being in the hospital is that the nursing staff will be managing your medication for you. But your vigilance is still required. While safety procedures are quite effective, remember that your nurse is probably administering medications to an entire floor of patients. Occasional medication errors can and do occur.

When your medication nurse arrives, does she check your wrist ID band or ask for verbal verification of your name? Have her describe each of the medications she presents. For example, "This is your blood pressure medicine. This is your antibiotic." If a medication seems unfamiliar or inappropriate, don't take it. Have the nurse recheck the medication order with the doctor or speak to him yourself. In the worst-case scenario, you'll take the medication a little later than intended.

On the day of your discharge, you will probably be somewhat fatigued and anxious to get home, but there is much to learn. Make sure your doctor or nurse carefully reviews any new prescriptions or changes in your medication regimen with you. Be especially alert for any discontinued medications. Write these on a separate sheet of paper so you can destroy them promptly once you arrive home. And last but not least: Ask your nurse what dosages you have already received that day. Have her help you calculate what you will need to take for the rest of the day so you can avoid repeating or skipping doses.

Medication alert: Not recommended for older adults

According to Dr. Barbara Bell, medical director of the Geriatric Assessment Unit at Abington Memorial Hospital, geriatricians view some 20 drugs, including selected tranquilizers, antidepressants and muscle relaxants, as generally inappropriate for use in older adults. "These drugs were first cited by a panel of geriatric experts who flagged them for use in nursing home residents," says Bell. "Later, the recommendation was broadened to apply to all older adults. Of course, every rule has its exceptions, and there are undoubtedly situations when the use of these drugs is acceptable. If you are taking any of these, the best course of action is to discuss your particular situation with your doctor."

Tranquilizers
Valium (diazepam): Due to an increase in body fat in older patients, this drug remains on board for long periods and can cause prolonged side effects, says Bell.
Librium (chlordiazepoxide): Similar to Valium, this drug has a long half-life (the time required for half the amount of a drug to be eliminated by natural processes from the body) and nasty side effects in the elderly, including EKG changes and rapid heartbeat.
Miltown (meprobamate): Also has a long half-life.

Sleeping aids
Dalmane (flurazepam); Nembutal (pentobarbital); Seconal (secobarbital): All three have a long half-life. Shorter-acting agents are available for use in the elderly.

Antidepressants
Elavil (amitriptyline): This drug has many undesirable side effects in older patients, including dry mouth, urinary retention, confusion and low blood pressure when standing, which can cause dizziness and dangerous falls. "Newer antidepressants are safer and just as effective, if not more effective," says Bell.

Anti-inflammatory/pain relievers
Indocin (indomethacin); Butagesic (phenylbutazone): These drugs can result in stomach upset.

Anti-diabetic agent
Diabinese (chlorpropamide): This drug also has a long half-life. "If a person developed low blood sugar on this drug, he would probably have to be hospitalized, since it would take time for it to clear out of the body," says Bell.

Muscle relaxants
Soma (carisoprodol); Flexeril (cyclobenzaprine); Robaxin (methocarbamol); Norflex (orphenadrine): These drugs have dangerous side effects such as confusion, and can also increase fall risks in older patients.

Blood thinner
Persantine (dipyridamole): "This used to be a widely used drug," says Bell. "However, studies show that its effectiveness is questionable."

Pain relievers
Darvon (propoxyphene): Darvon has bad side effects and is probably not much more effective than Tylenol, says Bell.
Talwin (pentazocine): Also has dangerous side effects.

Vasodilators
Vasodilan (isoxsuprine): Questionable efficacy.

Anti-nausea agent
Tigan (trimethobenzamide): "More effective drugs are available for this purpose," says Bell.

—Joyce Brazino

CHAPTER 20

The Lowdown on Life-Care

From personal desires to personal care, what continuing care retirement communities can offer today's seniors

For Eleanor Elkin, growing old is a potpourri of life's greatest gifts. It's autonomy and camaraderie. It's exhilaration and intellectual stimulation. It's safety and peace of mind.

Elkin lives at Center City Philadelphia's Logan Square East, a glowing example of a growing trend in elder care: continuing care retirement communities. Also called life-care communities, CCRCs are senior living facilities that are typically segmented into three distinct tiers—independent living (much like a regular apartment with senior-friendly amenities), assisted living (for those who can still care for themselves but might need help with physical tasks such as bathing) and nursing care. For a rather large sum of money, one may live out the rest of one's life in a CCRC, moving from one tier to the next as age assesses its physical and mental tolls.

Pennsylvania, along with New Jersey, Ohio and California, are hotbeds of life-care communities. With more than 60 CCRCs within a 40-minute drive of Philadelphia, this region has stepped up to bat to serve forward-thinking seniors. And it's a good thing. According to the American Association of Retired Persons (AARP), the fastest-growing population in the United States is over 85 years of age. Of even greater consequence, a person who reached 65 in 1992 could expect to live an average of 17 more years.

Today Elkin, 80, is healthy. She lives in her own apartment, one of 327 independent-living units at Logan Square East. It has two bedrooms and sleeps six, a tremendous convenience when her grandchildren come down from Massachusetts to visit her. She has emergency call bells in both of her bedrooms and bathrooms, and handrails in her bathtub and shower. For her monthly rental fee—$2,300, including utilities—Elkin also gets 24-hour security, one meal a day, weekly housekeeping and linen service, and transportation. Also on the premises of her high-rise are several doctors affiliated with Pennsylvania Hospital, a beauty salon and a full-service bank.

Quality Managed Care!

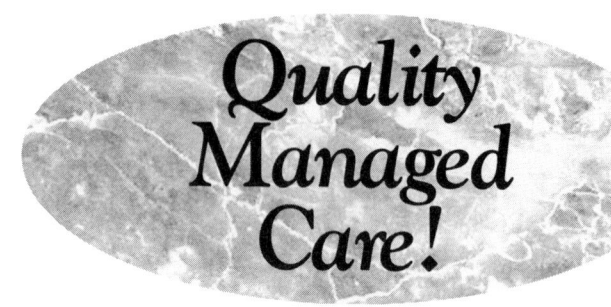

The future of health care and managed care is uncertain. But, the future of **_Quality Managed Care_** at Cathedral Village is very clear.

How can we make this statement with such certainty? The reasons are simple and direct.

- As one of the first Accredited Continuing Care Retirement Communities, Cathedral Village has helped to develop managed care.

- Cathedral Village has 17 years experience as a managed care provider.

- We emphasize quality, individualized care and personal attention.

- Health care is provided by experienced gerontologists who include our physicians and professional nurses.

Quality Managed Care at Cathedral Village means more than just visits to physicians or nurses. We encourage preventive health care through use of our fitness center, swimming water aerobic classes, nutritious meals, and many other services that maintain good health and a wonderful quality of life.

Call or visit today to learn the true meaning of _Quality Managed Care._

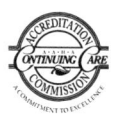

Cathedral Village

Equal Housing Opportunity

600 East Cathedral Road / Philadelphia, PA 19128 / (215) 487-1300
Cathedral Village is a Nonprofit, Nondenominational Continuing Care Retirement Community

Elkin moved into Logan Square East—the only three-tier facility in Center City—with her husband in 1988. They looked at several CCRCs and chose Logan Square East in part because of its location. After years of living in large homes in the suburbs, they wanted the convenience of urban apartment dwelling, with the added security of a community environment. The central issue to them, however, was the quality health care Logan Square East offered. Her husband's health was failing, and when Eleanor needed someone to help him out of bed in the morning, or sit with him when she had to leave on errands, all she had to do was pick up the phone. After a couple of years at Logan Square East, he was placed in the skilled-care unit of the 24-story tower.

"I don't know if I could have handled it if I was in a regular apartment," Elkin says of her husband's bouts with strokes and diabetes. "All I had to do was get in the elevator to visit him."

Since her husband's death five years ago, Elkin's life has not slowed down. She walks to downtown shops, museums, the Academy of Music. She participates in activities and events arranged by Logan Square East, such as concerts, movies, lectures and day trips to places like New York City and Longwood Gardens. She volunteers in the skilled-care center, and she presides over the Residents' Council. Most important, she says, she enjoys the friendships she shares with many of Logan Square East's largely educated, cultured residents.

"I didn't know a soul when I moved here," she remembers. "But I've found my own kindred spirits. I go visit my friends. And then it's nice to come back home and close the door. It's a good life."

And if Elkin's life ever becomes not so "good" because of advancing age, she can move into Logan Square East's personal-care or nursing-care center.

A difficult decision

The advantages of CCRC living are obvious. But making the move is not an easy choice for many older adults. Studies have shown that 85 percent of elderly individuals prefer to remain in their own homes. And while most were formerly living on their own, about 30 percent of those moving into senior living facilities were previously living with their adult children, says Annie Lundgren, coordinator of the older adult counseling program at the Family and Community Service of Delaware County in Media.

Typically, Lundgren says, there's guilt associated with the realization that one can no longer take care of Mom or Dad. So the waiting game begins—and a crisis often occurs. Dr. Barry Rovner, director of geriatric psychiatry at Jefferson Medical College, points to certain red flags that, if caught, can help short-circuit such a problem. Is vision, mobility or memory failing? Is the person having difficulty taking medications and preparing meals? Does he or she need supervision when going outdoors? Once the situation has been evaluated and the decision made, it's often easier on everyone—especially the senior relative.

It's a decision that Eleanor Elkin tried to help her parents make in the late '60s. "I couldn't convince them that it was a good idea," she laments. "But I did convince myself."

Good health carries clout

With so many elderly seeking suitable living arrangements—the minimum age for entry is usually 62 or 65—CCRCs can be choosy. And many of them choose healthy over sick applicants. In other words, they want individuals to come into independent living on the ground floor. After all, the cost to maintain a sick individual in nursing care far outpaces any rate increases that may be assessed (sometimes the rates stay the same) as an individual moves from his or her own apartment to a nursing-care unit.

Unfortunately, foresight is not always the thing that puts an elderly person on a CCRC's doorstep. "They're often not ready for the move," says Anneta Kraus, president of Geriatric Planning Services in Media, "because they look at it as their last stop. But then bad things start to happen to them." A spouse dies. A hip breaks. The memory starts to slip. And by the time they apply for admission to a CCRC, it's often too late. According to Kraus, more than half of all CCRCs accept only well elderly, whom they can place in independent units.

The Quadrangle, which is operated by Marriott Senior Living Services—the second-largest provider of housing and care for the elderly in the country—is one of these. A complex of red brick buildings on 74 acres of suburban greenery in Haverford, The Quadrangle has 349 independent-living accommodations, 36 assisted-living dwellings and 43 skilled-nursing units. The waiting list for some of the independent-living units is a couple of years, and getting one's name on it requires a deposit of $1,000. Currently, an applicant who needs medical supervision is immediately turned away. Part of the reason for this is space. The Quadrangle is contractually obligated to provide personal and/or nursing care to hundreds of healthy residents, should they become sick or otherwise impaired. With only 79 such units—which run at 100 percent occupancy—The Quadrangle is now expanding its assisted-living and nursing facilities and will add a state-of-the-art Alzheimer's wing.

The Main Line's ManorCare at Devon, on the other hand, accepts new residents directly into any of its three tiers, space permitting. With 100 independent, 50 personal-care and 121 skilled-nursing units, space is not normally an issue. Yet even at ManorCare, says marketing director Cathryn Schenk, "the goal is to keep people as independent as possible for as long as possible." According to Schenk, about 35 percent of those who start out in ManorCare's independent-living units eventually move on to its nursing facility. The progression, she says, is a natural one: "It allows for a better quality of life and a smoother transition."

What price happiness?

When one applies for admission to a three-tier facility, a medical assessment is done to determine his or her limitations and needs, and what type of accommodations would suit him or her best. But that's not all. CCRCs also examine applicants' financial health. At Logan Square East, they review critical numbers, including an applicant's age, assets and monthly income versus projected health care expenses. At Martins Run, in Media, actuarial tables are used to predict life span in accordance with an analysis of income and assets. At The Quadrangle, they assess an applicant's ability to pay the entrance and monthly fees over a 20-year period. According to the AARP, only five percent of Americans who are over the age of 65 live in skilled long-term facilities. And the exorbitant cost—an average of about $35,000 annually—is the main barrier to entry. The expense of developing the properties and meeting stringent government regulations, owners say, keeps costs high.

Most CCRCs require an initial entrance fee, which averages nearly $146,000 for an individual. This money doesn't buy property; rather, it buys a sort of "you're-in-good-hands" insurance policy. Add to this monthly rental charges, which average about $1,500. Given these numbers, CCRCs are wise to question applicants' ability to pay. Once a resident runs out of money, Medicaid will take over the cost. But because these facilities can charge higher rates for private-paying residents than they receive through Medicaid, many—about half the CCRCs in this region—refuse Medicaid payments. Even at those that accept Medicaid, an applicant who can pay out-of-pocket stands a better chance of being admitted than one who cannot.

Most CCRCs accept Medicare, which pays for some skilled-nursing care for up to 100 days for persons who are over 65 and need intensive nursing care following hospitalization. While some three in four CCRCs incorporate the cost of limited nursing and medical care into the rent, fees for doctors' visits, diagnostic workups and certain treatments are often extra. Some CCRCs, like Logan Square East, require residents to buy supplemental insurance policies to cover extra medical costs.

Contracts and fee arrangements vary widely among three-tier facilities. Generally, an extensive contract covers shelter, residential services, amenities and unlimited long-term nursing care. In effect, this type of contract spreads the risk of catastrophic health care costs among all the residents of the community, sick and healthy alike. A modified contract includes shelter, residential services, amenities and limited nursing care; supplemental care may be purchased on a monthly or per diem basis. A fee-for-service contract covers shelter, residential services and amenities. Long-term nursing care costs extra, but entrance and monthly fees are typically lower.

At Cathedral Village, situated on 35 acres in Montgomery County, entrance fees range from $43,000 to $180,000, and monthly fees from $1,460 to $3,165. Residents may choose from among 277 independent living units, ranging from studios to two-bedroom units. There is also a 148-bed skilled-nursing facility with a dedicated Alzheimer's unit.

Logan Square East is unique in the fact that its life-care contract includes such care with virtually no price increase from a residential apartment—which costs $1,400 per person to $3,600 per couple—to the skilled-nursing facility, other than medication, supplies and extra meals. Residents pay a one-time entrance fee ranging from $48,512 to $189,806, depending on the apartment style and type of contract chosen. For those who prefer to pay less up front, Logan Square East offers a declining refund plan. If a resident leaves for any reason, upon reoccupancy of the apartment Logan Square East will refund—to the individual or his/her estate—the entrance fee less 2 percent for each month of residence. A second type of declining refund plan requires a higher entrance fee, which is 75 percent refundable should a resident leave for any reason.

One of the pricier life-care communities, The Quadrangle assesses entry fees ranging from $81,000 to $313,000, depending on the apartment size and number of occupants. Monthly rental fees run from $1,634 (single occupancy) to $5,100 (double occupancy). Three payment plans are available. An individual can choose to pay a higher entrance fee (90 percent refundable upon his or her departure) coupled with a lower monthly payment; a lower entrance fee (90 percent refundable upon his or her departure) coupled with a higher monthly fee; or a lower monthly fee coupled with a moderate entrance fee that is amortized over a five-year period, after which no refund is given.

ManorCare at Devon is one of the few life-care communities that doesn't charge an entrance fee. An independent-living apartment costs $2,100 to $5,500 monthly, depending on the style and whether it's for single or double occupancy; personal-care units are $2,700 $4,500; and skilled-nursing units are $199 a day.

The expense of CCRC living puts it out of reach for many Americans. One exception to the rule, however, is Kearsley Retirement Community. Located on 13 acres in the Wynnefield section of Philadelphia, Kearsley is America's oldest retirement community. It is also one of the only facilities that provides the three-tier option to low-income individuals. There's no entrance fee, monthly charges are assessed on a sliding scale according to residents' ability to pay, and Medicaid is accepted. Having recently completed a $15.1 million expansion, Kearsley now offers 87 independent-living units, 60 personal-care units and 84 nursing-care beds.

Though its prices are relatively low, says Valerie A. Deorio, Kearsley's public relations coordinator, its intensive fund-raising efforts enable Kearsley to offer quality care to its residents. Medical care is provided by Thomas Jefferson University Hospital, and nurses work around the clock. Also on the premises are physical, speech and occupational therapists.

The final analysis

Like Eleanor Elkin, most older individuals who decide on their own to move into life-care communities enter into independent-living arrangements. But regardless of your needs—residential autonomy, personal assistance or full nursing care—there are key areas to probe when choosing the CCRC that's best for you. For most prospective residents, the principal concerns are affordability, proximity to family, quality of care and the neighborhood, says Karen Mudd, director of communications at the Philadelphia Corporation for Aging.

But, she adds, you might also contact your local area agency on aging (each county has one) for additional information and recommendations. Also, monitor comments by regulatory agencies. The Pennsylvania Department of Health regulates CCRCs' nursing-care divisions, the Department of Public Welfare the assisted-living sectors; the Department of Insurance certifies that the CCRC is, on the whole, financially sound. You can also get a listing of all CCRCs certified by the Continuing Care Accreditation Commission. The CCAC scrutinizes four areas—governance and administration, resident life, health care and finance. CCAC's seal of approval has been given to nearly 200 of the 1,000 or so three-tier facilities in the country.

But you can also do your own investigative work. Visit different life-care communities. Look at the qualifications of the people who run them. Find out what the nursing staff-to-patient ratio is (the average ranges from 1-to-6 to 1-to-9 during daytime hours). Ask about the activities program. And once you've gotten the information together, ask yourself, "Is this where I want to be if I ever become very sick?"

For Eleanor Elkin, the answer was yes when she found Logan Square East. "There is peace of mind in knowing that when I need more care, I will still be here. This whole place is my home."

CCRC Checklist

Here are some of the questions you should ask about each facility you consider:

___
Is the facility convenient?
___
Will your physician continue to treat you there?
___
Can the facility handle your special needs?
___
Are physical, occupational and other special therapists available at the facility?
___
What is the nursing staff-to-patient ratio?
___
Does the facility participate in Medicaid and/or Medicare?
___
Can you afford the facility's fees?
___
How long is the waiting list, if one exists?
___
Does the facility have a good reputation among health-care professionals?
___
Does the staff pay close attention to the residents and treat them respectfully?
___
Does the quality of care appear consistent even during "off times," like evenings and weekends?
___
Does the staff answer call bells promptly?
___
Are the residents clean, dressed and well-groomed?
___
Are the residents encouraged to leave their rooms and participate in social activities?

Is there a regular schedule of activities?

Are the visiting hours convenient for your family and friends?

Are outings planned on a regular basis?

Are residents' rooms pleasant?

Is there a residents' council? If so, what types of issues has it handled lately?

Are the stairs and hallways clear of obstacles, well-lit and equipped with handrails?

Are spills cleaned immediately?

Do all areas appear, and smell, clean?

Do residents enjoy the food?

Are accommodations made for special diets?

Is there a registered dietitian on staff?

Are smoke detectors appropriately located and functioning properly?

Are fire drills held according to schedule?

Resources

Educational materials

Contact the following organizations for valuable informational materials:

American Association of Retired Persons (AARP): 717-238-2277. *Nursing Home Life: A Guide for Residents and Families; Making Wise Decisions for Long-Term Care.*

Pennsylvania Association of Non-Profit Homes for the Aging (PANPHA): 717-763-5724. *Come to Life! What to Look for and Expect From Today's Non-Profit Homes for the Aging.*

American Association of Homes and Services for the Aging (AAHSA): 202-783-2242. *Choosing a Nursing Home: A Guide to Quality Care.*

Northwest Interfaith Movement: 215-843-5600. *Nursing Homes in Philadelphia: A Directory and Consumer Guide.*

Alzheimer's Association: 1-800-621-0379. *The Family Guide to Alzheimer's Care in Residential Settings.*

Associations and services

Keep the following phone numbers handy during your survey of facilities:

ALZHEIMER'S INFORMATION CLEARINGHOUSE: 1-800-367-5115

AMERICAN ASSOCIATION OF HOMES AND SERVICES FOR THE AGING (AAHSA): 202-783-2242

AMERICAN ASSOCIATION OF RETIRED PERSONS (AARP): 1-800-424-3410; AARP PENNSYLVANIA STATE OFFICE: 717-238-2277

BETTER BUSINESS BUREAU OF EASTERN PENNSYLVANIA: 215-448-6100

CHILDREN OF AGING PARENTS (CAPS): 215-945-6900, 1-800-227-7294

FAMILY AND COMMUNITY SERVICE OF DELAWARE COUNTY: 610-566-7540

GERIATRIC PLANNING SERVICES: 610-566-6686

LONG-TERM CARE CONSORTIUM OF THE MAIN LINE: 610-525-0896

RETIREMENT AND TRANSITION ELDERCARE SERVICES: 610-527-4578

County offices for the aging

Pennsylvania

BUCKS COUNTY AREA AGENCY ON AGING: 215-348-0510

CHESTER COUNTY DEPARTMENT OF AGING SERVICES: 610-344-6350

DELAWARE COUNTY OFFICE OF SERVICES FOR THE AGING: 610-713-2100

MONTGOMERY COUNTY OFFICE OF AGING AND ADULT SERVICES: 610-527-7962; NORRISTOWN BRANCH: 610-278-3601

PHILADELPHIA CORPORATION FOR AGING: 215-765-9040

New Jersey

ATLANTIC COUNTY INTERGENERATIONAL SERVICES: 609-645-7700, EXT. 4700

BURLINGTON COUNTY OFFICE ON AGING: 609-265-5069

CAMDEN COUNTY OFFICE ON AGING: 609-310-8900

CUMBERLAND COUNTY OFFICE ON AGING: 609-453-2225

GLOUCESTER COUNTY OFFICE ON AGING: 609-384-6910

SALEM COUNTY OFFICE ON AGING: 609-769-4150

Delaware

NEWCASTLE COUNTY DIVISION OF SERVICES FOR THE AGING AND ADULTS WITH PHYSICAL DISABILITIES: 1-800-223-9074

—Joan P. Capuzzi

Section

For Your Information

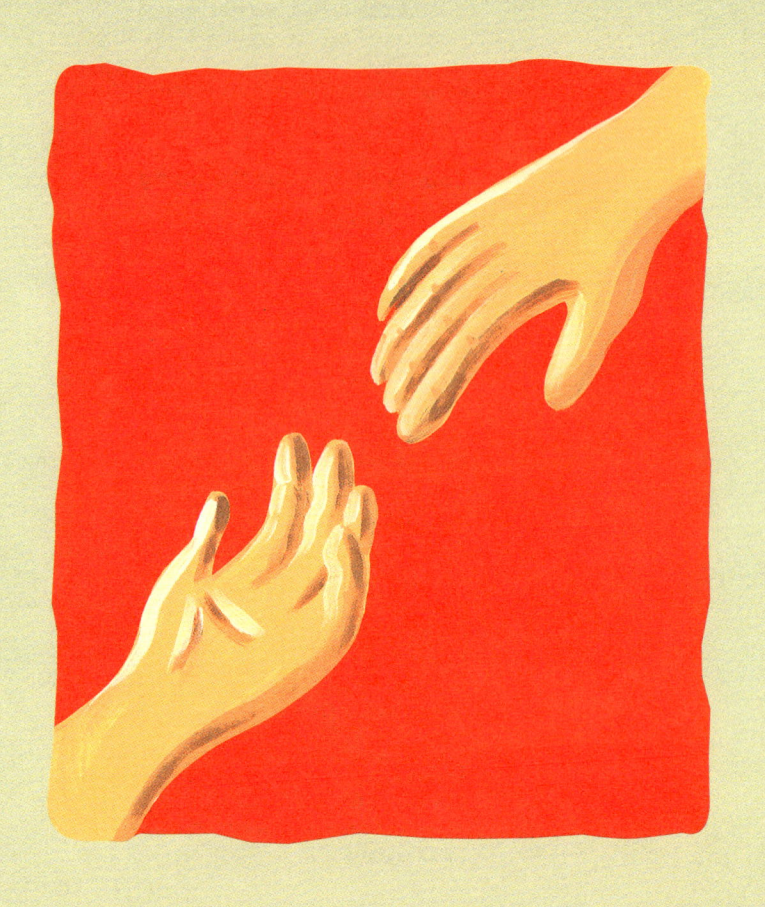

Nine

Chapter 21
   Home Sweet Home
   Help that makes house calls

Chapter 22
   The Road Back
   Resources for rehabilitation services

Chapter 23
   We've Got Your Number
   Special programs, groups and health services

Choose your home care provider as if your life depended on it.

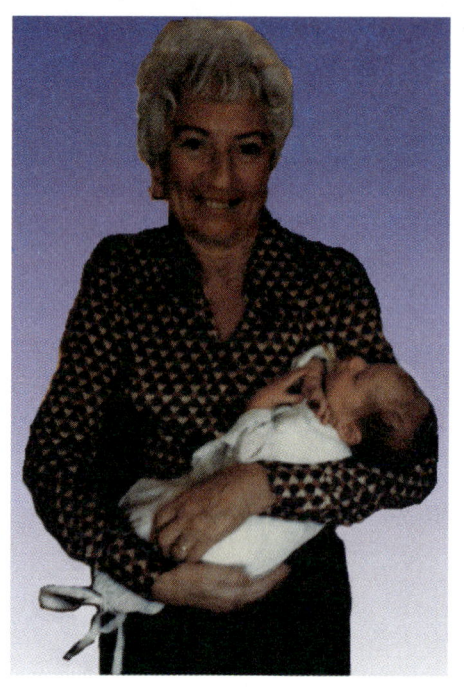

ProCare Health Services

Licensed and bonded. Highly-trained. Criminally-checked. 24-hour response time. Quality care for people in their own homes. Includes nursing (R.N., L.P.N.), home health aids, live-ins, rehab, P.T., O.T., S.T. Medicare certified. Serving the entire Delaware Valley.

610-645-7515

Joint Commission on Accreditation of Healthcare Organizations

CHAPTER 21

Home Sweet Home

Help that makes house calls

When you're sick in a hospital, help is as close as the nurse call button. But once you get home, there is a whole range of services you may need that are not always easy to find. This chapter is a sampling of resources for the homebound patient. In general, when people talk about *home health care* they're referring to skilled nursing care provided by licensed professionals such as registered nurses and various kinds of therapists. When people use the terms *home care, homemaker care* or *personal care*, they're describing those who help with dressing, feeding, bathing, housekeeping, meal preparation and errands—the kinds of services performed by nonprofessional but trained home health aides or homemakers. You'll find both of these kinds of services at a home care agency. On a full-time, part-time or live-in basis, they provide nurses, aides and companions not only for the elderly, but for anyone physically disabled, ill or injured who needs assistance with personal needs, treatments and therapies.

Home-Care Agencies

Aid for Friends
215-464-2224
Serving Greater Philadelphia with meals, friendship, emergency financial aid and advocacy.

Bayada Nurses
1-888-681-1000
A JCAHO-accredited home-care agency founded in 1975, with 30 area offices serving Philadelphia and surrounding counties, all of New Jersey and parts of Delaware. Specializes in RNs, LPNs, aides, homemakers and live-in companions providing

services 24 hours a day, at fixed hourly or daily rates. Medicare and private insurance accepted.

Central Health Services
215-664-7711

Offers complete in-home care, including nurses, homemakers and companions; child care; IV therapy; rehabilitation; and elder care. Insurance accepted.

Community Health Affiliates
610-642-7696

A member of the Jefferson Health System, which includes Bryn Mawr Hospital, Lankenau Hospital, Paoli Memorial Hospital, Great Valley Health, Thomas Jefferson University Hospital and Bryn Mawr Rehabilitation. Provides visiting nurses, home support services and hospice care. Medicare, Medicaid and private insurance accepted.

Episcopal Community Services
215-351-1400

Provides free RN-supervised home-care services, including Meals on Wheels, to Supplementary Security Income recipients and lower-income individuals in Philadelphia. Some health-aide services are available on a sliding-fee scale for those ineligible for the free services.

Family Care Associates
215-431-3141

Provides full-service pediatric home health care, including neonatal health care, therapies for medically fragile children, photo therapy, support services, continuous care for babies and help with developmentally delayed children and adults. Both nurses and home health aides available. Serves Philadelphia, surrounding counties and South Jersey.

Fox Chase Cancer Center Home Health Services
215-728-3011

Provides nursing support; physical, speech and occupational therapy; medical social services; home health aides; laboratory services; and intravenous therapies. Also provides nursing support, medical social services, pastoral counseling, home health aides, medical equipment and supplies for patients in the terminal stages of disease. Accepts many insurance plans.

Friends Life Care at Home
215-628-8964

Serving Greater Philadelphia area seniors 65 and older with round-the-clock professional health and support services, including nurses, home aides, companions, meals and emergency response system.

Help-U-Care
215-673-5965

For anyone requiring non-medical help with personal needs, including newborn/child care and the disabled. Homemakers, companions and home health aides work under the supervision of visiting nurses. Hourly or live-in fees.

Home Health Care for Jewish Family and Children's Services of Philadelphia
215-545-3290

Nursing and social-work services for the elderly and homebound.

Home Health Corporation of America
610-272-1717

Provides nurses, aides and companions; respiratory, IV, physical, occupational and speech therapies; medical equipment; and pediatric services. Medicare, Medicaid and private insurance accepted.

Homemaker Service of the Metro Area
215-592-0002

A United Way member agency providing RNs, LPNs and home health aides; physical, speech and respiratory therapists; and medical social workers. Medicare, Medicaid and private insurance accepted.

Homestaff of Delaware Valley
215-696-4191

Provides nurses and aides; physical, speech and occupational therapists; and medical social workers. Adult and pediatric services. Medicare, Medicaid, Blue Cross and private insurance accepted.

Hospital Homecare
215-923-0411

Affiliated with Chestnut Hill Hospital, Pennsylvania Hospital and Episcopal Hospital. Provides private nurses (in the hospital or at home); aides, therapists and nannies; and medical equipment. Insurance accepted.

Interim Health Care
215-664-6720

Provides nurses, aides, live-ins, therapists and homemakers. Medicare certified.

JEVS (Jewish Employment and Vocational Service) Attendant Care Program
215-728-4411

Clients must be residents of Northeast Philadelphia or Bucks or Montgomery counties, between 18 and 59, disabled and in need of assistance with personal care. Services are free to those on medical assistance or Supplemental Security Income, and offered on a sliding scale to others.

Jewish Family and Children's Service of Southern New Jersey
609-662-8611

Provides trained aides and homemakers through the Carl Auerbach Friends of JFCS on a short-term basis (up to 12 weeks).

Liberty Health System
1-800-676-1161
215-690-2500 OR 1-800-676-1161

JCAHO-accredited full-spectrum care including medical treatment, nurses and household aides. Medical equipment, respiratory and infusion therapy also available by calling 1-800-345-8611. Insurance accepted. A special new mother/new baby program matches a new mother with a Liberty professional who assists the mom and teaches her to care for her baby. Also available are trained personnel to care for a child who's sick or when school unexpectedly closes (215-690-2532).

Allegheny University Hospitals Homebound Services
215-927-HOME

Geriatric physician and nurse-practitioner teams provide physical exams, ongoing health care, routine lab testing, caregiver support and guidance and physical therapy.

Neighborhood Home Health
215-755-6464

Provides RNs, aides, therapists and medical social workers for homebound patients who are referred by their physicians.

Nursefinders
610-667-2901 OR 610-638-2044

Provides home health care and private-duty hospital and nursing home staff. RNs, LPNs, aides and live-ins. Medicare, Medicaid and private insurance accepted.

Olsten Kimberly QualityCare
215-563-8100

Provides nurses and aides specializing in pediatrics, neonatal care and infusion therapy. Medicare and Medicaid certified.

Premier Medical Services/SRT Med Staff
215-676-9090

Provides RNs, LPNs and home health aides. Insurance accepted.

ProCare Health Services
(610) 645-7515

Serving the Delaware Valley with home physical and occupational therapy, chemotherapy, stomal therapy and pediatrics.

Protocall
215-664-8700

Provides nurses, aides and live-ins and speech, physical and IV therapists. Special asthma control and diabetes programs. May be covered by insurance.

Vintage Health Care Service
215-684-8024

Provides RNs; aides; and physical, occupational and speech therapists. Medicare and Medicaid certified.

The Visiting Nurses Association of Greater Philadelphia
215-473-7600

One of the oldest nonprofit home health-care agencies in the nation provides health professionals, homemaker services and hospice in Philadelphia and lower Bucks, eastern Montgomery and Delaware counties. Medicare certified, and services for uninsured and underinsured patients.

Post-Hospitalization Home Care

Many hospitals provide short-term (two to eight weeks) home care services for patients covered by insurance—Medicare, Medicaid, Blue Cross and others. Services usually include nursing care; home health aides; hospice care; maternal/child health care; physical, speech and occupational therapists; medical social workers; and medical equipment. (See hospital listings, Chapter 8.)

Equipment/ Home Services

Beckett Apothecary
215-726-9964

Delivery and repair of home medical equipment. Basic Medicare and Medicaid, as well as most insurance.

Caremark Connection
215-985-4020

Specimen collections, chemotherapy administration, blood transfusions, inhalation therapy, mid-line insertions and counseling for homebound patients. Insurance accepted.

Vision Care

Dr. E. David Pollock, O.D.
215-379-4990

Offers complete vision care at home, including glaucoma testing, vision examination, all optical services, lenses and frames, and low-vision aids. Medicare accepted.

Dental Care

Dentistry-To-You
215-784-9984

Comprehensive dental care for homebound patients or those in nursing homes. With portable equipment, Kenneth B. Siegel, D.M.D., can do everything from extractions to root canals to crowns.

Mobile Dental Services
215-732-7053

Dentures and repairs in private homes. Limited to Northeast Philadelphia and Montgomery and Bucks counties. Reasonable fees; cash or checks only.

CHAPTER 22

The Road Back
A survey of rehabilitation services

In the world of health care, hospitals fall into two broad categories. General hospitals, as implied, treat a wide range of illnesses. Specialty hospitals, on the other hand, deal with very specific needs. In this section we focus on places geared toward physical problems—recovery from an injury or debilitating illness, like a stroke or cancer. Check out any referral carefully and discuss with your personal physician whether it's the appropriate place for you. Many general hospitals also have rehabilitation services. See the listings in Chapter 8.

Physical Rehabilitation

Bryn Mawr Rehabilitation Hospital

414 PAOLI PIKE, MALVERN; 610-251-5400. DOCTORS ON ACTIVE STAFF: 12. NUMBER OF BEDS: 141. ACCREDITATION: JCAHO, CARF.

Specialized treatment programs: brain injury, stroke (including young stroke), neurological disorders, spinal cord injury, MS, orthopedics, arthritis, Guillain-Barre.
Clinical services: physical, occupational and speech therapy; aquatic, equestrian and horticultural therapy; therapeutic recreation; psychology services.
Outpatient health and wellness programs: adapted driver education, vocational rehab, amputee clinic, occupational rehab medicine.

Bryn Mawr Rehab is a member of the Jefferson Health System.

Chestnut Hill Rehabilitation Hospital

8601 STENTON AVENUE, WYNDMOOR; 215-233-6200. DOCTORS ON ACTIVE STAFF: 4. NUMBER OF BEDS: 88. SPECIAL GOURMET MENU: $10 PER MEAL. ACCREDITATION: JCAHO, CARF.

Specialized treatment programs: comprehensive rehabilitation for stroke, arthritis, orthopedic injury, amputation, cancer, joint replacement.
Medical rehabilitation services (inpatient and outpatient): physical medicine, internal medicine, physical and occupational therapy, therapeutic recreation, speech-language pathology, psychology and case management.
Outpatient health and wellness programs: wheelchair clinic, prosthetic and orthotic clinic, wound care, SAFE (Senior Activity and Functional Evaluation), WorkForce for worker injuries, Arthritis Information and Management (AIM) Club, stroke club, 55-Plus and Fit.

Chestnut Hill Rehabilitation Hospital, a service of Chestnut Hill HealthCare, offers a rehabilitation unit at Grand View Hospital in Sellersville, Bucks County, to provide services to people in Bucks and Montgomery counties.

HealthSouth Rehabilitation Hospital of New Jersey

14 HOSPITAL DR., TOMS RIVER, N.J.; 908-244-3100, 1-800-54-REHAB, EXT. 5222. DOCTORS ON ACTIVE STAFF: 7. NUMBER OF BEDS: 155. ACCREDITATION: JCAHO, CARF.

Specialized treatment programs: Joint Replacement Program, Deconditioned Program, Stroke Program, Surgical Orthopedic Program, Prosthetic Training Program, Brain Injury Program, Degenerative Neurological Disorder Program (Acute or Chronic), Pre-Prosthetic Amputee Program, Spinal Disorders Program.
Outpatient health and wellness programs: audiology, breast rehabilitation, hand therapy, occupational therapy, orthopedic rehabilitation, behavioral health and wellness, work injury rehabilitation, physical therapy, speech therapy, biofeedback, comprehensive rehab day hospital, brain injury day treatment, psychology, pediatric therapy, TMJ, arthritis, back injuries, burns, chronic pain, developmental disorders, neurological disorders, peripheral nerve injuries, sports injuries, traumatic injuries, Return to Work program, psychophysiological conditions.

Magee Rehabilitation

SIX FRANKLIN PLAZA (16TH AND RACE STREETS), PHILADELPHIA; 215-587-3000. DOCTORS ON ACTIVE STAFF: 9. NUMBER OF BEDS: 96. ACCREDITATION: JCAHO, CARF.

Specialized treatment programs: Riverfront Outpatient and Day Hospital Center; Lifetime Follow-up Clinic; Electronically Stimulated Standing, Walking and

Cycling; Swallowing Disorders Clinic; Horticultural Therapy; Wheelchair Sports and Recreation; HireAbility (employment agency for the disabled); Legal Clinic for the Disabled; Work Fitness®; Magee at Methodist; Skintegrity (pressure ulcer management); Confidence (incontinence management); Mild Head Injury Center; Riverside Care at Magee (substance abuse treatment); Community Peer Support programs.
Physical rehab services: stroke, spinal cord injury, brain injury, orthopedic fracture and replacement, amputation, geriatrics, pain management, work-related injury.

Magee is the region's original provider of physical and cognitive rehabilitation and is home to the nation's first CARF-accredited brain injury program.

MossRehab

1200 West Tabor Road, Philadelphia; 215-456-9900, 1-800-CALL-MOSS. Doctors on active staff: 61 (88.5% *board-certified*). Number of beds: 152. RNs per bed: 1.6. Accreditation: JCAHO, CARF.

Specialized treatment programs: Drucker Brain Injury Center, MossRehab Stroke Center, Regional Amputee Center, orthopedic rehabilitation, Kardon Center for Pediatric Rehabilitation, Regional Spina Bifida Center for Adults, Einstein-MossRehab Arthritis Center, Einstein-MossRehab Joint Replacement Center, MossRehab-Einstein Limbs with Restricted Motion Program.
Physical rehab services: physical, occupational and speech therapy; therapeutic recreation; psychological services; electrodiagnostic center; gait and motion analysis laboratory; motor-control analysis laboratory; prosthetics and orthotics service; day hospital, subacute rehab.
Outpatient health and wellness programs: fitness and exercise programs for people with physical disabilities; hand rehabilitation; rehabilitation for orthopedic disorders, neurological impairment, general edema and lymphedema; Driving School; Back School.

MossRehab, a part of Albert Einstein Healthcare Network, is the region's largest provider of medical rehab services and has outpatient centers in Olney, Northeast Philadelphia and Jenkintown.

Mount Sinai Hospital

4th and Reed streets., Philadelphia; 215-339-3456. Doctors on active staff: 36 (*70% board-certified*). Number of beds: 220. Accreditation: JCAHO, CAP.

Physical rehab services: Inpatient, outpatient and day hospital programs for stroke, head injury, amputation, arthritis, chronic pain, neurologic illness and orthopedic problems. Also offers occupational and sports medicine. All patients can use Easy Street Environments®, a therapy environment simulating a city street.

Skilled Nursing Facility: 40-bed unit for patients who no longer require acute hospital care but need services such as wound care, colostomy care, insulin injection and IV therapy.

Mount Sinai, part of The Graduate Health System, also offers free health lectures for the community.

Other Rehab Services

The Cancer Rehabilitation Center
8080 OLD YORK ROAD, ELKINS PARK; 215-782-8760

Staff composed of physical therapists, an occupational therapist, a social worker and a psychologist. Accreditation: APTA, PPTA. A unique outpatient facility established to provide physical therapy, conditioning and strengthening programs to treat cancer patients physically and emotionally. Specialized treatment programs: pain management, strengthening and endurance training, services for postoperative stiffness and shoulder problems, lymphedema management, medically supervised weight reduction, home exercise, aerobics, functional assessments for disability determinations, counseling, psychological evaluation, return-to-work programs.

The Philadelphia Center for Aquatic Rehabilitation
3600 GRANT AVENUE, PHILADELPHIA; 215-677-0400

Staff composed of five physical therapists, ten physical therapy assistants and aides and two exercise specialists. Aquatic physical therapy services: most advanced techniques used for patients recovering from work, orthopedic and sports-related injuries. Land-therapy services: outpatient services using equipment for strengthening and conditioning. Activities of daily living and back and neck care are emphasized. Outpatient treatment using fully equipped Work Conditioning Center aids in quick return to work with less risk of reinjury; emphasizes job skills and FCEs.

ReMed Recovery Care Centers
CORPORATE OFFICE, 625 RIDGE PIKE, BUILDING C, CONSHOHOCKEN; 610-834-1300

Staff composed of five doctors and 47 specialists. Number of beds: 74. Accreditation: CARF. Provides post-acute, community-based rehabilitation to people with brain injuries and other neurological impairments. Behavioral programs in Malvern and Valley Forge offer therapy in a safe, structured environment; community re-entry services supervise apartment living, teaching skills for daily living; community apartment living programs are a less-structured support for apartment living in Malvern and Philadelphia; Living Community in Malvern provides long-term rehab with supportive therapy; Community Services Network in Bryn Mawr has day treatment and outpatient services; Program for Adults With Autism; Speech Pathology Consultants, Inc. (affiliated company); all programs incorporate substance-abuse treatment when needed. ReMed is Pennsylvania's largest provider of post-acute brain injury rehab.

CHAPTER 23

We've Got Your Number

A potpourri of services geared toward a particular audience

Special Programs

Annual Physicals

The Executive Health and Wellness Center of Allegheny University Hospital
Two Logan Square, Suite 1800, Philadelphia; 215-299-3800

Aimed at the busy executive, this center provides fast and personally designed annual physicals, including all the latest testing equipment under one roof. A total workup covers detailed personal history and physical exam, the complete spectrum of laboratory tests, X-rays, gynecologic exams, cardiovascular stress test, flexible sigmoidoscopy and a fitness/nutrition assessment. Treatments with a variety of specialists also provided.

Brain/Body Connection

International Behavioral Medical Center (IBMC)
300 West Basin Road (Route 141), New Castle, Del.; 302-328-2262

This outpatient hospital practices the therapies of behavioral medicine as its primary treatment modality. Its interdisciplinary approach to disease brings together a broad range of disciplines—things like imagery, biofeedback, massage therapy, stress reduction, exercise, medical psychology and more—to deal with illnesses related to daily living. IBMC considers its strengths to be in heart disease, chronic pain and muscle disorders, gastrointestinal and addiction problems, allergies, sexual dysfunction, PMS and pharmacotherapy disorders. All major insurance is accepted.

Brain Waves

The Mastery Program
491 Allendale Road, Suite 222, King of Prussia; 610-337-4550

A seven-week outpatient treatment program, medically directed by Dr. Carl Sonder,

Helen's kids have seen a change in her lately.

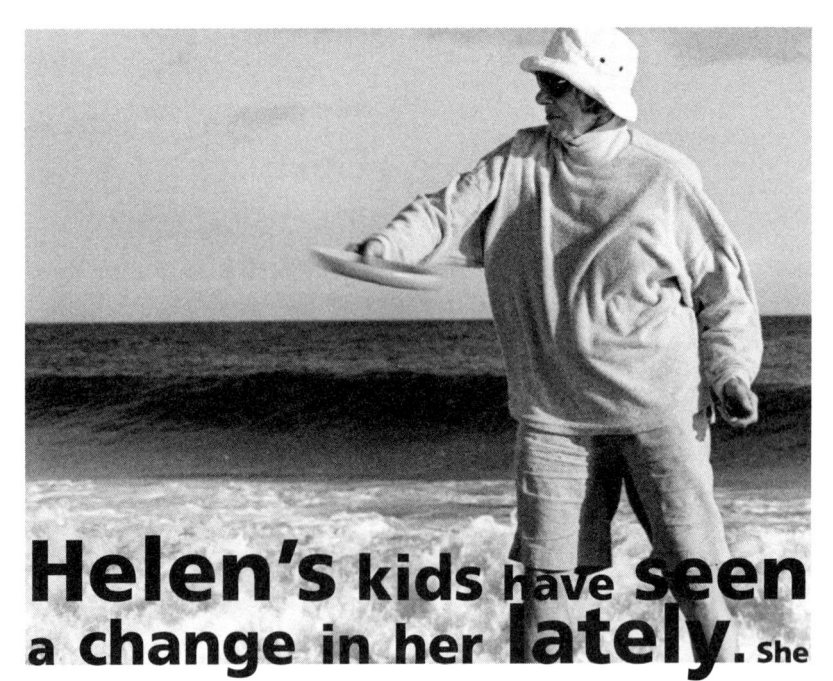

She can remember her fifth birthday, but forgets what day it is today. At Genesis ElderCare℠, we assess the individual needs of the elderly and their families and provide health care services through a network of people, places and programs. We do all we can to prolong people's independence and help them live a full life. If you're concerned about an elderly loved one, or have questions about eldercare, call the Genesis ElderCare Line at 1-800-699-1520.

Genesis ElderCare℠

a board-certified psychiatrist, for depression, anxiety, stress-related medical disorders, post-traumatic stress disorders and some substance abuse cases. Treatment involves a combination of cognitive behavior psychotherapy and brain-wave biofeedback. Patients are hooked up to a computer that monitors electrical activity of the brain and are taught how to change their patterns without drugs. The Mastery Program claims an 80 percent success rate. Medical treatment is available for patients who prefer it.

Eating Disorders

Arbor Counseling Center
110 NORTH ESSEX AVENUE, NARBERTH; 610-664-5858

Specializing in the treatment of eating disorders among both men and women, including problems with anorexia, bulimia, binge eating disorder and compulsive overeating. Individual, group and nutrition therapies focus on how eating disorders help people endure rather than change themselves, their relationships and the circumstances of their lives. Directed by Leonard Levitz, Ph.D., the founding clinical director of The Renfrew Center, and Merrily Karpell, Ph.D.

Headaches

Comprehensive Headache Center at The Germantown Hospital
ONE PENN BOULEVARD, PHILADELPHIA; 215-951-8926

Some 45 million people suffer from recurring headaches, and while there is no cure, doctors can control the pain and related symptoms in up to 90 percent of them. The Headache Center is a research and treatment facility dedicated solely to the headache sufferer. Patients are evaluated medically by a neurologist, then seen and tested by a psychologist or psychiatrist. Treatment includes medication, behavior modification, biofeedback, diet changes and psychological and physical therapies.

Heart Health

Benjamin Franklin Center for Health
PUBLIC LEDGER BUILDING, 6TH AND CHESTNUT STREETS, PHILADELPHIA; 215-829-8660

The Benjamin Franklin Center for Health is a Center City internal medicine, risk reduction and wellness center offering medical services to individuals, business and industry. The Center provides comprehensive corporate health services including an executive health program, health assessment programs for employees and a full range of preventive and occupational health services tailored to each corporation's needs. Risk reduction services include programs for heart disease prevention and rehabilitation, cancer screening and prevention, pulmonary rehabilitation, weight management and nutrition and exercise. Ongoing comprehensive care is available on-site through the center's full-service internal medicine private practice.

Learning Problems
Vision Development Center
919 East Germantown Pike, Suite 4, Plymouth Meeting; 610-279-8900

Many children diagnosed as having learning difficulties, attention deficit/hyperactivity disorder or trouble concentrating may, in fact, be suffering from a vision disability. Visual disorders stem from an improper interplay of signals between the eye and the brain. While they cannot be corrected by glasses, they can be detected by special tests and corrected with specific visual exercises. Optometrist Arthur S. Seiderman, O.D., M.A., F.A.A.O., F.C.O.V.D., co-author of *20/20 Is Not Enough*, evaluates and treats patients having trouble in school with an optometric visual and perceptual therapy program he's developed.

Sick Kids
Under the Weather
602 South Bethlehem Pike, Ambler; 610-643-9460

This state-licensed day-care facility provides a haven for sick children between the ages of six weeks and 12 years who are unable to attend their school or regular day-care center due to illness. The center is specially designed to reduce the spread of illness. Medical care is provided by nurses and pediatricians from Ambler Pediatrics. Children are supervised full time, and the center is filled with books, games and activities. Open Monday-Friday, 8 a.m.-5:30 p.m.

Women's Mental Health
The Renfrew Center
475 Spring Lane, Philadelphia; 1-800-RENFREW

This opened in 1985 as the country's first residential center for women with eating disorders such as anorexia, bulimia and compulsive overeating. Building on its expertise in eating disorders and the emphasis on the participation of each individual in her own treatment, Renfrew has now extended its services to include treatment for women struggling with depression, anxiety, post-traumatic stress disorder or substance abuse. Programs include residential, day, intensive outpatient, group, individual, family and nutritional counseling. Educational programs include seminars on a wide range of women's issues and a speakers bureau.

Workplace Violence
Corporate Crisis Intervention Network
The Woods, Suite 719, 987 Old Eagle School Road, Wayne; 1-800-221-6776

David Reed, formerly of the Marriage Council, is executive director of this organization, which does strategic management of traumatic stress in the workplace. Included in its evaluation service is the design and implementation of a crisis intervention program to be used when something causes a major emotional upset at work. Its psychological trauma experts are on 24-hour alert and can be reached via a toll-free hotline in case of a critical incident of violence or physical endangerment.

Smoking Cessation and Treatment Programs

Smoking is the most preventable cause of death in our society. While the number of smokers in the country has certainly decreased, one wonders why there are any left at all given how horrifying the statistics are. The good news is that it's never too late to quit—and you don't have to tough it out alone. Here are some programs to help you. Many are covered by insurance—check with your carrier.

American Cancer Society
215-985-5400

Call for schedule.

American Lung Association
1-800-LUNG-USA

Learn how to deal with your cravings to smoke and get the support you need to quit for good. Call for schedule and locations.

Associates for Health and Guidance
215-473-8900

Learn to hypnotize yourself, practice methods of behavior modification, try electro-acupuncture and acupressure, or use nicotine replacement therapy. The staff here will even make you a personalized relaxation tape. Call for an appointment.

Free and Clear
1-800-292-2336

A personalized smoking cessation program. Includes contact with an assigned specialist five times throughout the year. The toll-free Quitline offers additional guidance and support. $160 for a one-year program.

Smoke Enders
1-800-828-4357

A learning technique based on behavior modification, taking into consideration weight control, physical withdrawal symptoms, etc., with the object of reaching complete "freedom" from the smoking habit. $325 for six-week seminar. Self-study Learn-to-Quit Kit is $129. Discounts for corporate seminars and some insurance plans. Call for schedule and locations.

Smoke Stoppers
1-800-843-6247

A national organization offering three treatment options. 1. Group Program: Maximum interaction with an instructor, group support and intensive behavior modification and lifestyle management. $100-$165 for eight sessions. 2. Staying-Stopped Program: Support program with a flexible format that gives the participant the "how tos" of smoking cessation. Ideal for those thinking about quitting, ready to quit or relapsing. $75-$125 for five sessions. 3. Self-Help Program/Kit: A 26-day program designed for self-study, including behavior modification, relapse prevention and lifestyle management development. Participants have access to a toll-free telephone support service. $49-$69. Call for information, locations and schedules.

TAO-Eager to Quit
215-241-4709

A four-week program offering varied treatment methods: not ready (readiness preparation), gradual withdrawal, withdrawal with a nicotine replacement product and "cold turkey." $150 for four sessions. Call for schedule and locations.

Dr. Steven Rosenberg
ELKINS SQUARE MALL, SUITE 206, OLD YORK AND
CHURCH ROADS, ELKINS PARK; 215-782-8414

A psychologist and hypnotherapist who has used hypnotism to help more than 25,000 stop smoking. In addition, he gives his patients a "smoke-breaker" kit with herbal tablets he's developed to ease nicotine withdrawal. $75 per session.

For additional listings of the many smoking cessation programs held at area hospitals, see Chapter 8.

Support Groups

These listings include many of the organized self-help and support groups in the Delaware Valley. In addition, most local hospitals have regularly scheduled support groups too—check the hospital listings, Chapter 8. Meeting times and dates tend to change, so for current information, it's a good idea to check first. The National Self-Help Clearinghouse number is 212-642-2944.

Abortion Counseling

Amnion Crisis Pregnancy Center
610-525-1557

One-on-one counseling for women experiencing post-abortion stress.

AIDS

Philadelphia Community Health Alternatives/AIDS Task Force of Philadelphia
215-545-8686

An anonymous HIV test site in Center City. Case management program provides services to people living with HIV and AIDS. A variety of support groups are available. Also check independent hospital listings.

AIDS Psychotherapy
215-567-2260

Dr. Mary V. Cochran conducts sessions, by appointment, in Center City for both men and women, and consults with service providers. Fees are on a sliding scale.

Alcoholism

Al-Anon
215-222-5244

For the relatives and friends of alcoholics. More than 175 regular meeting places in the Delaware Valley. Call for locations.

Alateen
215-222-5244

For teenagers whose lives have been affected by someone else's drinking.

Alcoholics Anonymous
215-574-6900

The world's most successful program for people who want to stop drinking. More than 1,700 ongoing meeting places in the Delaware Valley. Call for information.

ALS

National ALS Association
215-643-5434

Support groups in Philadelphia, New Jersey and Delaware. Call for specific locations.

Alzheimer's

Alzheimer's Association, Southeastern Pennsylvania Chapter
215-925-6019 (INSIDE PHILADELPHIA); 1-800-559-0404 (PENNSYLVANIA, OUTSIDE PHILADELPHIA AREA); 609-346-8883 (NEW JERSEY)

Provides information, emotional support and referrals. Operates Safe Return program to locate people who have wandered away from home: For $25, a person's identifying data is added to a computerized registry of Alzheimer's sufferers. The association will notify a network of police agencies and hospitals when a victim is reported missing.

Alzheimer's Disease Clearing House
1-800-367-5115

Sponsored by the Pennsylvania Department of Aging and the Pennsylvania Council on Aging. For caregivers or others interested in support groups, care and information.

National Institute of Aging's Information Line on Alzheimer's Disease and Forgetfulness
1-800-438-4380

Arthritis

The Arthritis Foundation
215-665-9200

Various meeting places scattered throughout the Delaware Valley for those suffering from any form of arthritis. Family and friends invited.

Autism

The Center for Autistic Children (CAC)
215-878-3400

Groups for parents and friends.

Bereavement

Abington Memorial Hospital
1200 OLD YORK ROAD, ABINGTON; 215-576-2700

Compassionate Friends
215-952-6777

For parents who have lost a child. Several meeting places. Call for locations.

Counseling Network for Loss and Transition
215-624-8190

For people who are grieving the death of a loved one.

Delaware County Memorial Hospital Hospice Program
501 NORTH LANSDOWNE AVENUE, DREXEL HILL; 610-394-1016

For adult children who have lost a parent, and a general loss group.

Elkins Park Free Library
CHURCH ROAD NEAR OLD YORK ROAD., ELKINS PARK; 215-635-5000

For adults who have lost a parent.

Fox Chase Cancer Center
7701 Burholme Avenue, Philadelphia; 215-728-2668

Groups for adults and children ages 5 to 18.

Mercy Catholic
Misericordia Division, 5301 Cedar Avenue, Philadelphia; 215-748-9440

Montgomery Home Care/Hospice
25 West Fornance Street, Norristown; 610-270-2711

Unite

For parents who've lost a baby during pregnancy or shortly after birth. Program is available at most area hospitals; check Chapter 8.

Breast-Feeding

La Leche League
610-666-0359

An international organization offering breast-feeding information and support for mothers. Call for information about your local group.

Cancer

American Cancer Society
215-985-5400 in Philadelphia and Montgomery counties; 717-553-6144 for Pennsylvania listings; 908-297-8000 for New Jersey

Sponsors a great variety of support groups for cancer patients, families and caregivers at many locations.

Philadelphia Candlelighters
215-884-0413 or 610-431-7295

For the families of children diagnosed with cancer and survivors of childhood cancer and other catastrophic childhood illnesses. Meetings held at members' homes.

Cardiac

Cardiac Support Group
215-643-4330

For individuals with heart disease and their family and friends, led by a professionally trained psychologist. Meets third Monday of each month at Abington Memorial Health Center.

Zipper Club
215-887-6644

For those who have had any sort of heart problem (heart attack, angioplasty, open-heart surgery, etc.) Support groups are run in conjunction with 38 area hospitals. Family and friends are invited.

Caregivers

CAPS (Children of Aging Parents)
215-945-6900

National information and referral service. Sponsors support groups for middle-aged children and caregivers dealing with elderly parents or relatives. Meetings deal with medical, legal and financial matters. Also sponsors educational outreach programs.

Diabetes

American Diabetes Association
610-828-5003; 908-469-7979 IN NEW JERSEY;
1-800-DIABETES

Offers a complete listing of the various support groups for those with juvenile or adult-onset diabetes. Family and friends are welcome. Free educational information on Type I and Type II diabetes.

Disabled Issues

Coalition of Active Disabled of Chester County
610-436-6502

Advocacy, referral and support services.

Epilepsy

Epilepsy Foundation of Southeastern Pennsylvania
215-627-4442

Sponsors self-help groups, guest speakers, informative lectures, employment assistance programs and community outreach and education programs for epilepsy patients, family and friends.

Delaware Valley Parents of Children With Epilepsy
215-789-2142

For the parents of epileptic children. Education and support.

Guillain-Barre Syndrome

Guillain-Barre Syndrome Foundation International
610-667-0131

Focuses on education, support and research. Family and friends are invited to meetings. Also publishes newsletters and educational materials and holds international symposia.

Huntington's Disease

Huntington's Disease Society of America
610-413-1844

Offers has a complete listing of groups for those suffering from the disease, their family, and friends. Also check specific hospital listings, Chapter 8.

Laryngectomee

Support groups are available to people who've had their larynxes removed:

Delaware County Memorial Hospital
501 North Lansdowne Avenue, Drexel Hill; 610-259-7021

Fox Chase Cancer Center
7701 Burholme Avenue; 215-728-2668

Montgomery Hospital Rehab
1330 Bowell Street, Norristown; 610-337-4677

Lung Disease

The American Lung Association of Southeastern Pennsylvania
1-800-LUNG-USA

A nonprofit organization offering support and information for those with various kinds of lung diseases.

Lupus

Lupus Foundation
215-877-9061 in Philadelphia; 610-649-9202 for more Delaware Valley locations

Sponsors various groups for sufferers, family and friends. Also check area hospitals.

Mental Illness

Project SHARE
215-751-1800

Managed by former mental patients. Provides support, information, referral and technical assistance to patients nationwide.

Multiple Sclerosis

National Multiple Sclerosis Society
215-271-1500, 1-800-548-4611

Greater Delaware Valley chapter runs meetings for sufferers, families, and friends. Also check specific hospital listings, Chapter 8.

Narcotics

Narcotics Anonymous
215-934-3944

For those ready to confront a narcotic addiction. Meets at more than 50 area hospitals.

Organ Transplants

National Transplant Assistance Fund
610-527-5056

Offers advice, support groups, alternative payment opportunities and public education for all transplant patients and their families and friends.

Obsessive-Compulsive Behavior

Obsessive-Compulsive Support Group
215-842-4010

A group designed to help people dealing with this condition is held at Allegheny University.

Ostomy

Philadelphia Ostomy Association
215-483-1818

Refers to various area support groups dealing with specific ostomies.

Parkinson's Disease

National Parkinson's Association, Philadelphia Chapter
215-893-2440

Has a thorough listing of support groups. Also check area hospitals, Chapter 8.

Spinal Cord Injury

Support groups sponsored through various hospitals. Check Chapter 8.

Stroke

Support groups for people recovering from strokes, and their families and friends, are held at various hospitals. Check Chapter 8.

Survivors of Suicide

Survivors of Suicide, Inc.
215-745-8247

Various programs for people who have lost a loved one or a friend to suicide.

Elderly Self-Care

Bayada Nurses
1-888-681-1000

A JCAHO-accredited home-care agency founded in 1975, with 30 area offices serving Philadelphia and surrounding counties, all of New Jersey and parts of Delaware. Specializes in RNs, LPNs, aides, homemakers and live-in companions providing services 24 hours a day, at fixed hourly or daily rates. Medicare and private insurance accepted.

Episcopal Community Services
215-351-1400

Provides free RN-supervised home-care services, including Meals on Wheels, to Supplemental Security Income recipients and lower-income individuals in Philadelphia. Some health-aide services are available on a sliding-scale fee for those ineligible for the free services.

Jewish Family and Children Service
215-545-3290; 609-662-8611 IN NEW JERSEY

Has worked with Philadelphia and suburban elderly since 1953. All home care is provided in coordination with a social worker, on a sliding-scale fee, from two to 20 hours a week, with occasional overnight service. In the Cherry Hill area, JFCS provides homemakers through the Carl Auerbach Friends of JFCS.

Northwestern Home Services
215-755-6464

A private Medicare-certified agency with 15 years of experience providing primary-care RNs who work mainly with Medicare referrals.

Philadelphia Geriatric Center
215-456-2900

Health and social services for Jewish elderly and their families. Recreational and religious activities. Also, full-care nursing home.

The Ralston-Penn Center
215-662-2746

Medical, nursing and social assistance for the elderly. Focuses on improving the quality of life of seniors. The various programs include a post-stroke nursing consultation program and a geriatric psychiatry program.

Senior Outreach Services
610-446-6442

A nonprofit agency providing home care in the western suburbs. Rates are generally $8 to $10 an hour.

Share the Care Respite Program
215-487-1750

Run by Intercommunity Action, Inc. Provides health aides in East Falls, Germantown, Roxborough, Andorra and Manayunk. Hourly rates are $8 to $10, with a minimum of two hours weekdays and three hours weekends.

Supportive Older Women's Network (SOWN)
215-477-6000

Organizes community self-help groups that help older women cope with health issues, social issues and widowhood.

Surrey Services for Seniors
610-647-6404

Volunteers and a small paid staff provide home care and chore services, on a sliding-scale fee, to elderly people on the Main Line between Bryn Mawr and Malvern. Formerly known as the Surrey Club, it also sponsors social programs for the elderly.

The Visiting Nurse Association of Greater Philadelphia
215-473-7600

One of the oldest nonprofit home health-care agencies in the nation, dating to 1886. The Medicare-certified agency provides health professionals and homemaker services in Philadelphia and the surrounding counties. It also offers services to uninsured and underinsured patients.

Diagnostic Centers — Alzheimer's Disease

For support groups, see "Support Groups" on page 269.

Abington Memorial Hospital, 215-881-5640

Allegheny University Hospitals, Center City, 215-762-6660

Allegheny University Hospitals, East Falls, 215-842-4070

Alzheimer's Association, 215-925-6019

Ambulatory Geriatric Evaluation Service, 610-435-2277

Crozer-Chester Medical Center, 610-447-6060

Doylestown Hospital, 610-345-2200

Albert Einstein Medical Center, 215-456-7890

Foerderer Evaluation Program, 215-662-2746

Institute of Pennsylvania Hospital, 215-471-2862

Thomas Jefferson University Hospital, 215-955-8033, 215-955-8780

Jeanes Vital Age, 215-663-0575

Lifespan Adult Health Center, 610-536-6016

Paoli Memorial Hospital, 610-648-1206

Pennsylvania Hospital, 215-829-3000

Philadelphia Geriatric Center, 215-456-2900

Prime Health Medical Offices, 215-333-3500

St. Mary's Hospital, 215-757-5800

Temple University Hospital, 215-707-8902

University of Pennsylvania Medical Center, 215-662-4000

University of Pennsylvania Medical Center Cognitive Neurology Program, 215-662-3606

University of Pennsylvania Medical Center King of Prussia Facility, 610-337-8882

Nursing Home Care

AgeWise Family Services
1250 GLENBURNIE LANE, DRESHER, PA.; 610-659-2111

Contact: Susan P. Weiss, Roberta Rosenberg.

Columbus Life Management, Inc.
20106 VALLEY FORGE CIRCLE, KING OF PRUSSIA;
1-800-229-5116

Clients undergo complete health-care assessment emotional and social evaluations to help them identify the appropriate home health care or nursing-home options. Trained experts act as professional, objective advocates and liaisons in dealing with long-term care needs. They also monitor and manage client services.

Comprehensive Health and Human Services Inc./Eldercare
8329 HIGH SCHOOL ROAD, ELKINS PARK; 215-635-6849

Contact: Sheila R. Bergman.

Comprehensive Health and Human Services Inc./Eldercare
435 East Lancaster Avenue, #211, Wayne; 610-688-5579

Contact: Barbara R. Feinstein.

Elder-Service, Inc.
301 North York Road, Suite 105, Warminster; 215-442-1800

Contact: Mary K. Evereroeck.

Geriatric Planning Services
2 South Orange Street, Suite 201, Media; 610-566-6686

Contact: Anneta Kraus.

Intervention Associates
P.O. Box 572, Wayne; 610-254-9001

Contact: Marsha Solmssen, Marion Thompson.

Retirement and Transition, Inc.
1049 West Lancaster Avenue, P.O. Box 451, Bryn Mawr; 610-527-4578

Contact: Helena A. Stewart. R.N., MSD.

Star Systems Consultation and Training, Inc.
Madison House, Suite D-122, 3900 City Avenue, Philadelphia; 215-477-2211

Contact: Janice Brown.

Supportive Care Services, Inc.
507 West 9th Street, Wilmington, Del.; 302-655-5518

Contact: Thomas J. Posatko.

Hot Numbers

These are some of the more widely used national hotline numbers. Try them if you are looking for information, referrals, counseling or technical assistance.

Aging
Medicare Telephone Hotline, 1-800-638-6833
National Council on Aging, 1-800-424-9046

AIDS
National AIDS Clearinghouse, 1-800-458-5231
National AIDS Hotline, 1-800-342-2437

Alcoholism and Drug Dependence
National Council on Alcoholism and Drug Dependence, Inc., 1-800-nca-call

Alzheimer's
Alzheimer's Association Toll-Free Information and Referral Service, 1-800-272-3900

Arthritis
Arthritis Foundation Information Line, 1-800-283-7800

Cancer
AMC Cancer Information and Counseling Line, 1-800-525-3777
American Cancer Society's Cancer Response system, 1-800-acs-2345
American Institute for Cancer Research, 1-800-843-8114
Cancer Information Service, 1-800-4-cancer

Care for the Dying
Choice in Dying, 1-800-989-will
Compassion in Dying, 206-624-2775
Hemlock Society USA and Patients Rights Organization USA, 1-800-247-7421
National Hospice Organization Hospice Helpline, 1-800-658-8898

Children
American SIDS Institute, 1-800-232-sids
National Child Abuse Hotline, 1-800-422-4453
National Resource Center on Child Abuse and Neglect, 1-800-2-ask-aha

Cystic Fibrosis
Cystic Fibrosis Foundation, 1-800-344-4823

Diabetes
American Diabetes Association, 1-800-ada-disc

Down's Syndrome
National Down's Syndrome Congress, 1-800-232-6372

Hearing Problems
DEAFNESS RESEARCH FOUNDATION, 1-800-535-3323
EAR FOUNDATION, 1-800-545-4327
HEARING AID HELPLINE, 1-800-521-5247
HEARING HELPLINE, 1-800-327-9355

Lead Poisoning
NATIONAL LEAD INFORMATION CENTER,
1-800-LEADFYI

Liver and Kidney
AMERICAN LIVER FOUNDATION'S HEPATITIS LIVER
DISEASE HOTLINE, 1-800-223-0179
NATIONAL KIDNEY FOUNDATION, 1-800-622-9010

Lung Illness
ALLERGY INFORMATION REFERRAL LINE,
1-800-822-ASMA
ASTHMA AND ALLERGY FOUNDATION OF AMERICA,
1-800-7-ASTHMA

Lupus
AMERICAN LUPUS SOCIETY INFORMATION LINE,
1-800-331-1802
LUPUS FOUNDATION OF AMERICA INFORMATION LINE,
1-800-558-0121

Marijuana Therapy
ALLIANCE FOR CANNABIS THERAPEUTICS, 202-483-8595

Mental Illness
NATIONAL FOUNDATION FOR DEPRESSIVE ILLNESS,
1-800-248-4344
NATIONAL MENTAL HEALTH ASSOCIATION,
1-800-969-6642
PANIC DISORDER, 1-800-64-PANIC

Miscellaneous Diseases
AMYOTROPHIC LATERAL SCLEROSIS ASSOCIATION,
1-800-782-4747
ANOREXIA/BULIMIA: RENFREW CENTER, 1-800-RENFREW
HUNTINGTON'S DISEASE SOCIETY OF AMERICA,
1-800-345-4372
NATIONAL OFFICE OF RARE DISEASES, 1-800-999-6673
NATIONAL TEMPORAL BONE HEARING AND BALANCE
PATHOLOGY RESOURCE REGISTRY, 1-800-822-1327
THE VESTIBULAR DISORDERS ASSOCIATION,
1-800-837-8428

Multiple Sclerosis
National Multiple Sclerosis Society, 1-800-944-4151

Sexual Problems
Impotence Information Center, 1-800-843-4315
STD Hotline, 1-800-227-8922

Sickle-Cell Anemia
Sickle-Cell Disease Association of America, 1-800-421-8453

Stroke
American Heart Association Stroke Connection, 1-800-553-6321
National Stroke Association, 1-800-367-1990

Vision Problems
Prevent Blindness America, 1-800-221-3004

Women
Women's Help America Group, 1-800-222-4767
Women's International Pharmacy, 1-800-279-5708

Local Organizations

Ambulance Services
Action Ambulance Co., 215-244-3900
American Medical Response, 215-537-2120
Bridesburg Civic and Town Watch, 215-288-8545
Burholme First Aid Corps, 215-745-1550
MetTrans Delaware Valley, 215-922-6006
Northeast First Aid Corps, 215-624-7024
Rhawnhurst Bustleton Ambulance Association, 215-698-9111
Wissahickon Community Ambulance Association, 215-482-6400
Wissonoming First Aid Corps, 215-332-1509
Wynne-Brook Community Ambulance Association, 215-473-4043

Diseases and Disorders
Action AIDS, 215-981-0088
Alzheimer's Association, 215-568-6430
American Cancer Society, 215-985-5400
American Diabetes Association, 610-828-5003
Arthritis Foundation, 215-665-9200
Asthma and Allergy Foundation, Southeastern Pennsylvania Chapter, 610-630-8050

Center for Advancement in Cancer Education, 610-642-4810
City of Hope, 215-731-9000
Community AIDS Hotline, 215-985-2437
Crohn's and Colitis Foundation, 215-396-9100
Cystic Fibrosis Research Foundation, 215-587-2800
Delaware Valley Transplant Program, 1-800-543-6391
Easter Seals Society, 215-879-1000
Elm LifeLine (cancer counseling and support programs), 609-654-4044
Epilepsy Foundation of Philadelphia, 215-627-4442
Guillain-Barre Syndrome Foundation International, 610-667-0131
Heart Association, 215-735-3865
Hemophilia Foundation, 215-885-6500
Juvenile Diabetes Foundation, 215-567-4307
Lupus Foundation of Delaware Valley, 610-649-9202
National Kidney Foundation, Delaware Valley Chapter, 215-923-8611
National Multiple Sclerosis Society, 215-271-2400
Operation VENUS (venereal disease), 215-567-6969
Ostomy Association of Philadelphia, 215-483-1818
Overeaters Anonymous, 215-698-1701
Parkinson's Disease and Movement Disorder Center, 215-545-8406
Philadelphia Community Health Alternatives (HIV screening and treatment), 215-545-8686
Philadelphia Help Group (herpes), 215-763-2247
Reye's Syndrome Foundation, 215-677-1730
Scleroderma Federation of the Delaware Valley, 609-678-6707
Sickle-Cell Anemia, Volunteers in Aid of, 215-877-3485
Spina Bifida Association, 215-676-8950
Tourette's Syndrome Association, Pennsylvania 1-800-446-6356
United Cerebral Palsy Association, 215-242-4200
Zipper Club (cardiac surgery and heart information), 215-887-6644

Hospice Programs

Bryn Mawr Hospital Hospice Program, 610-526-3265
Albert Einstein Medical Center Hospice, 215-456-7155
Holy Redeemer Hospice, 215-671-9200
Hospice of Pennsylvania Hospital, 215-829-7820
Penn Care at Home, 215-662-8996
Wissahickon Hospice, 215-247-0277

Suicide
CONTACT, 215-879-4402; 609-667-3000
SUICIDE AND CRISIS INTERVENTION CENTER, 215-686-4420
SURVIVORS OF SUICIDE, 215-545-2242

Visual Impairment
ASSOCIATED SERVICES FOR THE BLIND, 215-627-0600
BLINDNESS AND VISUAL SERVICES, 215-560-5700
BLIND RELIEF FUND OF PHILADELPHIA, 215-222-7613
FEDERATION OF THE BLIND OF PENNSYLVANIA, 215-988-0888
FIGHT FOR SIGHT CHILDREN'S SERVICE AT WILLS EYE HOSPITAL, 215-928-3240
LIBRARY FOR THE BLIND AND PHYSICALLY HANDICAPPED, 215-925-3213
LIONS EYE BANK OF DELAWARE VALLEY, 215-627-0700
PENNSYLVANIA COUNCIL OF THE BLIND, 215-238-1410

Women's Services
SEE CHAPTER 14 FOR SPECIFIC LISTINGS.

Professional Profile Section

As an additional source to our readers, the following health professionals have elected to list their services. These listings are paid advertisements and the information they contain has been furnished by the doctors and other medical practitioners. PHILADELPHIA Magazine's Guide to Good Health is not responsible for the credentials, affiliations, associations or other claims provided and does not endorse or recommend any medical professionals on the basis of their advertisement in this space. The listings appear in alphabetical order by specialty and name.

Acupuncture

C.M.D. ACUPUNCTURE CENTER AND HERB STORE
Chenghui Zhu, L.A.
1644 Bridge St., Philadelphia, PA 19124; (215)744-8260 and 1405 Joel Dr., Ambler, PA 19002; (215)646-3153.
26 years experience of Acupuncture, Chinese medicine and herbology. Specializing in relieving pain, quitting smoking, losing weight and controlling diseases, sterility, GYN disorders.

Rong-Bao Lu, M.D.
Acupuncture and Pain Control
1218 Walnut St., Rm. 901, Philadelphia, PA 19107; (215)546-7806.
Trained in China and USA. Free consultation. Arthritis, back/neck pain, headache, migraines, car accidents, sports injuries, nervousness, insomnia, PMS, weight control, smoking, stress, allergies. Foreign language spoken: Chinese.

Marshall H. Sager, D.O.
One Bala Plaza, Ste. 133, Bala Cynwyd, PA 19004; (610)668-2400.
University trained, licensed, certified medical acupuncture physician combining acupuncture, osteopathic manipulation, and Western medicine. Smoking, pain control, arthritis, backs, migraines, allergies, tendinitis, colitis, PMS, fatigue, stress.

MARLTON PAIN CONTROL AND ACUPUNCTURE CENTER
Wan B. Lo, M.S., Ph.D., D.O.
Pain Control
Evesham Commons, Ste. 301, 525 Rt. 73 S., Marlton, NJ 08053; (609)596-1005.
Board-certified. Specializing in traditional Chinese art of acupuncture. 25 years experience in treating arthritis, rheumatism, allergies, tendinitis, stress, smoking, weight, chronic pain, etc. Foreign language spoken: Chinese.

Alzheimer's Disease

THE MEMORY INSTITUTE
Dr. Steven D. Targum
Vascular Dementia
1015 Chestnut St., Ste. 1303, Philadelphia, PA 19107; (215)923-8378.
Multi-site research and treatment center which evaluates promising new medications for Alzheimer's disease. Free memory screenings and treatment programs are available to qualified individuals.

Asthma

S. David Scott, Ph.D., M.D.
2 Chesney Lane, Erdenheim, PA 19038; (215)233-9494.
A practice dedicated exclusively to diagnosing and treating asthma. Excellent results achieved for 12 years using personal attention, innovative therapy, and home monitoring. All ages.

Artificial Limbs/Orthopedic Braces

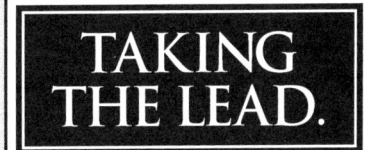

TAKING THE LEAD.

Since 1977 Harry J. Lawall & Son, Inc., has remained in the forefront of our industry by providing the latest high-tech, conventional, and sports prosthetics and orthotics.

HARRY J. LAWALL & SON, INC.
Prosthetics and Orthotics

(215) 338-6611
8028 Frankford Ave., Philadelphia, PA
Offices located in Cape May Court House, NJ
Vineland, NJ • Lawrenceville, NJ • Wilmington, DE
Newton Square, PA • Philadelphia, PA • Willow Grove, PA

Audiology

MAIN LINE AUDIOLOGY CONSULTANTS, P.C.
Kathy Landau Goodman, President, M.S.P.A., C.C.C., F.A.A.A, Edwin J. Winner, M.S., C.C.C.-A., F.A.A.A., Associate Director of Audiology, Michael J. Davenport, M.A., C.C.C.-A., Emmalyn Bernhardt, M.S., C.C.C.-A
822 Montgomery Ave., Ste. 318, Narberth, PA 19072; (610)667-EARS(3277).
Personalized caring service with state-of-the-art technology, diagnostic hearing evaluations by licensed audiologists, hearing aid evaluations, musicians' earmolds, swim molds, assistive listening devices.

HEARING TECHNOLOGY ASSOCIATES
Gail B. Brenner, M.A., CCC-A
1015 Chestnut St., Ste. 300, Philadelphia, PA 19107; (215)413-0800.
Specializing in digitally programmable hearing instruments. Hearing testing. Hearing aid fitting and dispensing. All makes repaired. Custom hearing protection. Assistive listening and alerting devices. Tinnitus management (ear/ head noises).

Breast Surgery

Dahlia M. Sataloff, M.D., F.A.C.S
1800 Lombard St., Ste. 901, Philadelphia, PA 19146; (215)735-4699.
Comprehensive, state-of-the-art care for benign and malignant disorders of the breast by board-certified breast surgeon. Surgical services available at the Graduate and Pennsylvania Hospitals.

Cardiology

ALLEGHENY UNIVERSITY OF THE HEALTH SCIENCES, THE HEART HOSPITAL AT ALLEGHENY UNIVERSITY
Susan Brozena, M.D., F.A.C.C., Farooq A. Chaudhry, M.D., F.A.C.C., Marc Cohen, M.D., F.A.C.C., Ami Iskandrian, M.D., Steven P. Kutalek, M.D., F.A.C.C., William G. Kussmaul III, M.D., F.A.C.C., Francis Marchlinski, M.D., F.A.C.C., David Naide, M.D.
Allegheny University Hospitals, Center City formerly The Heart Hospital at Hahnemann University Hospital, Broad and Vine Sts., Philadelphia, PA 19102; 1(800)PRO-HEALTH.
Listed above are the clinical chiefs and directors at Philadelphia's first Heart Hospital, who along with more than 100 other board-certified cardiologists, provide the full spectrum of state-of-the-art cardiac services, including catheterization, nuclear cardiology, electrophysiology, echocardiogram, arrythmia services and treatment of heart failure and transplant.

ALLEGHENY UNIVERSITY OF THE HEALTH SCIENCES, THE HEART HOSPITAL AT ALLEGHENY UNIVERSITY HOSPITALS
Herbert A. Fischer, M.D., F.A.C.C., William S. Frankl, M.D., F.A.C.C., Charles Gottlieb, M.D., F.A.C.C., Ami Iskandrian, M.D., Francis Marchlinski, M.D., F.A.C.C., Steven Meister, M.D., F.A.C.C., Alexis B. Sokil, M.D., William A. Van Decker, M.D., Nelson M. Wolf, M.D.
Allegheny University Hospitals, East Falls Formerly The Heart Hospital at Medical College of Pennsylvania Hosptial
3300 Henry Ave., Philadelphia, PA 19129; 1-(800)PRO-HEALTH.
Listed above are the clinical chiefs and directors at Philadelphia's newest Heart Hospital, who along with almost 100 other board-certified cardiologists, provide the full spectrum of state-of-the-art cardiac services, including catheterization, nuclear cardiology, electrophysiology, echocardiogram, and arrythmia services.

CARDIOLOGY CONSULTANTS OF PHILADELPHIA
P.M. Procacci, M.D., F.A.C.C., Mark F. Victor, M.D., F.A.C.C., Daniel J. McCormick, D.O., F.A.C.C., Veronica A. Covalesky, M.D., F.A.C.C., Dean G. Karalis, M.D., F.A.C.C., Michael A. Deangelis, M.D., Stanley Spitzer, M.D., F.A.C.C., Ted M. Parris, M.D., F.A.C.C., Garo S. Garibian, M.D., F.A.C.C., Kevin G. Robinson, M.D., F.A.C.C., Daniel Mason, M.D., F.A.C.C., Kevin J. Kasper, M.D., F.A.C.C., Andrew Fireman, M.D., Gilbert Grossman, M.D., Jacob Goldstein, M.D., Kenneth J. Forman, M.D., Paul Grena, D.O.
1703 S. Broad St., Ste. 300, Philadelphia, PA 19148; (215)463-5333; 227 N. Broad St., Ste. 200, Philadelphia, PA 19107; (215)564-3050; 700 Cottman Ave., Philadelphia, PA 19111; (215)745-4100; 525 Jamestown Ave., Ste. 208, Philadelphia, PA 19128; (215)482-1607; 1 Abington Plaza 401, Old York Rd. and Township Line Rd., Jenkintown, PA 19046; (215)885-1173.
We at Cardiology Consultants of Philadelphia are a group of physicians dedicated to providing the highest quality, most up-to-date, and comprehensive cardiac care in the Philadelphia area.

Let Penn and Presbyterian add Muscle to your Heart Treatment

Treating all aspects of heart disease at two convenient locations:

- 34th and Spruce Streets, University of Pennsylvania Medical Center
- 39th and Market Streets, Presbyterian Medical Center

The Cardiovascular Center

The University of Pennsylvania Health System

KELLY CARDIOVASCULAR GROUP
James G. Kitchen III, M.D., F.A.C.C., Michael J. Dougherty, M.D., F.A.C.C., James F. Burke, M.D., F.A.C.C., Donald F. Yih, M.D., F.A.C.C., Frank C. McGeehin, III., M.D., F.A.C.C., John W. Shuck, M.D., F.A.C.C., Thomas P. Phiambolis, M.D., F.A.C.C., Joseph G. Lewis, M.D., F.A.C.C., Maribel Hernández, M.D., F.A.C.C., John D. Blannett, M.D., Otto F. Müller, M.D., F.A.C.C., Martin J. O' Riordan, M.D., Richard H. Hunn, M.D.
Primary and Interventional Cardiology
Suite 365 Lankenau Medical Bldg. East, Wynnewood, PA 19096; (610)649-7625; 1503 Lansdowne Ave., Darby, PA 19023; (610)586-4100.

Our practice specializes in diagnosis, treatment, and prevention of disorders of the heart and blood vessels. Affiliated with Lankenau and Fitzgerald Mercy Hospitals.

MAIN LINE ARRHYTHMIA AND CARDIOLOGY CONSULTANTS, P.C.
Peter R. Kowey, M.D., Roger A. Marinchak, M.D., Seth J. Rials, M.D., Ph.D., Roland A. Filart, M.D.
Electrophysiology, Cardiac Rhythm Problems
Lankenau Medical Office Bldg. East, Ste. 556, 100 Lancaster Ave., Wynnewood, PA 19096-3425; (610)649-6980.
Physicians are trained in treatment of all heart disorders with advanced training in rhythm disorders. Specializing in electrophysiology, pacemakers/internal defibrillators, catheterization, ablation, unexplained fainting.

Cardiothoracic Surgery

ALLEGHENY UNIVERSITY OF THE HEALTH SCIENCES, THE HEART HOSPITAL AT ALLEGHENY UNIVERSITY HOSPITALS
Stanley Brockman, M.D., Verdi DiSesa, M.D., Inder P. Goel, M.D., Karl E. Grunewald, M.D., M.L. Ray Kuretu, M.D., J. March Maquilan, M.D., Rohinton J. Morris, M.D., Louis E. Samuels, M.D., Michael Strong, III, M.D.
Allegheny University Hospitals, Center City formerly The Heart Hospital at Hahnemann, Broad and Vine Sts., Philadelphia, PA 19102; 1(800)PRO-HEALTH.
These board-certified surgeons provide the full spectrum of state-of-the-art adult cardiothoracic surgery, including transplantation, at Philadelphia's first Heart Hospital.

ALLEGHENY UNIVERSITY OF THE HEALTH SCIENCES, THE HEART HOSPITAL AT ALLEGHENY UNIVERSITY OF HOSPITALS
Sariel Ablaza, M.D., Ray A. Blackwell, M.D., Anil Deshpande, M.D., Verdi DiSesa, M.D., W. Clark Hargrove III, M.D., James D. Sink, M.D., Haji Shariff, M.D., Glenn J.R. Whitman, M.D.
Allegheny University Hospitals, East Falls formerly The Heart Hosptial at Medical College of Pennsylvania Hospital, 3300 Henry Ave., Philadelphia, PA 19129; 1(800)PRO-HEALTH.
These board-certified surgeons provide the full spectrum of state-of-the-art adult cardiothoracic surgery at Philadelphia's newest Heart Hospital.

Peter R. Figueroa, M.D., F.A.C.S.
Vascular
Episcopal Hospital, 100 E. Lehigh Ave., MAB

CENTER FOR PREVENTIVE MEDICINE's
MEDICAL DIRECTOR

Howard Posner, M.D.

—*Nationally recognized authority on*

- **NUTRITIONAL MEDICINE**
- **HERBAL & VITAMIN THERAPY**
- **CLASSICAL HOMEOPATHY**

can help you if you suffer from—

Chronic Fatigue Syndrome • Yeast Infections
Infertility • Headaches • GI complaints • Allergies
Eczema • Arthritis • Hypertension • Prostatism
Cancer • Heart Disease • Acne • Depression

Total Family Care • Medicare Accepted
CENTER FOR PREVENTIVE MEDICINE
111 BALA AVE., BALA CYNWYD, PA 19004
(610) 667-2927

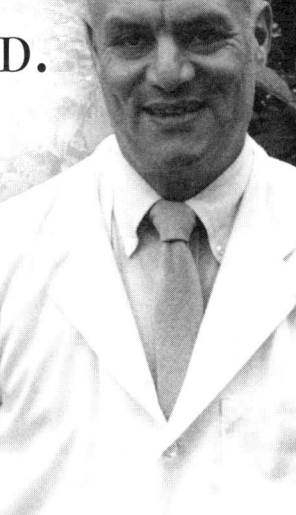

#302, Philadelphia, PA 19125; (215)427-7255. Surgical practice includes all aspects of heart surgery, i.e. coronary bypass, valve replacement and repair, pacemakers, defibrilators, aneurysm and lung, peripheral vascular surgeries. English and Spanish spoken.

MAIN LINE CARDIOTHORACIC SURGEONS, P.C.
Scott M. Goldman, M.D., F.A.C.S., Francis P. Sutter, D.O., F.A.C.S., Brian P. Priest, M.D.
2220 Lankenau Medical Science Bldg., 100 Lancaster Ave., Wynnewood, PA 19096; (610)896-9255.
Board-certified. State-of-the-art techniques include heart valve repair vs. replacement surgery without blood supply interruption to the heart, blood conservation preventing transfusions.

Steven J. Weiss, M.D.
5401 Old York Rd., Klein Bldg., Suite 206, Philadelphia, PA 19141; (215)324-5508.
State-of-the-art cardiothoracic surgical team. Special expertise in warm heart surgery, valve repair instead of replacement, high-risk and reoperative bypass surgery using a microscope.

Cardiovascular Diseases

CARDIOVASCULAR RISK INTERVENTION PROGRAM
Daniel J. Rader, M.D., Gregg Fromell, M.D., Christopher Friedrich, M.D., Ph.D.
Ground Rhoads, Hospital of the University of Pennsylvania, Philadelphia, PA 19104; (215)349-5640.
The program evaluates patients with high cholesterol, high triglyceride levels, low HDL, or history of heart disease or stroke but "normal" cholesterol.

Chiropractic

David W. Nadler, D.C., C.C.S.P.
Back and Neck Specialist
3475 W. Chester Pk., Ste. 140, Newtown Sq., PA 19073; (610)353-3888.
Board-certified. Sports, chiropractic and pain management. Advanced methods, non-surgical and drug-free approach; gentle, safe adjustments; state-of-the-art therapy equipment.

Colon/Rectal Surgery

Dr. Lowell D. Meyerson
Proctology
7516 City Line Ave., Philadelphia, PA; (215)877-3639 and Allegheny University Hospitals; Elkins Park Campus, 50 E. Township Line Rd., Elkins Park, PA; (215)379-0444.
Board-certified. Emphasis on office procedures for hemorrhoid treatment and cancer screening of colon and rectum. Laser surgery.

STEPHEN C. SILVER, M.D. ASSOCIATES
Stephen C. Silver, M.D., F.A.C.S., Taro Arai, M.D.
Ste. 201, 1010 W. Chester Pk., Havertown, PA 19083; (610)446-7882.
Practice limited to prevention and treatment of diseases of the colon and rectum. Special expertise in sphincter-saving operations for colorectal cancer and inflammatory bowel disease.

Community Health/Education

FRANKFORD HOSPITAL
Knights and Red Lion Rds., Philadelphia, PA 19114.
A community teaching hospital with two inpatient sites in Northeast Philadelphia, Frankford provides medical, surgical, obstetric, pediatric, rehabilitation, cancer center, wellness and trauma center services.

MONTGOMERY HOSPITAL MEDICAL CENTER
1301 Powell St., Norristown, PA 19404; (610)270-2000.
Montgomery Hospital Medical Center offers: 24-hour emergency department, Montgomery Cancer Center; diabetes treatment, short stay unit, sleep study program, state-of-the-art nursery, LDRP suites, and women's center.

RIDDLE MEMORIAL HOSPITAL
1068 W. Baltimore Pike, Media, PA 19063; (610)566-9400.
"We're dedicated to your good health." For a program, call (610)891-3560.

Medical College of
Pennsylvania and Hahnemann
University Hospital System
is now

ALLEGHENY UNIVERSITY HOSPITALS

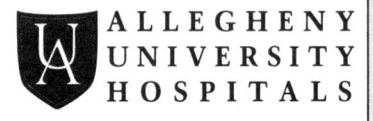

1-800-PRO-HEALTH[SM]
(1-800-776-4325)

Cosmetic Skin Surgery

CENTER FOR REJUVENATION OF AGING SKIN.
110 Chesley Dr., Media, PA 19063; (610)565-3300 and (610)892-0300.

Board-certified physicians provide complete evaluation and treatment for sun damaged and aging skin problems. Skin rejuvenation including laser for wrinkles, collagen, Gortex, liposuction, sclerotherapy for spider veins, facial peels, hair transplants. Skin care products.

Cosmetic/Plastic/ Reconstructive Surgery

Scott A. Brenman, M.D., F.A.C.S.
Hand Surgery
800 Spruce St., 10th Floor, Philadelphia, PA 19104; (215)829-7290.

Certified by the American Board of Surgery and Plastic Surgery, Dr. Scott Brenman provides comprehensive personalized care for the cosmetic surgical treatment of the face, breasts and body. Reconstructive surgery and hand surgery also performed.

MARK P. SOLOMON, MD

PLASTIC AND
RECONSTRUCTIVE SURGERY

HAS RELOCATED HIS PRACTICE TO

ONE BALA PLAZA
SUITE 639
BALA CYNWYD, PA 19004

TEL: 610.667.7070 FAX: 610.664.6664

CERTIFIED, AMERICAN BOARD
OF PLASTIC SURGERY

Marc S. Cohen, M.D., F.A.C.S, Nancy G. Swartz, M.D.
Ophthalmic Plastic and Cosmetic Surgeons
Wills Eye Hospital, Newtown, PA 19047; (215)772-0900; Pavilion of Voorhees, Ste. 101, 2301 Evesham Rd., Voorhees, NJ 08043; (609)772-0900; 1500 Tilton Rd., Northfield, NJ 08225; (609)772-0900.

Board-certified ophthalmologists educated at Wills Eye Hospital. Trained in Beverly Hills. Specializing in cosmetic eyelid surgery. Named by Philadelphia Magazine in "Top Doctors" issue.

COOPER PLASTIC SURGERY ASSOCIATES
Arthur S. Brown, M.D., Lenora R. Barot, M.D., Martha S. Matthews, M.D.
702 E. Main Street, Moorestown, NJ 08057; (609)342-3114.

Cosmetic and reconstructive surgery-facial, hand, and breast; liposuction; laser surgery; microsurgery; birth defects; biomedic skin care. Affiliated with Cooper Hospital. Other offices in Camden, Washington Twp.

COSMETIC AND PLASTIC SURGERY CENTER
James W. Slavin, M.D., Director
Abington Medical Plaza, Ste. 218, 1235 Old York Rd., Abington, PA 19001; (215)572-7200.
Full range of plastic, reconstructive and cosmetic surgery. First to offer Endermologie, a proven, non-surgical technique for fat/cellulite reduction. Dr. Slavin, board certified with over 25 years of experience, pioneered Alpha-Hydroxy Acids, used worldwide for skin rejuvenation.

Richard L. Dolsky, M.D., Cosmetic Surgery of Philadelphia
191 Presidential Blvd., Ste. 105., Bala Cynwyd, PA 19004; (610)667-3341.
President of the American Academy of Cosmetic Surgery and certified by the American Boards of Plastic Surgery, Otolaryngology, and Cosmetic Surgery, Richard Dolsky is internationally recognized for his contributions to cosmetic plastic surgery. He has been repeatedly named a Top Doc in Philadelphia Magazine. Dr. Dolsky's specialties include facial surgery, rhinoplasty, laser surgery, liposuction, and breast contouring. The initial consultation is complimentary.

Larry Jonas, M.D.
Lankenau MOB East, Ste. 65, Wynnewood, PA 19096; (610)649-9099.

Plastic and reconstructive surgery. Lankenau and Paoli Hospital; specializing in cosmetic surgery, breast surgery, liposuction and skin cancer surgery. Certified, American Board of Plastic Surgery.

Ronald A. Lohner, M.D.
888 Glenbrook Ave., Bryn Mawr, PA 19010; (610)527-4833.

Board-certified plastic surgeon at Bryn Mawr and Lankenau Hospitals, specializing in all aspects of aesthetic and reconstructive surgery, with special interest in cosmetic and laser procedures.

J. Brien Murphy, M.D.
Reconstructive Surgery
888 Glenbrook Ave., Bryn Mawr, PA 19010; (610)527-4833.

Attending plastic surgeon at Bryn Mawr, Children's and Lankenau hospitals; specializing in all aspects of cosmetic and reconstructive surgery with emphasis on breast, pediatric and laser surgery.

R. Barrett Noone, M.D.
Reconstructive Surgery
888 Glenbrook Ave., Bryn Mawr, PA 19010; (610)527-4833.
Chief of Plastic Surgery and Surgery Department Chairman at Bryn Mawr Hospital. Dr. Noone specializes in all aspects of cosmetic surgery and in breast reconstruction.

PHILADELPHIA INSTITUTE OF COSMETIC SURGERY
Zaki S. Ftaiha, M.D., Ellen A. Mahony, M.D.
15 North Presidential Blvd., Ste. 200, Bala Cynwyd, PA 19004; (610)664-5500.
Cosmetic, reconstructive and hand surgeon. Specializing in the unique needs of women, assisting those who wish to maximize their potential as women.

Mark P. Solomon, M.D., F.A.C.S.
One Bala Plaza, Ste. 639, Bala Cynwyd, PA 19004; (610)667-7070.
Dr. Solomon has over a decade of experience in plastic surgery. Board-certified and former Chief of Plastic Surgery at MCP, he has relocated his practice to Bala Cynwyd. His latest testbook on male cosmetic surgery has just been published.

Roslyn Coskery Souser, M.D., F.A.C.S.
Cosmetic Surgery
44 Haverford Rd., Ardmore, PA 19003; (610)642-9300 and 1558 McDaniel Dr., West Chester, PA 19380; (610)431-4055.
Dr. Souser is a board-certified plastic surgeon with over 20 years of experience. She's caring and competent and treats each patient as an individual.

Counseling

PENN COUNCIL FOR RELATIONSHIPS
4025 Chestnut St., Philadelphia, PA 19104; (215)382-6680.
A non-profit clinical, training, and research organization providing couple, individual, family and sex therapy. Nine locations throughout the Greater Philadelphia area. Sliding fee scale.

Dental

DENTAL RESOURCE GROUP, LTD.
Burton E. Balkin, D.M.D.
Implantology/Implant Dentistry
632 Montgomery Ave., Narberth, PA 19072-2031; (610)664-6700.
Dr. Balkin is board certified by the American Board of Oral Implantology/Implant Dentistry. The practice provides comprehensive dental implant treatment, including consultation, diagnosis, implant insertion surgery, implant prostheses and bone regenerative procedures.

David P. DiGiallorenzo, D.M.D.
Periodontics, Oral Implantology
191 Presidential Blvd., Ste. BS-17, BalaCynwyd, PA 19004; (610)664-3230.
State-of-the-art therapy including oral implantology, non-surgical and reconstructive periodontics, advanced case types, head and neck pain. Asleep or awake. Complimentary consultation. Italian spoken.

Richard S. Tobey, Jr., D.M.D., M.S
Prosthodontics, Periodontics
1601 Walnut St., Medical Arts Bldg., Ste. 822, Philadelphia, PA 19102; (215)557-7979.
For the highest level of care in a warm, personal environment, Dr. Tobey's practice specializes in dental implantology, dental reconstruction, periodontics and cosmetic dentistry, as well as quality general care. Foreign languages spoken: French.

ROSENBERG, GIAN-GRASSO ASSOCIATES
Edwin S. Rosenberg, B.D.S., H.DIP., DENT., D.M.D., Joseph E. Gian-Grasso, D.M.D., Farshid Sanavi, D.M.D., Ph.D., James Torosian, D.M.D., Barry Kayne, D.D.S.
Periodontics and Implant Dentistry
Ste. 1408, 1500 Locust St., Philadelphia, PA 19102-4314; (215)732-4450.
This comprehensive dental practice specializes in periodontics and implant dentistry. Drs. Edwin S. Rosenberg and Joseph Gian-Grasso are Board-Certified Diplomats of the American Board of Periodontology. Dr. Rosenberg is President of the Academy of Osseointegration.

Dermatology

ALLEGHENY UNIVERSITY OF THE HEALTH SCIENCES
Island Avenue Medical Practice, Ellen Burov, M.D.
2901 S. Island Ave., Philadelphia, PA 19153; (215)365-7900.
Dr. Burov's practice includes general and cosmetic dermatology, skin cancer diagnosis and treatment and laser surgery (tattoo removals and treatment of vascular lesions.) Her special interests include contact dermatitis and nail diseases.

ALLEGHENY UNIVERSITY OF THE HEALTH SCIENCES
Josepha Bueno DeVaro, M.D.
One Bala Plaza, 231 St. Asaphs Rd., Ste. 117, Bala Cynwyd, PA 19004; (610)660-7000.
Dr. Bueno DeVaro's practice includes general office dermatology, skin cancer diagnosis and

treatment, hair and nail disorders and cosmetic dermatology. Her special interests include dermatologic disease in the immunocompromised patient and women's dermatology.

Anne Marie Angeles, M.D.
Dermatology and Dermatologic Surgery
1440 McKean St., Philadelphia, PA 19145; (215)334-2238.
Board-certified. General Dermatology. Surgery for pigmented and non-pigmented lesions, skin cancers, warts. Chemical peels, sclerotherapy (spider veins). Laser surgery and laser skin resurfacing.

Arthur K. Balin, M.D., Ph.D., F.A.C.P.
MOHS Micrographic Surgery and Cutaneous Oncology, Dermatologic Cosmetic Surgery
2129 Providence Ave., Chester, PA 19013; (610)876-0200. New Media office scheduled to open Winter, 1996; (610)565-3300.
Board certified in 6 specialties. Skin cancer and aging skin specialist, MOHS micrographic surgery for skin cancer. Cosmetic skin surgery, hair transplants for balding, laser resurfacing for wrinkles, liposuction, lipoinjection, collagen.

Thomas D. Griffin, M.D., Graduate Dermatology Associates

Dermatopathology
1005 Pepper Pavilion, One Graduate Plaza, Philadelphia, PA 19146; (215)893-2717.
Specializing in cosmetic dermatology. Recognized as a Top Doc in hair transplantation. Performs laser resurfacing of wrinkles, acne scars, chemical peel, collagen, skin cancer surgery.

Loretta A. Pratt, M.D.
2129 Providence Ave., Chester, PA 19013; (610)876-0200, Media office (610)565-3300.
Board certified dermatologist specializing in skin problems of women. Individualized complexion evaluation, therapy for acne, aging, sun-damaged skin, laser for wrinkles, facial peels, collagen, sclerotherapy for spider veins.

Dermatopathology

JOHNSON & GRIFFIN DERMATOPATHOLOGY ASSOCIATES, P.C.
Waine C. Johnson, M.D., Thomas D. Griffin, M.D., Jacqueline Junkins-Hopkins, M.D.
137 S. Easton Road, Box 8, Glenside, PA 19038; (215)886-3074.
Specializing in the accurate interpretation of

The Joy of a Child Lasts a Lifetime...
Make this dream a reality for you or someone you love.

Practice Dedicated to the Treatment of Female and Male Infertility.

JEROME H. CHECK, M.D.

We offer a devoted, caring, knowledgeable staff with hours convenient to patient's needs.

Specializing In:
- In Vitro Fertilization
- GIFT • ZIFT • ICSI
- Ovulation Induction
- Therapeutic Artificial Insemination
- Hormonal Therapy

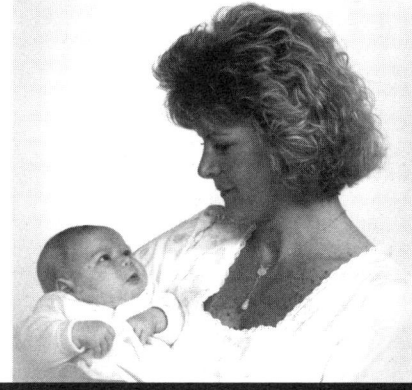

MARLTON, NJ	MELROSE PARK, PA	NEWARK, DE
609-751-5575	215-635-4400	302-633-0500
8002 E Greentree Commons	7447 Old York Road (Route 611)	620 Stanton Christiana Road
COOPER INSTITUTE FOR REPRODUCTIVE HORMONAL DISORDERS, P.C.	REPRODUCTIVE AND MEDICAL ENDOCRINE ASSOCIATES, P.C.	DELAWARE CENTER FOR INFERTILITY AND GYNECOLOGIC ENDOCRINOLOGY, P.A.
COOPER CENTER FOR IN VITRO FERTILIZATION, P.C.		

MOST INSURANCES ACCEPTED

skin biopsies performed by dermatologists, surgeons and primary care physicians. Consultations performed on biopsy slides.

Family Practice

Dr. Warren Mark Cohen, Ltd.
Emergency Medicine/Diagnostic Radiology
Jamestown Medical Bldg., Ste. 103, 525 Jamestown Ave., Philadelphia, PA 19128; (215)482-8556-7.
True Family/Holistic practice of medicine. Board-certified with three major specialties. Female physician associate for women's health needs.

FAMILY PRACTICE ASSOCIATES ALDEN PARK
John A. Heydt, M.D., Martin S. Lipsky, M.D. Russell C. Maulitz, M.D., Ph.D., Marc C. Newman, M.D., Marna R. Sternbach, M.D.
Cambridge Bldg., Suites 109-110, 2967 W. Schoolhouse Lane, Philadelphia, PA 19144; (215)844-2880; 6607 Ridge Ave., Philadelphia, PA 19128; (215)482-0550.
This practice offers primary care for the entire family. The physicians have special expertise in geriatrics, sports medicine, counseling, women's health, child and adolescent medicine. The physicians are all board-certified faculty at Allegheny University of the Health Sciences. They offer same day appointments and have day and evening hours.

Robert G. Rothberg, D.O.
Rheumatology
616 South Ave., Secane, PA 19018; (610)544-3991.
40 years family practice, concerned, involved, conscientious, warm family doctor. Still makes house calls, mostly by bicycle.

Gastroenterology

CROHN'S & COLITIS FOUNDATION OF AMERICA
521 Bustleton Pike, Feasterville, PA 19053; (215)396-9100.
A voluntary non-profit organization to raise funds for research for Crohn's disease and ulcerative colitis and provide education/support services for patients and their families.

GRADUATE HOSPITAL GASTROENTEROLOGY ASSOCIATES, P.C.
George Ahtaridis, M.D., Steven Greenfield, M.D., S. Philip Bralow, M.D., Jeffrey N. Retig, M.D., Anthony Infantolino, M.D., David Katzka, M.D., Donald Caskell, M.D.
Esophageal/Pancreatic/Liver Disease
Pepper Pavilion, 1800 Lombard St., Ste. 100, Philadelphia, PA 19146; (215)893-2532, and 2300 S. Broad St., Ste. 202, Philadelphia, PA 19148; (215)336-9420, and 47 Copley Road, Upper Darby, PA 19082; (610)352-4426.
In addition to general gastroenterology, we offer areas of subspecialization so that patients with atypical or complicated gastrointestinal problems may also receive expert care.

THOMAS JEFFERSON UNIVERSITY DIGESTIVE DISEASE CENTER
132 S. 10th St., 480 Main Bldg., Philadelphia, PA 19107; (215)955-8900.
State-of-the-art facility dedicated to the diagnosis, treatment and research of gastrointestinal and liver disorders. Our board-certified physicians are proficient in all diagnostic and therapeutic endoscopic/laser procedures.

General and Oncologic Surgery

Thomas G. Frazier, M.D.
Breast Disease
101 Bryn Mawr Ave., Ste. 201, Bryn Mawr, PA 19010; (610)520-0700.
Specializing in oncologic and general surgery, emphasizing diseases of the breast. Offering superb personal care using state-of-the-art techniques in diagnosis and treatment.

General Practice

Vincent E. Baldino, D.O., P.C., Joseph Mangel, D.O., Michael J. Attanasio, D.O.
Family Medicine/Internal Medicine
1701 Ritner St., Philadelphia, PA 19145; (215)336-2145 and 5737 Chester Ave., Philadelphia, PA 19143; (215)726-1411.
Board certified physicians specializing in family and internal medicine. All ages accepted and most insurances accepted. Please call for appointment-evening and Saturday hours available.

General Surgery

John D. Angstadt, M.D.
Laparoscopic Surgery, Oncologic Surgery
101 Bryn Mawr Ave., Ste. 201, Bryn Mawr, PA 19101; (610)520-0700.
Specializing in general and oncologic surgery with particular emphasis in laparoscopic surgery. Offering excellence in patient care using state-of-the-art technique.

ASSOCIATED SURGEONS, P.C.
Colon and Rectal Surgery, Vascular Surgery
21 W. Fornance St., Norristown, PA 19401; (610)279-3300.
A multispecialty surgical group offering the latest techniques in general, colon and rectal, breast, vascular, thoracic and laparoscopic

surgery. We participate with most major insurances.

Gordon S. Clement, M.D., F.A.C.S., John J. Flanagan, Jr., M.D.
General Thoracic Surgery
21 W. Fornance St., Norristown, PA 19401; (610)279-3300.
Board-certified surgeons offering full treatment options of laparoscopic hernia repair and other laparoscopic procedures. Laparoscopic surgical procedures often have less pain and faster recovery times.

John J. Flanagan, Jr., M.D.
Vascular Surgery
21 W. Fornance St., Norristown, PA 19401; (610)279-3300.
Treatment and evaluation of both arterial and venous disease by board-certified surgeon. Outpatient sclerotherapy for venous varicosities and spider veins is offered.

David Rose, M.D.
Laparoscopic Surgery
101 Bryn Mawr Ave., Ste. 201, Bryn Mawr, PA 19101; (610)520-0700.
Specializing in general and oncologic surgery with particular emphasis in laparoscopic surgery. Offering excellence in patient care using state-of-the-art technique.

THOMAS JEFFERSON UNIVERSITY DEPARTMENT OF SURGERY
1025 Walnut St., Ste. 605 College, Philadelphia, PA 19107; (215)955-6411.
Board-certified surgeons specializing in cardiothoracic, colon and rectal, pediatric, general, transplant, trauma, and vascular surgery. Setting the standards for surgical care for over a century and half.

VALLEY FORGE SURGICAL ASSOCIATES, LTD.
Wasfy F. Fahmy, M.D., F.A.C.S., F.I.C.S., Deborah M. Rosa, M.D., F.A.C.S.
Peripheral, Thoracic and Endoscopic Surgery
750 S. Main St., Ste. 300, Phoenixville, PA 19460; (610)935-7772.
Fellows of American College of Surgeons and International College of Surgeons.

Geriatrics

SENIOR HEALTH ASSOCIATES FROM PHILADELPHIA GERIATRIC CENTER AND TEMPLE UNIVERSITY HEALTH SYSTEM
Martin Leicht, M.D., Alan Malkin, M.D.,

One out of every two women past menopause has osteoporosis.

~

Don't wait for a fracture to find out if you're the one.

The good news is that osteoporosis is preventable and treatable. The Women's Center at Montgomery Hospital Medical Center, 1330 Powell Street, Norristown, now offers a safe, painless and non-invasive test that takes only minutes to complete. The test can determine the current status of your bones and help your doctor assess your risk of developing osteoporosis. To learn more about osteoporosis testing and treatment options call:

~ 610-270-BONE ~

Linda P. Clark, M.D., Robert Gordon, M.D., Susan Denman, M.D., Charles Bongiorno M.D., Rebecca Wang, M.D., Helen Feit, M.D., Heidi Wittels, M.D.
Internal Medicine

Friends Hall Physicians Bldg., 7604 Central Ave., Philadelphia, PA 19111-2401; (215)742-2100; PGC Campus, 5301 Old York Rd., Philadelphia, PA 19141-2996; (215)324-5303.

Physicians who specialize in caring for seniors. Including: preventive medicine, internal medicine, arthritis, rehabilitation, diabetes, heart disease, intestinal disorders, Alzheimer's disease and memory disorders.

Gynecologic Oncology

Joel Noumoff, M.D., Randolph Deger, M.D.
Division of Gynecolgic Oncology, Crozer-Chester Medical Center, One Medical Center Blvd., Upland, PA 19013; (610)876-9640.

Through our advanced specialty training, we possess the special skills needed for the care of women with pre-malignant conditions of the ovaries, fallopian tubes, uterus, cervix, vulva and vagina. We emphasize a collaborative relationship with the patient and her primary physician.

Hair Replacement

COS MED HAIR TRANSPLANT AND TREATMENT CENTER
General Manager -Ernesto Altomari
7425 Old York Rd., Melrose Park, PA 19027; (215)635-5580, 1 (800)99-COS-MED.

Specializing in hair transplants and hair replacement units. National Hair Loss Educator and Board-Certified General Surgeon dedicated to high quality hair loss solutions at competitive prices. Free consultations available.

Hand Surgery

HAND SURGERY AND THERAPY ASSOCIATES
William H. Kirkpatrick, M.D.
Surgery and Rehabilitation of the Hand and Upper Extremity

Bryn Mawr Medical Office Bldg., N., 830 Old Lancaster Rd., Ste. 301, Bryn Mawr, PA 19010; (610)527-9000.

Board-certified in Orthopaedic and Hand Surgery. Practice devoted exclusively to injuries and problems of the hand and upper extremity. Specialties: carpal tunnel syndrome,

---

Starkey TYMPANETTE Micro-Canal Hearing Instrument

We accept physician's referrals for hearing assessment...

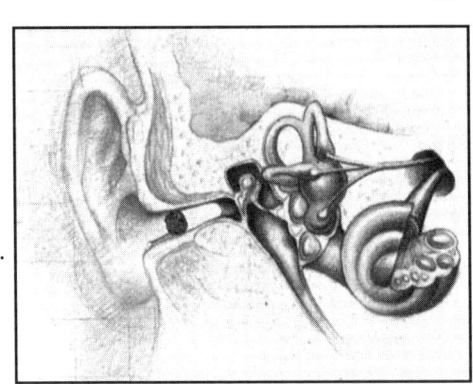

...and participate in all major health plans.

Contact a location nearest you:

JACOBSON'S HEARING AID CENTER	JENKINTOWN HEARING AID CENTER
108 S. 16th Street	179 Washington Lane
Philadelphia, PA 19102	Jenkintown, PA 19046
James Saad B.C./H.I.S. Richard Saad	Peter Ryan B.C./H.I.S.
Philadelphia: (215) 563-2403	Philadelphia: (215) 886-2268
New Jersey: (800) 869-4327	Fax: (215) 886-6016

arthritis, wrist pain, sports injuries, tendon and ligament injuries, fractures, nerve disorders, chronic pain. Clinical Asst. Professor of Orthopaedic Surgery, Jefferson Hospital; Attending Surgeon, Bryn Mawr Hospital. Hand Therapy provided on-site by Bryn Mawr Rehab.

Hearing Aids

JENKINTOWN HEARING AID CENTER INC.
Peter Ryan, B.S., B.H.I./H.I.S.
Hearing Assessment/Ear Evaluation
179 Washington Ln., Jenkintown, PA 19046; (215)886-2268, Fax (215)886-6016.
Board-certified hearing instrument specialists. Specific areas of expertise: micro canal hearing instruments, hearing testing, video otocopy, real ear measurement. We specialize in 100% Digital Hearing systems "Senso" by Widex. Foreign Language: American Sign Language.

Hepatic and Biliary Diseases

ALBERT EINSTEIN CENTER FOR LIVER DISEASE AND TRANSPLANTATION
Liver Surgery and Transplant
5401 Old York Rd., Ste. 509, Philadelphia, PA 19141; (215)456-8242.
Multidisciplinary, comprehensive care of the patient with liver disease, including major liver surgery and transplantation. Dedicated medical, surgical, and nursing staff to fit patients' needs—with a personal touch.

Home Health Care

HOMEMAKER SERVICE OF THE METROPOLITAN AREA, INC.
801 Arch St., Ground Floor, Philadelphia, PA 19107; (215)592-0002.
Medicare certified home care agency providing homemaker/home health aides, nursing, speech, physical and occupational therapies and social services to medically and physically disabled people.

PROCARE HEALTH SERVICES, INC.
140 Tunbridge Rd., Haverford, PA 19041; (610)645-7515.
Provides complete staffing of nurses, aides, homemakers, I.V., physical, occupational and speech therapy as well as pediatric services. Call 24 hours a day. Medicare, Medicaid, HMO's and private insurance accepted.

VISITING NURSE ASSOCIATION OF GREATER PHILADELPHIA
Hospice
Monroe Office Center, 1 Winding Dr., Philadelphia, PA 19131; (215)473-7600.
The Visiting Nurse Association of Greater Philadelphia, founded in 1886, provides home health care and hospice services throughout southeastern Pennsylvania and southern New Jersey to patients of all ages. (215)473-7600; Toll Free: 1(800)862-1180.

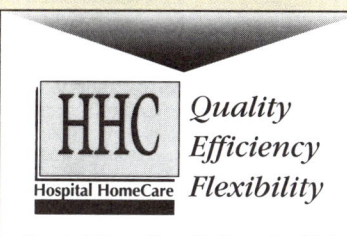

HHC — Hospital HomeCare
Quality
Efficiency
Flexibility

Hospital Home Care, Medicare-Certified, accredited with commendation by JCAHO, provides superior healthcare in a home setting - from skilled services for newborns to rehabilitation therapy for the elderly.

Providing Quality Home Healthcare Through the Generations

1-800-228-3299

Hypnotherapy

Lori S. Lewis, M.Ed., A.C.H., Certified Clinical Hypnotherapist
The Becoming Center, 250 N. Bethlehem Pk., Ambler, PA 19002; (215)407-1342.
Hypnotherapy for mind/body integration. Smoking cessation, eating disorders, insomnia, pain control, stress reduction. Also specializing in shyness, self-esteem, and self-confidence problems.

Infectious Diseases

ALLEGHENY UNIVERSITY OF THE HEALTH SCIENCES
Matthew E. Levison, M.D., Donald Kaye, M.D., Oksana M. Korzeniowski, M.D., Caroline Johnson, M.D., Allan Tunkel, M.D., Marla J. Gold, M.D., Judith A. O'Donnell, M.D., Allison Sigler, M.D., John Molavi, M.D, Craig Wood, M.D., Emily Blumberg, M.D., Amy Fuchs, M.D.
Allegheny University Hospitals, Center City formerly Hahnemann University Hospital, Broad and Vine Sts., Philadelphia, PA 19102; (215)762-8055; Allegheny University Hospitals, East Falls formerly Medical College of Pennsylvania Hospital, 3300 Henry Ave., Philadelphia, PA 19129; (215)842-6975.
Internationally recognized specialists provide diagnosis and treatment of infectious and tropical diseases. Clinics provide expert HIV-related health and support services. In addition, at Allegheny East Falls, a Travel Health Center

provides immunizations, health care and advice on travel precautions abroad.

DELAWARE VALLEY I.D. ASSOCIATES
Jerome Santoro, M.D., F.A.C.P., Mark Ingerman, M.D., F.A.C.P., Lawrence L. Livornese Jr., M.D., F.A.C.P.
Travel Health
Lankenau Medical Bldg. E., Ste. 467, Wynnewood, PA 19096; (610)896-0210.
Three-member group practice of board-certified infectious disease specialists with special interest in travel health immunization, Lyme disease, and disease caused by infectious agents.

Infertility

MAIN LINE FERTILITY AND REPRODUCTIVE MEDICINE
William H. Pfeffer, M.D., Michael J. Glassner, M.D.
1 Lankenau Medical Bldg. E., Ste. 563, 100 Lancaster Ave., Wynnewood, PA 19096; (610)649-0500; Paoli Pointe, Ste. 100, 11 Industrial Blvd., Paoli, PA 19301; (610)993-8200.
Specializing in infertility and gynecologic care in a personalized, informed and warm atmosphere. Advanced laparoscopic/hysteroscopic and microscopic surgery, insemination, IVF and GIFT. Many insurance plans accepted.

PENNSYLVANIA REPRODUCTIVE ASSOCIATES
Stephen L. Corson, M.D., Frances R. Batzer, M.D., Benjamin Gocial, M.D., Maureen Kelly, M.D., Jacqueline N. Gutmann, M.D., Leonore Huppert, M.D., Andre Denis, M.D., Louis Manara, M.D.
Spruce Bldg., Suite 786, Pennsylvania Hospital, 800 Spruce St., Philadelphia, PA 19107; (215) 829-5095; 5217 Militia Hill Rd., Plymouth Meeting, PA 19462; (610) 834-1140.
Focused on IVT, GIFT, ICSI, cryopreservation, Egg Donor Program, Gestational Carrier Program. Psychological counseling and support groups.

PHILADELPHIA FERTILITY INSTITUTE
Stephen L. Corson, M.D., Frances R. Batzer, M.D., Benjamin Gocial, M.D., Maureen Kelly, M.D., Jacqueline N. Gutmann, M.D.
815 Locust St., Philadelphia, PA 19107; (215)922-2206 and 5217 Militia Hill Rd., Plymouth Mtg., PA 19462; (610)834-1230 and 820 Town Center Dr., Ste. 120, Langhorne, PA 19047; (215)757-4440.
Philadelphia Fertility Institute. Focused on reproductive assessment and treatment of infertility, endocrine disorders, endometriosis, pelvic pain, ovulation induction, artificial insemination, IVF/GIFT and gynecologic surgery.

Internal Medicine

BENJAMIN FRANKLIN CENTER FOR HEALTH OF PENNSYLVANIA HOSPITAL
Steven A. Silber, M.D., F.A.C.P., Bradley W. Fenton, M.D., Adam C. Sobel, M.D.
Preventive Medicine
620 Chestnut St., Philadelphia, PA 19106; (215)829-8660.
Offering a multidisciplinary approach to disease prevention and rehabilitation. Programs include: Internal medicine private practice, risk reduction, cardiac and pulmonary rehabilitation, executive health, weight management.

FAMILY PRACTICE ASSOCIATES ALDEN PARK
Russell C. Maulitz, M.D., Ph.D.
Cambridge Bldg., Suites 109-110, 2967 W. Schoolhouse Lane, Philadelphia, PA 19144; (215)844-2880.
Dr. Maulitz, a board certified physician in internal medicine, offers general medicine for adults desiring consultative or ongoing empathetic care.**Michael Kirschbaum, D.O.**

Cardiology, Cardiovascular Medicine
G.S.B. Bldg., Suite 400, City and Belmont Aves., Bala Cynwyd, PA 19004; (610)667-8558.
Board-certified, Deborah trained, Fellow American College of Cardiology, textbooks published, nationally known, highest quality support staff. Consultation, stress testing, treatment of all cardiovascular problems. Weekdays, evenings.

Allan Koff, D.O. F.A.C.O.I., F.A.C.P., L.T.D., Marvin Schatz, D.O., F.A.C.O.I.
Klein Prof. Office Bldg., 5401 Old York Rd., Ste. 503, Philadelphia, PA 19141; (215)457-7188 and 9622 Bustleton Prof. Bldg., Ste. 1, Philadelphia, PA 19115; (215)969-5333 and Graduate Health System, Parkview Hospital, Physician's Medical Office Bldg., 1331 E. Wyoming Ave., Ste. 4110; (215)533-0909.
Focusing not only on symptoms, but on the total health of our patients. We involve the patient in a course of evaluation and treatment options.

Edward B. Ruby, M.D.
Endocrinology, Diabetes
1015 Chestnut St., Ste. 910, Philadelphia, PA 19107; (215)955-7285.
Patients seen chiefly have endocrine disorders, diabetes or metabolic disorders. This includes pituitary, thyroid, adrenal, calcium, lipid and metabolic bone disease. Bone densitometer on premises.

PHILADELPHIA HEALTH ASSOCIATES, UNIVERSITY CITY MEDICAL CENTER
Pediatrics, Dermatology, Podiatry, Surgery

3550 Market St., Philadelphia, PA 19104; (215)823-8660, and Bourse Bldg. Medical Center, 5th and Market Sts., 7th Fl., Philadelphia, PA 19106; (215)625-9100.

Multi-specialty medical group comprised of physicians and nurse practitioners providing primary care to seniors, adults, adolescents, and children, with an emphasis on preventive care.

Lipid and Endocrine Disorders

THE LIPID DISORDERS CENTER AT ALLEGHENY UNIVERSITY HOSPITALS EAST FALLS
David M. Capuzzi, M.D., Ph.D., John M. Morgan, M.D., Diane Morano, M.S., R.D., C.D.E.
Formerly Medical College of Pennsylvania Hospital, 3300 Henry Ave., Philadelphia, PA 19129; (215)842-6734.

The major center in the tri-state area for the evaluation, prevention and treatment of cholesterol, diabetic and metabolic disorder; addressing genetic and lifestyle issues; providing premium medical and nutritional care; superior physician training; certified laboratory and exceptional clinical research.

Mammography and Breast Ultrasound

Diagnostic Breast Center
101 Bryn Mawr Ave., Ste. 201, Bryn Mawr, PA 19101; (610)520-0900.

Providing women with mammogram and breast ultrasound studies using state-of-the-art techniques and equipment.

Medical Group Practice

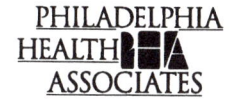

PHILADELPHIA HEALTH ASSOCIATES

Adult, Pediatric, Adolescent Medicine, and Specialty Care

University City Medical Center
(215) 823-8660

Bourse Building Medical Center
(215) 625-9100

— Evening Hours —

Appointments • Urgent Care

Medical Oncology

Sally D. Lane, M.D., Mary Denshaw Burke, M.D.
Hematology
5735 Ridge Ave., Ste. 103, Philadelphia, PA 19128; (215)487-3070.

Our practice provides general medical oncology and hematology services by board certified physicians in a friendly and personal setting. Convenient to public transportation in Roxborough.

Menopause

Philadelphia Menopause Group, Frances R. Batzer, M.D., Maureen Kelly, M.D., Jacqueline N. Gutmann, M.D., Stephen L. Corson, M.D., Benjamin Gocial, M.D.
815 Locust St., Philadelphia, PA 19107; (215)922-2206; 5217 Militia Hill Rd., Plymouth Mtg., PA 19462; (610)834-1230; 820 Town Center Dr., Suite 120, Langhorne, PA 19047; (215)757-4440.

Focused on individual evaluation of hormonal status, HRT, osteoporosis, bone density evaluation, cardiovascular risks, support groups, nutrition, exercise counseling. Routine gynecology, surgery.

Nephrology

ALLEGHENY UNIVERSITY OF THE HEALTH SCIENCES
Allegheny University Hospitals, Center City formerly Hahnemann University Hospital, 1427 Vine St, 7th fl., Philadelphia, PA 19102; (215)762-7848, Charles Swartz, M.D., Robert Chvala, M.D., Kwan E. Kim, M.D., Patricia Lyons, M.D.; Allegheny University Hospitals, East Falls formerly Medical College of Pennsylvania Hospital, 3300 Henry Ave., Philadelphia, PA 19129; (215)842-6988, Ziauddin Ahmed, M.D., Bonita Falkner, M.D., Jean Lee, M.D., Sandra P. Levinson, M.D., Steven J. Peitzman, M.D.; Clinical Nephrology Associates; 205 N. Broad St., Ste. 600, Philadelphia, PA 19107; (215)762-8345; 1440 McKean St., Philadelphia, PA 19145; (215)334-2237, Joseph H. Brezin, M.D., Larry Krevolin, D.O., M. Blanche Lim, M.D., Maria Mendez, M.D., Arthur R. Olshan, M.D., Ph.D., John F.Shulman, M.D.; W. Jersey Medical Plaza, 90 Brick Rd., Ste. 104, Marlton, NJ 08053; (609)596-7149; Woodbury Medical Center, 17 W. Red Bank Ave., Ste. 206, Woodbury, NJ 08096; (609)384-0147; 1809-13 Oregon Ave., Philadelphia, PA 19145; (215)551-4606, Joseph F. Girone, M.D.

Board certified specialists in high blood

pressure and kidney diseases including stones, urinary infections, kidney failure, dialysis and transplantation. Accepts most insurances and managed care plans. Foreign languages spoken include: Mandarin, Spanish, Koren, Bengali, Hini, Urdu, Yiddish.

KIDNEY DISEASE INTERVENTION PROGRAM
Alan Wasserstein, M.D., Director, Sidney Kobrin, M.D.
Hospital of the University of Pennsylvania, 3400 Spruce St., 210 White Bldg., Philadelphia, PA 19104; (215)662-3627.

The Kidney Disease Intervention Program at Penn treats patients with impairment of kidney function with low-protein diet to prevent progressive kidney failure.

STONE EVALUATION CENTER
Alan S. Wasserstein, M.D., Director
Hospital of the University of Pennsylvania, 3400 Spruce St., 210 White Bldg., Philadelphia, PA 19104; (215)662-3627.

The Stone Center performs metabolic evaluation in patients with kidney stones and offers complete dietary and lifestyle advice to prevent future stone growth or recurrence.

Neurology

EINSTEIN NEUROLOGY ASSOCIATES
Drs. M. Moster, J. Burke, M. Faynberg, G. Horowitz, M. McGlamery, N. Volpe, M. Zalewska.
5401 Old York Rd., Klein Bldg., Ste. 300, Philadelphia, PA 19141; (215)456-7190.

Board-certified physicians providing care in neurology including neuro-ophthalmology, neuromuscular, stroke, behavioral, epilepsy and pain. Neurodiagnostics: EEG, EMG, EP's, brain mapping and oculomotor-ENG.

GRADUATE NEUROLOGICAL CENTER, P.C.
Howard I. Hurtig, M.D., Matthew B. Stern, M.D., Michael R. Sperling, M.D., Joyce Liporace, M.D., Amy Colcher, M.D., Bryan DeSouza, M.D., Joseph Sirven, M.D.
Movement Disorders/Epilepsy
Ste. 900, Pepper Pavillion, 1800 Lombard St., Philadelphia, PA 19146; (215)893-2440.

The Parkinson's Disease and Movement Disorders Center and the Comprehensive Epilepsy Center specialize in the most advanced medical and surgical therapies.

Elliott Schulman, M.D.
Headache Management
Center for Headache Management, Crozer-Keystone Healthplex, Medical Office Pavilion, 196 W. Sproul Rd., Springfield, PA 19064; (610)604-9730.

Physician-led team dedicated to the treatment of headaches. Caring, professional staff responsive to individual patient needs. Emphasis on wellness and education. Offers headache support group, open to the community. Convenient access from tri-state area via the Blue Route.

DEPARTMENT OF NEUROLOGY, UNIVERSITY OF PENNSYLVANIA MEDICAL CENTER
Robert L. Barchi, M.D., Ph.D, Chair, Arthur K. Asbury, M.D., ViceChair, David E. Pleasure, M.D., Vice Chair, William J. Bank, M.D.,John E. Bevilacqua, M.D., Shawn J. Bird, M.D., Mark J. Brown, M.D.,Christopher M. Clark, M.D., Mark D'Esposito, M.D., John A. Detre, M.D., Marc A. Dichter, M.D., Ph.D, Roger E. Farber, M.D., John T.Farrar, M.D., Kenneth H. Fishbeck, M.D., Jacqueline A. French, M.D., Steven Galetta, M.D., Guila Glosser, Ph.D, Francisco Gonzales-Scarano, M.D., Murray Grossman, M.D., Ed.D, Dennis L. Kolson, M.D., Ph.D, Grant T. Liu, M.D., Joan E. Mollman, M.D., AmyA. Pruitt, M.D., Eric C. Raps, M.D., Martin Reivich, M.D., A.M. Rostami, M.D., Ph.D., Steven S. Scherer, M.D., Ph.D., Donald Schotland, M.D., Michael E. Selzer, M.D., Ph.D., Donald H. Silberberg, M.D., Mark M. Stecker, M.D., Ph.D., James W. Teener, M.D.
3 West Gates, 34th and Spruce Sts., Philadelphia, Pa 19104; (215)662-2700.

Penn's Department of Neurology, the first in the United States, provides care for patients with diseases of the brain, spinal cord, nerve or muscle.

Neurosurgery

ALLEGHENY UNIVERSITY OF THE HEALTH SCIENCES
Thomas A. Gennarelli, M.D., Perry Black, M.D., Leonard Bruno, M.D., Kenneth F. Casey, M.D., Thomas McCormack, M.D., Gerri McGinnis, Ph.D., Daniel K. O'Rourke, M.D., Gene Salkind, M.D., Alan R. Turtz, M.D.
Allegheny University Hospitals, Center City formerly Hahnemann University Hospital, Broad and Vine Sts., Philadelphia, PA 19102; (215)762-3131; Allegheny University Hospitals, East Falls formerly Medical College of Pennsylvania Hospital, 3300 Henry Ave., Philadelphia, PA 19129; Allegheny University Hospitals, Bucks County formerly Bucks County Hospital, 225 Newtown Rd., Warminster, PA 18974; Allegheny University Hospitals, Elkins Park formerly Elkins Park Hospital, 60 E. Township Line Rd., Elkins Pk., PA 19117; 1601 Walnut St., Ste. 908, Philadelphia, PA 19102.

The department maintains medical and surgical expertise in the practice of neurosurgery for treatment of cranial, spinal and peripheral nerve disorders including: brain tumors, brain injuries, brain infections and problems of cerebral circulation including aneurysm, AVM and stroke. Spinal disorders including stenosis, herniated disc, fracture, tumor and infection. The department performs specialized neurosurgery for epilepsy, Parkinson's Disease and hydrocephalus as well as stereotactic surgery and radiosurgery and can provide diagnostic neuropsychology, evaluate cognitive function and perform outpatient and intraoperative electrophysiologic testing and monitoring.

Division of Neurosurgery, University of Pennsylvania Medical Center, Eugene S. Flamm, M.D., Chief, Gordon H. Baltuch, M.D., Ph.D., Robert W. Hurst, M.D., Kevin D. Judy, M.D., Mark Kotapka, M.D., Paul J. Marcotte, M.D., Grant P. Stinson, M.D., Eric L. Zager, M.D.
5 Silverstein, 34th and Spruce Sts., Philadelphia, PA 19104; (215)662-3487.
The Division of Neurosurgery includes multidisciplinary programs in cerebrovascular disease, brain and cranial base tumors, spine, nervous system trauma, peripheral nerves, surgical treatment of epilepsy, interventional neuroradiology, and radiosurgery. Each member has an area of interest and expertise beyond his responsiblities to the general neurosurgical problems.

Nurse-Midwifery

PINE MIDWIFERY ASSOCIATES
Libby Cohen, C.N.M., Jane Silver Hoff, C.N.M.
Ob/Gyn
829 Spruce St., Ste. 407, Philadelphia, PA 19107; (215)625-9320.
Personalized gynecologic and prenatal care with time for questions and honest answers. Your birth, your choice-birthing suite or hospital, jacuzzi or epidural; caring midwifery support always. Evening hours downtown and in our City Line office.

OB/GYN

ABINGTON PERINATAL ASSOCIATES, PC
Linda K. Dunn, M.D., Frank J. Craparo, M.D., Richard A. Latta, M.D., Stephen J. Smith, M.D., Marc F. Rosenn, M.D.
Maternal-Fetal Medicine and Genetics
Abington Memorial Hospital,1235 Old York Rd.,

Care for Women
OF ALL AGES

❧ Board Certified in Obstetrics & Gynecology
❧ Specialty Training in High Risk Obstetrics
❧ Prenatal Care & Delivery ❧ Infertility
❧ Cancer Screening & Treatment
❧ Contraception & Menopause
❧ Treatment of Menstrual Disorders

NANCY K. BRIDGENS, DO

CHESTER VALLEY OBSTETRICS & GYNECOLOGY, INC.
649 North Lewis Road, Suite 240, Limerick, PA 19468
Phone (610) 495-0400   Fax (610) 495-5522

Convenient Location with Evening Hours Available.

Ste. 119, Abington, PA 19001; (215)576-4575.
One of Philadelphia's leading perinatal groups isn't in Philadelphia. Consultation and management services for women with complicated pregnancies and serious maternal illnesses. Comprehensive ultrasound services, prenatal diagnostic procedures (CVS, amnio, PUBS) and genetic counseling are offered. Foreign language spoken: Spanish.

CHESTER VALLEY OBSTETRICS AND GYNECOLOGY, INC.
Nancy K. Bridgens, D.O., F.A.C.O.O.G.
Perinatal Medicine
649 N. Lewis Rd., Ste. 240, Limerick, PA 19468; (610)495-0400.
Board-Certified obstetrical, gynecologist with specialty training in high risk obstetrics is dedicated to providing excellent individualized care to women of all ages. New patients welcome at our Limerick location.

GUILFOIL AND SULLIVAN OB/GYN ASSOCIATES
Daniel S. Guilfoil, M.D., Gail T. Sullivan, M.D.
2967 W. Schoolhouse Lane, Sts. 102-103, Philadelphia, PA 19144; (215)842-2244.
Maternity and gynecologic services for women of all ages. The doctors are committed to expert care with a personal approach, assuring patients a comfortable environment and individual care.

HEALTHPLEX OB/GYN
Mark Finnegan, M.D., John Burke, M.D., Ann Prodoehl, M.D., Joseph Sincavage, M.D.
Crozer-Chester Medical Center, Ste. 331, Upland, PA 19013; (610)867-0866; Ambulatory Care Pavilion, Ste. 208, 196 W. Sproul Rd., Springfield, PA 19064; (610)566-4061.
Caring, board-certified physicians make this OB/GYN office a place where women feel confident they are receiving state-of-the-art care.

MATERNITY AND WOMEN'S HEALTH
Earl Sands, M.D., Nicholas Chapis, M.D., Robert DiGregorio, D.O., Robert Neilson, M.D., Nancy Bridgens, D.O., Lee Zelley, M.D.
Pottstown Memorial Medical Center, 1600 E. High St., Pottstown, PA 19464; (610)327-7662.
Comprehensive services including obstetrics, gynecology, pregnancy, pre-natal care, family planning methods, contraception counseling, infertility, menopause, estrogen replacement, lamaze and refresher lamaze classes, VBAC classes.

Annette McDaniel-Turner, M.D., Patricia Hughes Jones, M.D.
241 S. 6th St., Ste. E, Philadelphia, PA 19106; (215)625-9594; 1 Bala Ave., Ste. 120, Bala Cynwyd, PA 19004; (610)667-4577.
Comprehensive Care-gynecologic surgery, obstetrical care. Specializing in menstrual disorders and fibroid uterus.

MEDPARTNERS/VANGUARD OB/GYN
Saul Jack, D.O., F.A.C.O.O.G.
Graduate Health Systems-City Ave. Hospital, Rowland Hall, 4190 City Ave., Ste. 411, Philadelphia, PA 19131; (215)871-1144.
Comprehensive gynecologic care including menopausal care and gynecologic surgery. Most insurances accepted.

NEMIROFF AND MELLEN ASSOCIATES
Richard L. Nemiroff, M.D., Drew Mellen, M.D.
301 S. 8th St., Ste. 3-D, Philadelphia, PA 19106; (215)829-5300.

PENN HEALTH FOR WOMEN
Michelle M. Battistini, M.D., Director, Todra L. Anderson, M.D., Michelle Berlin, M.D., Deborah A. Driscoll, M.D., Jane Fang, M.D., Valerie Weil Fornasieri, M.D., Laura Baum Holland, M.D., Samantha Pfeifer, M.D., Gita Singh, M.D., Richard Tureck, M.D., Andrea Boxer, Ph.D., Randi Cardonick, M.S., R.D.
Penn Medicine at King of Prussia, The Merion Bldg., Ste. 202A, 700 S. Henderson Rd., King of Prussia, PA 19406; (800)789-PENN.
Penn Health for Women specializes in: primary care, menopause, hormone replacement therapy, osteoporosis, gynecology, exercise, weight management, urinary incontinence, infertility, obstetrics, adolescent gynecology, and second opinions.

Jerrold M Snyder, D.O., F.A.C.O.O.G., Mortimer T. Nelson, M.D., F.A.C.O.G., F.A.C.S., Charlotte Dorko, C.R.N.P., R.N.C.
Oxford Square, Ste. 400, 360 Middletown Boulevard, Langhorne, PA 19047-1869; (215)750-7771.
Family centered obstetrics, gynecology, advanced laparoscopic surgery, hysteroscopy, laser surgery, endometriosis. We have a special interest in adolescent gynecology, perimenopause and menopausal management.

VAUGHN, RONNER AND ZADZIELSKI, INC.
Beverly M. Vaughn, M.D., Wanda Ronner, M.D., Elizabeth M. Zadzielski, M.D., Nina Mohammed, M.D., Jane A. Molinari, M.D.
700 Spruce St., Ste. B-01, Philadelphia, PA 19106; (215)829-7400.
All female OB/GYN practice affiliated with Pennsylvania Hospital. Providing comprehensive obstetric/gynecologic services, menopause management, and the latest in surgical techniques. Offices in Center City Philadelphia; Bala Cynwyd, PA; and Haddonfield, NJ.

Occupational Medicine
WORKWELL CLINICAL CARE ASSOCIATES

AT THE UNIVERSITY OF PENNSYLVANIA HEALTH SYSTEM

Carole N. Tinklepough, M.D.
700 S. Henderson Rd., Ste. 3043, King of Prussia, PA 19406; (610)768-9355.

Workwell is a full-service occupational medicine practice providing services including health examinations, drug and alcohol testing, workers compensation, injury treatment, case management and consultative services.

Oncology

FOX CHASE CANCER CENTER
Robert C. Young, M.D., F.A.C.P., President, Burton I. Eisenberg, M.D., F.A.S.C, Chairman, Surgical Oncology, Paul F. Engstrom, M.D., F.A.C.P., Senior Vice President, Population Science, Gerald E. Hanks, M.D., F.A.C.R., Chairman, Radiation Oncology, Robert F. Ozols, M.D.,Ph.D., Vice President, Medical Science.
7701 Burholme Ave., Philadelphia, PA 19111; (215)728-2570.

Fox Chase Cancer Center is one of 26 National Cancer Institute-designated comprehensive cancer centers in the nation. The Center's activities include basic and clinical research; prevention, detection and treatment of cancer; and community outreach.

UNIVERSITY OF PENNSYLVANIA CANCER CENTER
6 Penn Tower, 3400 Spruce St., Philadelphia, PA 19104; (800)383-UPCC.

A national leader in cancer care, this NCI-designated Comprehensive Cancer Center has 300 physicians and scientists specializing in cancer treatment and research.

Ophthalmology

EINSTEIN OPHTHALMOLOGY ASSOCIATES
Vincent K. Young, M.D.
5401 Old York Road, Klein Bldg., Ste. 205, Philadelphia, PA 19141; (215)456-7150.

Board-certified ophthalmologist providing comprehensive eye exams, treatment of eye disease, and eye surgery. Ophthalmology diagnostics: Contact lenses, low vision consultations, and optical shop.

KARP-GOLDMAN EYE ASSOCIATES, P.C.
Louis A. Karp, M.D., F.A.C.S., Stephen M. Goldman, M.D.
Ste. 100, Garfield Duncan Bldg., 700 Spruce

10,000 STEPS A DAY.

WHY SUFFER?

IT'S NO WONDER THAT 80 PERCENT OF AMERICANS WILL SUFFER FROM FOOT PAIN.

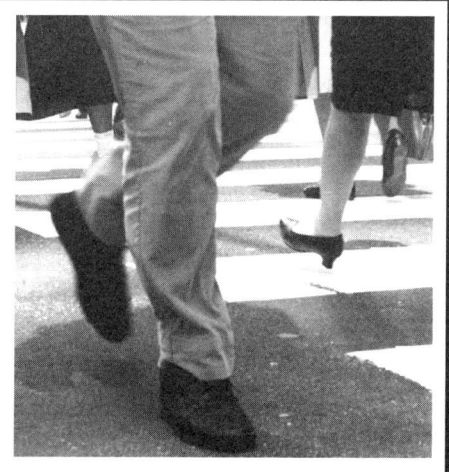

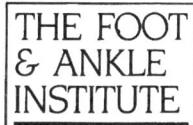

THE FOOT & ANKLE INSTITUTE
PENNSYLVANIA COLLEGE OF PODIATRIC MEDICINE™

- Personal attention and concern.
- The area's leading podiatric specialists.
- The latest diagnostic and treatment services.

8th & Race Sts. • Philadelphia, PA
215-238-6600

St., Philadelphia, PA 19106; (215)829-5311.
A general ophthalmology practice affiliated with Pennsylvania Hospital. Special interests: cataract and implant surgery, glaucoma management including laser and surgery, refractive surgery and contact-lens care.

KREMER LASER EYE CENTER
Frederic B. Kremer, M.D., George R. Pronesti, M.D., Allan E. Wulc, M.D., Peter V. Palena, M.D.
King of Prussia, Philadelphia, Pottstown, Hatboro; 1-800-694-EYES.
Specialists in laser refractive surgery for nearsightedness, farsightedness and astigmatism. Cataract surgery with no injections or stitches. Eye plastic surgery. Treatment for glaucoma and retina problems. Named in Philadelphia Magazine's Top Doctors issue.

Oral and Maxillofacial Surgery

E. Steven Moriconi, D.M.D.
Dental Implant Surgery, Temporomandibular Joint Surgery(TMJ)
609 Harper Ave., Jenkintown, PA 19046; (215)884-8263.
Board-certified in oral/maxillofacial surgery. Trained at University of Pennsylvania. Surgeon-in-Chief of dental division at Abington Memorial Hospital. 15 years experience and training in dental implant surgery, jaw surgery, TMJ.

Orthopedic Surgery

David J. Adams, M.D.
27 S. Bryn Mawr Ave., Bryn Mawr, PA 19010; (610)527-1762.
Temple graduate with 20 years experience in total joint-replacement surgery and general orthopedic care. Special expertise in spinal surgery.

Robert E. Booth, Jr., M.D.
Total Joint Replacement, Knee Revisions
Rothman Institute, 800 Spruce St., Philadelphia, PA 19107; (215)829-3458.
Practice specializes in problems of the knee and hip, with emphasis on surgical reconstruction of the knee. Foreign language spoken: French.

Nicholas A. DiNubile, M.D.
Sports Medicine, Arthroscopic Surgery
Office in Havertown, PA; (610)789-0150.
Practice focus: Knee disorders (injuries, rehabilitation, arthroscopy, surgery). Special advisor, President's Council on Physical Fitness and Sports. Orthopedist, Pennsylvania Ballet and Philadelphia 76ers. Faculty, Hospital of the University of Pennsylvania.

William D. Emper, M.D.
27 S. Bryn Mawr Ave., Bryn Mawr, PA 19010; (610)527-1762.
Practice of general orthopedic surgery specializing in sports medicine, arthroscopic surgery and joint replacement; surgery of the knee and shoulder. Team physician for Villanova University.

Gary Neil Goldstein, M.D.
Plastic Surgery and Hand Surgery
600 Somerdale Rd., #215, Voorhees, NJ 08043; (609)795-8884.
Only combined board-certified orthopedic and plastic surgeon in Philadelphia area. Specializing in carpal tunnel, cosmetic surgery and arthroscopic spine surgery.

Ronald B. Greene, M.D.
Arthroscopic Surgery, Joint Reconstruction
1525 Locust St., 2nd Floor, Philadelphia, PA 19102; (215)735-6104.
Arthroscopic surgery, including percutaneous lumbar disk surgery and TMJ arthroscopy; nerve compression syndromes, including carpal tunnel syndrome, and joint reconstruction and replacement.

JOYCE AND CAUTILLI PROFESSIONAL ASSOCIATION
Michael F. Joyce, M.D., Richard A. Cautilli, Sr., M.D., James V. Mackell, Jr., M.D., Richard A. Cautilli, Jr., M.D., George P. Cautilli, M.D., David A. Cautilli, M.D.
7922 Bustleton Ave., Philadelphia, PA 19152; (215)725-8500 and St. Mary Medical Office Bldg., Ste. 308, Langhorne, PA 19047; (215)702-9820 and St. Mary Wellness and Sports Care, Newtown, PA 18940; (215)702-9820.
Experienced professionals in adult and children's orthopaedics. Treating fractures; spine and foot problems. Subspecialty training in sports medicine, arthroscopy, hand surgery and joint replacement.

UNIVERSITY OF PENNSYLVANIA SHOULDER AND ELBOW SERVICE
Reconstructive Surgery of the Shoulder and Elbow
2 Silverstein Pavilion, 3400 Spruce St., Philadelphia, PA 19104; (215)349-8662.
The service includes four orthopedic surgeons specializing in the diagnosis and treatment of shoulder and elbow disorders, including rotator cuff injuries, unstable shoulders and elbows, arthoscopy and joint replacement.

Otolaryngology

ALLEGHENY UNIVERSITY OF THE HEALTH SCIENCES
Richard E. Hayden, M.D., F.A.C.S., Daniel G. Deschler, M.D., Steven E. Ladenheim, M.D., Raymond W. Lesser, M.D., F.A.C.S.,

Andrew M. Marlowe, M.D., Frank I. Marlowe, M.D., F.A.C.S., Matthew J. Nagorsky, M.D., F.A.C.S., Robert J. Wolfson, M.D., F.A.C.S., Seth Zwillenberg, M.D.
Head and Neck Surgery
Allegheny University Hospitals, Center City formerly Hahnemann University Hospital, 15th fl. S. Tower, Broad and Vine Sts., Philadelphia, PA 19102; (215)762-3700; Allegheny University Hospitals, East Falls formerly Medical College of Pennsylvania Hospital, 3300 Henry Ave., Philadelphia, PA 19129; (215)842-6569; Two Logan Sq., Ste. 1800, 18th and Arch Sts., Philadelphia, PA 19102; (215)762-4135; 1920 Chestnut St., Ste. 700, Philadelphia, PA 19103; (215)561-2546; W. Philadelphia Location, Myrin Bldg., Rm. 233, 39th and Market Sts., Philadelphia, PA 19104; (215)662-8230; N.E. Medical Center, 6579 Roosevelt Blvd., Philadelphia, PA 19149; (215)288-8300; Larchmont Medical Center, 210 Ark Rd., Bldg. #2, Mt. Laurel, NJ 08054; (609)235-0884.

As specialty care offices, this practice has a comprehensive array of diagnostic and support services, including head and neck surgery, facial plastic and reconstructive surgery, endoscopic sinus surgery, allergy testing, complete otologic testing for comprehensive evaluation of hearing loss, balance disorders, vertigo and voice evaluation including laryngeal videostroboscopy.

EAR, NOSE AND THROAT PROFESSIONAL ASSOCIATES
Max L. Ronis, M.D., F.A.C.S., Emil F. Liebman, M.D., F.A.C.S., Melvin L. Maslof, M.D., F.A.C.S.
Facial Plastic Reconstructive Surgery and Otology
2106 Spruce St., Philadelphia, PA 19103; (215)790-1553; 7906 Bustleton Ave., Philadelphia PA 19152; (215)342-9554; 850 W. Chester Pike, Havertown, PA 19083; (610)446-7960; 30 Washington Ave., Ste. E, Haddonfield, NJ 08033; (609)428-9314; 2835 S. Delsea Dr., Ste. D, Vineland, NJ 08360; (609)205-0800.

A University-based team with six decades combined experience. Each physician with special skills, including cosmetic surgery, sinus endoscopy, hearing disorders, allergy, pediatric/ENT and dizziness.

PROFESSIONAL OTOLARYNGOLOGY ASSOCIATES, M.D., P.A.
1307 White Horse Rd., Bldg. A, Voorhees, NJ 08043; (609)346-0200.

Practice limited to pediatric and adult diseases

Comprehensive Out Patient Physical Therapy and Rehabilitation Centers

Community Rehab Centers

Services
- Physical Therapy
- Hand Rehab
- Aquatic Rehab
- Fitness Programs
- On-site Employee Rehab and Prevention Programs

11 Convenient Locations in the Tri-State Area

Building Healthy, Active Lives

1•800•394•REHAB

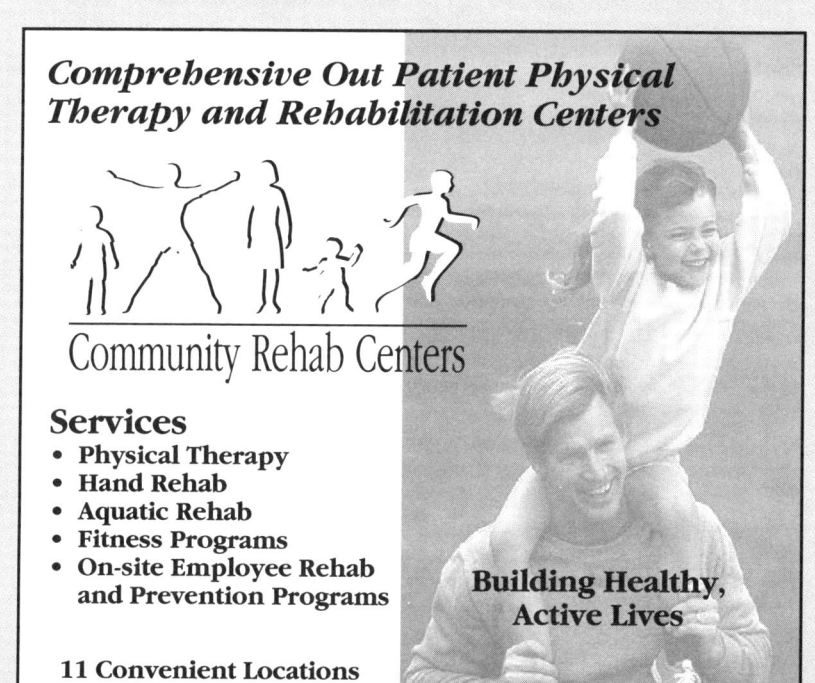

of the ears, nose and throat, facial plastic surgery, allergy, hearing and speech disorders, sleep disorders and snoring.

Robert Thayer Sataloff, M.D., D.M.A., Joseph R. Spiegel, M.D., F.A.C.S.
Neurotology, Voice
1721 Pine St., Philadelphia, PA 19103; (215)545-3322.
Board-certified ear, nose, and throat specialists. Dr. Sataloff's practice is limited to care of the professional voice and disorders of the ear-brain interface (hearing loss, tinnitus, dizziness, facial paralysis, acoustic neuroma, and other skull base tumors). He is Professor at Jefferson, Chairman of Otolaryngology at Graduate, and author of over 400 publications, including 13 books. Dr. Spiegel is Associate Professor at Jefferson, Vice Chairman at Graduate, and also a prolific author. He subspecializes in head and neck cancer, and sinonasal and swallowing disorders. He is also active in cosmetic/reconstructive surgery and general ear, nose and throat care. Both doctors treat adults and children.

WEDDINGTON ENT ASSOCIATES, INC.
Wayne P. Weddington Jr., M.D., William W. Banks, M.D.
827 E. Upsal St., Philadelphia, PA 19119; (215)438-3898 and Episcopal Hospital MAB Ste. 108, Front and Lehigh, Philadelphia, PA 19125; (215)427-7072.
Practice limited to general otolaryngology: ear nose and throat disorders and head and neck tumor surgery. Endoscopic sinus surgery and laser surgery available. By appt. only.

Pain Management

JEFFERSON PAIN CENTER
Evan D. Frank, M.D., Ph.D., Director.
Department of Anesthesiology, Thomas Jefferson University, Benjamin Franklin House, T-150, 834 Chestnut St., Philadelphia, PA 19107; (215)955-7300.
Board certified anesthesiologists and psychiatrist skilled in evaluation and triage of patients with chronic pain and cancer pain. Particularly skilled in interventional techniques for diagnosis and management of pain generators in back pain and neuropathic pain.

PROFESSIONAL PAIN MANAGEMENT ASSOCIATES, PA
Anesthesia
728 Black Horse Pike, Ste. C-6, Turnersville, NJ 08012.
We treat all types of pain: cancer, low back and neck, pancreatitis, RSD, headaches, neurapthics, etc., with the latest modalities and personalized care. Spanish and Korean spoken.

Pediatric Rehabilitation

CHILDREN'S SEASHORE HOUSE
3405 Civic Center Blvd., Philadelphia, PA 19104; (215)895-3600.
The nation's first hospital dedicated to helping children with physical and developmental disabilities and chronic illnesses achieve their full potential through excellence in patient care, research and training. Mark L. Batshaw, M.D., Developmental Pediatrics; Peggy S. Eicher, M.D., Dysphagia and Feeding Management; Susan E. Levy, M.D., Child Development and Learning Disabilities; Joyce E. Mauk, M.D., Autism and Severe Behavior Disorders; Marianne Mercugliano, M.D., Attention Deficit Hyperactivity Disorder, Stephanie Ried, M.D., Physical Medicine and Rehabilitation.

Pediatric Surgery

CHILDREN'S SURGICAL ASSOCIATES
Pediatric Urology
South Crossing Office Condominiums, 542 Lippincott Dr., Marlton, N.J. 08053; (609)342-3250.
Highly trained, extensively experienced, always mindful of the parent and the child, Children's Surgical Associates provides the finest operative care for your daughter or son.

PEDIATRIC CARDIOTHORACIC SURGERY
Thomas L. Spray, M.D., Chief, J. William Gaynor, M.D.
Pediatric Heart, Lung, and Heart and Lung Transplantation
Children's Hospital of Philadelphia, 34th St. and Civic Center Blvd., Philadelphia, PA 19104; (215)590-2708.
The Division of Cardiothoracic Surgery works with a multidisciplinary team of pediatric specialists in cardiology, anesthesiology, and critical care in the region's largest and most comprehensive program for children (birth through adolescence) with heart disease, and for adults with complex congenital heart disease. Specific areas of expertise include reconstructive surgery for complex congenital heart disease in newborns, surgical management of left ventricular outflow tract obstruction, and thoracic organ transplantation for end-stage or "inoperable" cardiovascular or pulmonary disease.

John P. Dormans, M.D., Director, Denis S. Drummond, M.D., Richard S. Davidson, M.D., John M. Flynn, M.D., John R. Gregg, M.D., Malcolm L. Ecker, M.D., Bong S. Lee, M.D.
Pediatric Orthopaedics
Children's Hospital office; (215)590-1527; King of Prussia office; (610)337-3232; Exton office; (610)594-9008; Voorhees, NJ office; (609)435-1300.

The Division of Orthopaedic Surgery provides diagnostic evaluation and treatment of all orthopedic conditions in children and adolescents, including spinal and foot deformities, sports injuries, tumors and chronic disorders. Office hours: Monday through Friday, 8:00 a.m. - 4:30 p.m.

N. Scott Adzick, M.D., Director, Timothy M. Crombleholme, M.D., Louise Schnaufer, M.D., Stephen J. Shochat, M.D., Perry W. Stafford, M.D., Paul T. Stockmann, M.D.
Pediatric General and Thoracic Surgery
The Children's Hospital of Philadelphia, 34th St. and Civic Center Blvd., Philadelphia, PA 19104; (215)590-2730; The Children's Hospital Specialty Care Center, Oaklands Corporate Center, 481 John Young Way, Exton, PA 19341; (610)594-9008; The Children's Hospital Specialty Care Center, Laurel Oak Corporate Center, 1040 Laurel Oak Road, Voorhees, NJ 08043; (609)435-1300.
A comprehensive service covering the surgical needs of children of all age groups with congenital malformations, endocrine disorders, vascular problems, tumors, injuries and various acquired conditions, including surgery and related endoscopy of the head and neck, thorax, abdomen, and extremities.

Leslie N. Sutton, M.D., Luis Schut, M.D., Ann-Christine Duhaime, M.D.
Pediatric Neurosurgery
The Children's Hospital of Philadelphia, 6th Floor Wood Bldg., 34th St. and Civic Center Blvd., Philadelphia, PA 19104; (215)590-2780.
Complete pediatric neurosurgical evaluation and care for congenital disorders of the brain and spine, tumors of the brain and spine, craniofacial anomalies, epilepsy surgery and rhizotomy.

John W. Duckett, M.D., Howard M. Snyder, III, M.D., Stephen A. Zderic, M.D., Douglas A. Canning, M.D., Seth Schulmann, M.D.
Pediatric Urology
Richard D. Wood Ambulatory Care Center, Children's Hospital of Philadelphia, 34th St. and Civic Center Blvd., Philadelphia, PA 19104; (215)590-2754.
Complete pediatric urological care and evaluation, including all renal, bladder, and genital abnormalities. The D.O.V.E. (dysfunctional outpatient voiding educations) Center provides comprehensive care for children with daytime and nighttime wetting.

David B. Schaffer, M.D., Chairman, James A. Katowitz, M.D., Graham E. Quinn, M.D., Richard W. Hertle, M.D., Katrinka L. Heher,

---

"We treat every patient as our only patient."

University of Pennsylvania

CANCER CENTER

- 300 full-time physicians and scientists
- Multidisciplinary evaluation centers and treatment programs
- National leader in cancer research, including clinical trials
- Hospital rated best in region for cancer treatment by U.S. News & World Report

1-800-383-UPCC

3400 Spruce Street • 6 Penn Tower • Philadelphia, PA • 19104

UNIVERSITY OF PENNSYLVANIA HEALTH SYSTEM
The future of medicine.℠

M.D., Martin C. Wilson, M.D.
Pediatric Ophthalmology
The Children's Hospital of Philadelphia, 1st floor Wood Ambulatory Care Bldg., 34th St. and Civic Center Blvd., Philadelphia, PA 19104; (215)590-2791; Children's Surgical Associates, Ltd., 583 Shoemaker Rd., King of Prussia, PA 19406; (610)337-3232; The Children's Hospital Specialty Care Center, Oaklands Corporate Center, 481 John Young Way, Exton, PA 19341; (610)594-9008; Children' Surgical Associates of N.J., Inc., Executive Mews Suite M65, 1930 E. Rt. 70, Cherry Hill, NJ 08003; (609)424-7749.

In addition to complete ophthalmological care for the full range of pediatric ophthalmological problems, the Division of Ophthalmology offers special testing not routinely available elsewhere. These include visual acuity testing for preverbal children, adult and pediatric visual fields, electroretinography, visual evoked responses, infrared oculography, ultrasonography and medical photography. In addition, there are complete oculoplastic and contact lens services.

William P. Potsic, M.D., Steven D. Handler, M.D., Ralph F. Wetmore, M.D., Lawrence W. C. Tom, M.D., Mitchell B. Ausin, M.D.
Pediatric Otolarygology
The Children's Hospital of Philadelphia, 1st floor Wood Ambulatory Care Bldg., 34th St. and Civic Center Blvd., Philadelphia, PA 19104; (215)590-3440; Children's Surgical Associates, Ltd., 583 Shoemaker Rd., King of Prussia, PA 19406; (610)337-3232; The Children' s Hospital Specialty Care Center, Oaklands Corporate Center, 481 John Young Way, Exton, PA 19341; (610)594-9008; The Children's Hospital Specialty Care Center, Laurel Oak Corporate Center, 1040 Laurel Oak Rd., Voorhees, NJ 08043; (609)435-1300.

Pediatric surgical specialty care in ear, nose and throat disorders.

Linton A. Whitaker, M.D., Scott P. Bartlett, M.D., Louis P. Bucky, M.D., Howard S. Caplan, M.D., Benjamin Chang, M.D., Don LaRossa, M.D., David W. Low, M.D., Peter Randall, M.D.
Pediatric Plastic and Reconstructive Surgery
The Children's Hospital of Philadelphia, 1st floor Wood Ambulatory Care Bldg., 34th St. and Civic Center Blvd., Philadelphia, PA 19104; (215)590-2208; The Children's Hospital Specialty Care Center, Oaklands Corporate Center, 481 John Young Way, Exton, PA 19341; (610)594-9008; The Children's Hospital Specialty Care Center, Laurel Oak Corporate Center, 1040 Laurel Oak Rd., Voorhees, NJ 08043; (609)435-1300.

Pediatrics

ALFRED I. DUPONT INSTITUTE CHILDREN'S HOSPITAL, DEPARTMENT OF ORTHOPAEDICS
J. Richard Bowen, M.D., Chairman, Kirk W. Dabney, M.D., S. Jayakumar, M.D., Richard Kruse, D.O., William G. Mackenzie, M.D., Dan E. Mason, M.D., Freeman Miller, M.D., Robert P. Stanton, M.D.
Orthopaedics
1600 Rockland Road, Wilmington, DE 19803; (302)651-5913.

One of the nation's largest orthopaedic programs for children and adolescents, offering a full range of inpatient, outpatient and emergency care. Specialized services are available for the treatment and correction of congenital and acquired orthopaedic conditions including clubfoot; hip dislocation; scoliosis and spinal disorders; fractures; dislocations and sports injuries; gait abnormalities; limb length discrepancies; upper extremity problems; cerebral palsy, and arthrogryposis.

THE CHILDREN'S REGIONAL HOSPITAL AT COOPER HOSPITAL/UNIVERSITY MEDICAL CENTER
Frank A. Briglia, M.D., M.P.H., Chief, Department of Pediatrics
Three Cooper Plaza, Ste. 520, Camden, NJ 08103; (609)342-2546.

A multi-specialty group providing comprehensive pediatric services for all children of southern New Jersey at three convenient locations. For appointments or referrals please call: Camden: (609)342-2001, Voorhees: (609)751-9339, Moorestown: (609)722-9001.

THE CHILDREN'S HOSPITAL OF PHILADELPHIA, GENERAL PEDIATRICS FACULTY PRACTICE
Rosemary Casey, M.D., Stephen Ludwig, M.D., Andria Barnes Ruth, M.D., Richard Rutstein, M.D., Kathy Zsolway, D.O.
34th St. and Civic Center Blvd., 2nd floor, Philadelphia, PA 19104.

Unique practice of academically trained physicians from the University of Pennsylvania faculty. Focused on all aspects of children's health. 24-hour availability.

Physical Disabilities

INGLIS HOUSE, A WHEELCHAIR COMMUNITY
2600 Belmont Ave., Philadelphia, PA 19131; (215)878-5600.

Inglis House is a long-term care facility for persons with physical disabilities, providing 24-hour nursing and other services. Adult day care and accessible apartments available.

Physical Therapy and Rehabilitation

COMMUNITY REHAB CENTERS
Corporate Headquarters, 115 W. Ave., Jenkintown, PA 19046; (800)394-REHAB.

Building Healthy, Active Lives... Comprehensive outpatient physical therapy and rehabilitation centers. 11 convenient locations in the Tri-state area including (in PA) Bryn Mawr, Media, Hunting Park, Mount Airy, Northeast Philadelphia, Southampton, Swarthmore, Flourtown, Bala Cynwyd; and Stratford, NJ and Newark, DE. Expert services include physical therapy, hand rehab, aquatic rehab, fitness programs, on-site employee rehab and prevention programs.

MAIN LINE MEDICAL EXERCISE
Sports Medicine and Orthopedic Rehabilitation
Main Line Health and Fitness Bldg., 931 Haverford Rd., Bryn Mawr, PA 19010; (610)527-7870.

Main Line Medical Exercise is a dynamic and comprehensive physical therapy facility featuring MedX testing and rehabilitative exercise equipment, proven to restore function and relieve pain from spinal injury.

MYOFASCIAL RELEASE TREATMENT CENTER
John F. Barnes, P.T.
Physical Therapy for Complex Chronic Pain and Dysfunction
10 S. Leopard Rd., Rts. 30 and 252, Suite One, Paoli, PA 19301; (800)FASCIAL, (610)644-0136.

Patients treated from around the world to resolve chronic pain using innovative, hands-on myofascial release. Specialty: fibromayalgia, back/neck pain, headaches, traumatic injuries. Whole-body approach to return you to pain-free, active lifestyle.

Podiatric Medicine and Surgery

CHESTNUT HILL PODIATRY ASSOCIATION
John P. Scanlin, D.P.M., Terence C. Dunn, D.P.M., Annalisa Fioriti, D.P.M.
Podiatric Surgery, Diabetic Foot Care
33 E. Chestnut Hill Ave., Ste. 204, Philadelphia, PA 19118; (215)247-0879.

Drs. Scanlin and Dunn are board-certified podiatric physicians and surgeons. Dr. Fioriti is board-eligible. Affiliated with Chestnut Hill and Germantown Hospitals. Specializing in total foot care for the entire family. Foreign language spoken: Italian.

THE BIRTHPLACE AT RIDDLE SPECIALIZES IN FAMILY GATHERINGS.

At Riddle Memorial Hospital, we take special care to ensure you and your family celebrate all the joys of childbirth. From our Perinatal Testing Center to childbirth education classes, our highly skilled staff covers every aspect of your pregnancy. The Birthplace at Riddle offers every comfort expectant parents could want in your own maternity suite. For a free video, call (610) 891-3600.

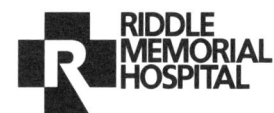

RIDDLE MEMORIAL HOSPITAL

1098 West Baltimore Pike • Media, PA 19063-5177

FIRST STEP PODIATRY
Robert P. Bloch, D.P.M., Michael P. Bernstein, D.P.M.
5555 Wissahickon Ave., Ste. T-O, Philadelphia, PA 19144; (215)849-2804; TLC Healthcare Center, 230 N. Maple Ave., Marlton, NJ 08053.
Board-certified (ACCPPS) for 24 years, providing our patients, infants to seniors, with complete conservative orthopedic and surgical care. Most insurances accepted.

THE FOOT AND ANKLE INSTITUTE, PENNSYLVANIA COLLEGE OF PODIATRIC MEDICINE
Eighth at Race St., Philadelphia, PA 19107; (215)238-6600.
The area's leading podiatric specialists. Full diagnostic and treatment services for foot problems. Departments include Podiatric Medicine, Surgery, Orthopedics, and Biomechanics, Sports Medicine, Pediatrics, Gait Study and Geriatrics.

Preventive Medicine

Howard Posner, M.D.
Holistic Health/Classical Homeopathy
111 Bala Ave., Bala Cynwyd, PA 19004; (610)667-2927.
Total family care with nutritional therapy. Classical homeopathy. Can help with arthritis, hypertension, heart disease, depression, acne, PMS, cancer, diabetes, allergies, obesity, infertility, digestive disorders, etc.

Professional Care Management

GENESIS ELDERCARE℠ COMMUNITY CARE MANAGEMENT
500 North Walnut Rd, Kennett Square, PA 19348; 1-(800)699-1520.
We offer in-home comprehensive geriatric assessments, care planning and cost options, assistance with arranging for eldercare services and on-going care coordination.

Prosthodontics

Joseph B. Breitman, D.M.D. and Associates
8021-B Castor Ave., Philadelphia, PA 19152; (215)728-1696.
Specializing in adult restorative dentistry-crowns, bridges, dentures and implant supported restorations. Post-doctoral residency training, 17 years at present location. Fellow of the International Congress of Oral Implantologists.

Psychiatry

Susan Poritsky, M.D.
Psychotherapy/Psychopharmacology
Suite 202, 234 Bryn Mawr Ave., Bryn Mawr, PA 19010; (610)525-0390, and 800 Spruce St., Pennsylvania Hospital, Philadelphia, PA 19107; (215)471-2413, and Institute of Pennsylvania Hospital, 111 N. 49th St., Philadelphia, PA 19139; (215)471-2413.
Board-certified psychiatrist, specializing in treatment of anxiety, depression, marital difficulties, women's issues, women's health. Psychotherapy and psychopharmacologic consultations.

UNIVERSITY OF PENNSYLVANIA HEALTH SYSTEM, DEPARTMENT OF PSYCHIATRY/PENN BEHAVIORAL HEALTH
3 Blockley Hall, Philadelphia, PA 19104-6021; (215)573-9563 Triage.
Board-certified physicians specializing in various mental health issues including: geriatrics, eating disorders, substance addiction, children and adolescence, family therapy, and mood disorders, also comprehensive inpatient services.

Psychology

BALA PSYCHOLOGICAL RESOURCES
Ellen Berman, M.D.*, Robert Garfield, M.D.*, Michael Reichert, Ph.D., Cynthia Shar, M.Ed., Dea Silbertrust, J.D., Ph.D., Associates
New Perspectives on Men, Women, and Relationships
One Bala Ave., Ste. 110, Bala Cynwyd, PA 19004; (610)667-4804.
Interdisciplinary group of experienced, licensed clinicians; individual, couple, family and group psychotherapy; men's and women's programs; relational issues, eating disorders, self-esteem; medication. *Top Docs, Family Therapy, Philadelphia Magazine, 1996.

Robert J. Berchick, Ph.D.
Cognitive Therapy
433 E. Street Rd., Warminster, PA 18974; (215)674-9445.
Specialist in depression, relationship difficulties and various anxiety disorders. Formerly served as Clinical Director for Dr. Beck's Center for Cognitive Therapy/University of Pennsylvania.

Psychotherapy

PSYCHIATRIC PHYSICIANS ASSOCIATION, INC.
Emanuel E. Garcia, M.D., Lewis Merklin, M.D., Bruce J. Levin, M.D., Richard F.

Limoges, M.D., Gary Flaxenburg, M.D., William O'Brien, M.D., Susan Shively, M.D., Eric Stake, M.D.
Impaired Professionals Evaluation; Medical and Legal Consultation
1525 Locust St., Philadelphia, PA 19102; (215)985-1230; fax: (215)985-1232.

Nearly 60 board-certified private practitioners throughout Tri-State area providing consultation, evaluation, diagnostic and treatment of emotional, behavioral and social problems for individuals, couples, families, or in workplace. Patient's problem matched with best therapist, in office most convenient for patient; prompt response assured.

Pulmonary/Critical Care Medicine

ALLEGHENY UNIVERSITY OF THE HEALTH SCIENCES
Eddy Bresnitz, M.D., Rosemary Cirelli, M.D., Arthur Combs, M.D., Bruce Davidson, M.D., Stanley B. Fiel, M.D., Barry Fuchs, M.D., Joanne Getsy, M.D., Jeffrey Glassroth, M.D., Rochelle Goldberg, M.D., Gregg Lipschik, M.D., Salvatore Mangione, M.D., Donald Raible, M.D., Edward Schulman, M.D., William Sexauer, M.D.,

Michael Sherman, M.D., Paul Siegel, M.D.
Allegheny University Hospitals, Center City formerly Hahnemann University Hospital, Broad and Vine Sts., Philadelphia, PA 19102; (215)762-7011; Allegheny University Hospitals, East Falls formerly Medical College of Pennsylvania Hospital, 3300 Henry Ave., Philadelphia, PA 19129; (215)842-6974.

This practice offers patients effective medical and surgical interventions for treatment-resistant lung disorders. Treatment programs include the Lung Health Center, adult cystic fibrosis program, asthma center, pulmonary rehabilitation program and pulmonary diagnostic laboratory.

Radiation Oncology

ALLEGHENY UNIVERSITY OF THE HEALTH SCIENCES
Luther W. Brady, M.D., Jorge Freire, M.D., Bizhan Micaily, M.D., Curtis Miyamoto, M.D., Fariba Asrari, M.D., Jeffrey Damsker, M.D.
Allegheny University Hospitals, Center City formerly Hahnemann University Hospital, Broad and Vine Sts., Philadelphia, PA 19102; (215)762-8409; Allegheny University Hospitals, East Falls formerly Medical College of Pennsylvania Hospital, 3300 Henry Ave.,

---

Reaching New Heights In Children's Health Care

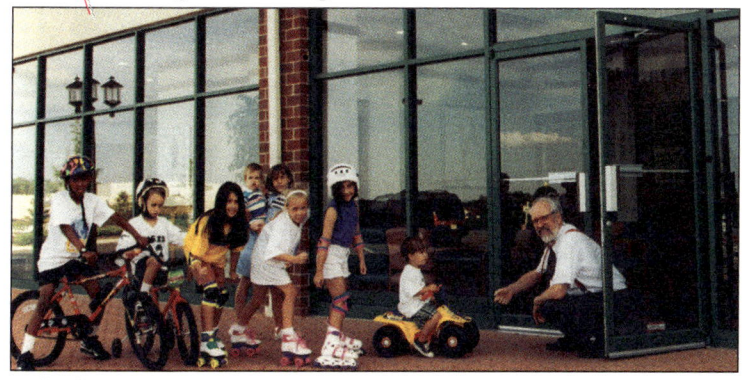

Dr. Sharrar greeting our outpatients at The Children's Regional Center at Voorhees.

Our Pediatric Medical & Surgical Specialists from The Children's Regional Hospital at Cooper provide a wide range of comprehensive services for infants, children and adolescents throughout Southern New Jersey at three conveniently located centers.

The Children's Regional Hospital at Cooper Hospital/University Medical Center

Three Cooper Plaza	Main Street	Moorestown Office Ctr.
Camden, NJ	Voorhees, NJ	Moorestown, NJ
609-342-2001	609-751-9339	609-722-9001

Philadelphia, PA 19129; (215)842-6585.
Conveniently located in Center City and East Falls and staffed with certified professionals, Allegheny University of the Health Sciences offers Delaware Valley Patients the most comprehensive Radiation Oncology services available.

Rachelle M. Lanciano, M.D.
Gynecology and Gastrointestinal Cancers
Delaware County Memorial Hospital, 501 N. Lansdowne Ave., Drexel Hill, PA 19206; (610)284-8240, Fax (610)284-8101.
Board-certified, Fox Chase affiliate, offers all Radiation Oncology services; high dose-low dose Brachytherapy (implants). Subspecializes in gynecologic and gastrointestinal cancers. Active participation in national cancer trials: RTOG, GOG, Fox Chase.

Reproductive Endocrinology

Michael D. Birnbaum M.D., P.C.
Gynecology
8118 Old York Rd., Elkins Park, PA 19027; (215)635-0545.
Fully trained reproductive endocrinologist offering a full range of infertility care including ovulation induction, intrauterine insemination and reconstructive pelvic surgery. Special expertise in operative laparoscopy, endometriosis, pelvic adhesions, pelvic pain and menopausal disorders.

Jerome H. Check, M.D.
Reproductive and Medical Endocrine Associates, P.C., 7447 Old York Rd., Melrose Park, PA 19027; (215)635-1567; Cooper Center for Reproductive Endocrinology, P.C., 8002E Greentree Commons, Marlton, NJ 08053; (609)751-5575; Delaware Center for Infertility and Gynecologic Endocrinology, P.A., 620 Stanton-Christiana Rd., Ste. 202, Newark, DE 19713; (302)633-0500.
Dr. Check is world-renowned for achieving successful pregnancies using various forms of infertility treatment, including ovulation induction, artificial insemination and hormonal therapy. He specializes in the use of all forms of assisted reproductive technologies, including in-vitro fertilization, micromanipulation, GIFT, ZIFT, and ET. A dedicated, caring knowledgeable staff. Hours and locations convenient for patients.

Services for the Aging

CATHEDRAL VILLAGE
600 E. Cathedral Rd., Philadelphia, PA 19128; (215)487-1300.
An innovative leader in retirement living. Compare our unparalleled services...flexible life style...all day casual dining...spectacular health club, indoor pool and fitness center.

Sleep Disorders

ALLEGHENY UNIVERSITY OF THE HEALTH SCIENCES
Joanne Getsy, M.D.
Pulmonary and Sleep Disorders
Allegheny University Hospitals, Center City formerly Hahnemann University Hospital, Broad and Vine Sts., Philadelphia, PA 19102; (215)762-3672.
Joanne Getsy, M.D., who is board-certified in Sleep Disorders Medicine, offers a comprehensive evaluation and treatment plan for all types of sleep disorders in adults.

ALLEGHENY UNIVERSITY OF THE HEALTH SCIENCES
Neurology and Sleep Disorders
June M. Fry, M.D., Rochelle Goldberg, M.D., A. Sinan Baran, M.D., Jodi A. Mindell, Ph.D.
Allegheny University Hospitals, East Falls formerly Medical College of Pennsylvania Hospital, 3200 Henry Ave., Philadelphia, PA 19129; (215)842-4250; Allegheny University Hospitals, Bucks County formerly Bucks County Hospital, 205 Newtown Rd., Ste. 202, Warminster, PA 18974.
Thorough, cost-effective sleep disorders diagnosis and treatment by board-certified specialists in an accredited sleep disorders center.

Sports Medicine

FAMILY PRACTICE ASSOCIATES ALDEN PARK
John A. Heydt, M.D.
Cambridge Bldg., Suites 109-110, 2967 W. Schoolhouse Lane, Philadelphia, PA 19144; (215)844-2880.
Dr. Heydt is a board-certified physician with a certificate of added qualification in sports medicine. He offers management of medical problems and non-surgical management of sports related injuries in competitive and recreational athletes.

ORTHOPAEDIC AND SPORTS MEDICINE SPECIALISTS OF THE MAIN LINE
Lawrence S. Miller, M.D., and David L. Rubenstein, M.D.
Sports Medicine, knee, shoulder, ankle and elbow reconstruction
100 E. Lancaster Ave., Ste. 650, Lankenau Medical Bldg. E., Wynnewood, PA 19096; (610)649-8055 and 3740 West Chester Pike, Newtown Sq., PA 19073; (610)356-9410.
Board-certified in Orthopedic Surgery and Fellowship- trained in Sports Medicine. Specializing in the diagnosis and treatment of sports related injuries. Doctors are associated

with Lankenau and Mercy Haverford Hospitals. Day and evening appts.

Surgical Oncology

James L. Weese, M.D.
The Graduate Hospital, Pepper Pavilion, Ste. 1006, 1800 Lombard St., Philadelphia, PA 19146; (215)893-2300.

Diagnosis and surgical treatment of patients with gastrointestinal, pancreatic, liver and biliary cancers; breast cancer; melanoma and soft tissue tumors.

Urology/Urologic Surgery

The Rosenblum Center for Urologic Care

Jeffrey Lee Rosenblum, M.D.
Board Certified, University Trained
Adult and Pediatric Urology

Providing total urologic care including the treatment of prostatic enlargement, urologic cancer, nerve-sparing techniques, impotence, incontinence, infertility, prosthetics, and stone disease.

**Medical Arts Building
80 W. Welsh Pool Road, Suite 100
Exton, PA 19341**
Located at the intersection of Routes 100 & 113
(610) 594-5444

JEFFERSON UROLOGY ASSOCIATES OF THOMAS JEFFERSON UNIVERSITY
Demetrius H. Bagley, M.D., Michael B. Chancellor, M.D., Leonard A. Frank, M.D., Leonard G. Gomella, M.D., Irvin H. Hirsch, M.D., S. Grant Mulholland, M.D., David A. Rivas, M.D., Stephen E. Strup, M.D.
111 S. 11th St., Ste. 6220, Philadelphia, PA 19107; (215)955-6963.

Nationally and internationally recognized urologists on the faculty of Jefferson Medical College who are experts in kidney stones, neuro-urology, incontinence, urologic cancer, male fertility, sexual function, general urology.

PHILADELPHIA UROSURGICAL ASSOCIATES, P.C.
Kristene E. Whitmore, M.D., David A. Gordon, M.D., Joseph G. Trapasso, M.D.
Female Urology, Urologic Oncology, Erectile Dysfunction
Graduate Hospital, 1900 Lombard St., Philadelphia, PA 19146; (215)893-2643.

Specializes in bladder problems, voiding dysfunction, impotence, infertility, prostate disease and cancer.

Important Phone Numbers

Records

Name _____ **Date of Birth** _____
Family Doctor _____
Family Doctor's Address/Phone _____
_____

Family Dentist _____
Family Dentist's Address/Phone _____
_____

Medications _____
_____

Allergies _____
_____

Name _____ **Date of Birth** _____
Family Doctor _____
Family Doctor's Address/Phone _____
_____

Family Dentist _____
Family Dentist's Address/Phone _____
_____

Medications _____
_____

Allergies _____
_____

Name _____ **Date of Birth** _____
Family Doctor _____
Family Doctor's Address/Phone _____
_____

Family Dentist _____
Family Dentist's Address/Phone _____
_____

Medications _____
_____

Allergies _____
_____

Name _____ **Date of Birth** _____
Family Doctor _____
Family Doctor's Address/Phone _____
_____

Family Dentist _____
Family Dentist's Address/Phone _____
_____

Medications _____
_____

Allergies _____
_____

Index of Advertisers

Advertiser	Page	Reader Service #
Alfred I. duPont Institute of the Nemours Foundation	198 & 231	1
Allegheny University of the Health Sciences	82 & 288	2
Cathedral Village	242	3
Chester Valley Obstetrics and Gynecology, Inc.	299	4
Children's Hospital of Philadelphia	204	5
Children's Regional Hospital at Cooper Hospital	309	6
Children's Seashore House	211	7
College of Podiatric Medicine	301	8
Community Rehab Center	303	9
Fox Chase Cancer Center	16	10
Frankford Hospital	178	11
Genesis Eldercare	264	12
Graduate Hospital Gastroenterology Associates	8	13
Harry Lawall & Son, Inc.	285	14
Hospital Home Care	295	15
Independence Blue Cross/PA Blue Shield/ AmeriHealth in New Jersey & Delaware	2 & 195	16
Jefferson Center for Women's Medical Specialties	164	17
Jenkintown Hearing Aid Center/Jacobson's Hearing Aid Center	294	18
Kremer Laser Eye Center	60	19
Montgomery Hospital	293	20
Philadelphia Fertility Institute	186	21
Philadelphia Health Associates	297	22
Howard Posner, M.D.	287	23
Procare Health Services	252	24
Reproductive & Medical Endocrine Associates	291	25
Riddle Memorial Hospital	307	26
The Rosenblum Center for Urologic Care	311	27
Mark P. Solomon, M.D., F.A.C.S.	289	28
Temple University Hospital	40	29
Thomas Jefferson University Hospital – Dept. of Surgery	46	30
University of Pennsylvania Health System – Cardiovascular Center	286	31
University of Pennsylvania Health System – Cancer Center	305	32
University of Pennsylvania Health System	94	33
University of Pennsylvania Health System – Penn Health Aware Line	25-37	34

Index

A
Abington Memorial Hospital, 120-21, 141, 159
Abuse, 144, 188-89
Accidents. *See* Emergencies
ACE (Acute Care of Elders) Unit, 70
ADHD, 203, 205-10, 219
Adolescent Clinic of Children's Hospital, 62
Adolescent medicine, 62
Aged adults. *See* Elderly adults
AIDS, 190-92
Albert Einstein Breast Cancer Center, 66
Albert Einstein Medical Center, 75, 95-96, 141
Alfred I. duPont Institute, 136-37
Allegheny University Hospitals, Bucks County, 110-11
Allegheny University Hospitals, Center City, 62-63, 71, 96-97, 141
Allegheny University Hospitals, East Falls, 71-72, 77, 97, 141
Allegheny University Hospitals, Elkins Park, 121
Allergy and immunology specialists, 49-50
ALS Clinical Services Center, 62-63
ALS (Lou Gehrig's disease), 62-63
Alzheimer's disease, 276-77
Ambulance services, 281
American Cancer Society, information service of, 21
Anesthesiology specialists, 49-50
Angiography, 86
Angioplasty, balloon, 87
Antidepressants, 215, 220-22
Anxiety
　drugs for, 218-19
　warning signs of, 215-16
Assault, 188-89
Asthma attacks, 144
Atlantic City Medical Center, 125-26
Attention deficit/hyperactivity disorder, 203, 205-10, 219

B
Balance Center, The, 63
Balance disorders, 63
Balloon angioplasty, 87
Basal cell carcinoma, 18, 39
Beebe Medical Center, 137
Behavioral medicine, 263, 265
Belmont Center for Comprehensive Treatment, 224-25
Bipolar disorder, drugs for, 219-20
Birth defects, 63-64
Birthing Suite, The, 73
Bladder cancer, signs of, 21
Bladder Health Center, The, 78
Bleeding, 144, 146, 174
Board certification of physicians, 42
Bone loss. *See* Osteoporosis
Bone marrow transplant centers, 64
Brain injury, 65
Brandywine Hospital, 114-15
Breast cancer, 65-66, 166-68
　hormone replacement therapy and, 181-82
　screening for (*See* Mammography)
　signs of, 20
　women's health services for, 190
Breast cancer programs, 65-66
Breast cancer surgery specialists, 57
Breast-feeding, eating for, 154
Bryn Mawr Hospital, 121-22, 159
Bryn Mawr Rehabilitation Hospital, 65, 78, 259
Bucks County Hospital. *See* Allegheny University Hospitals, Bucks County
Burdette Tomlin Memorial Hospital, 131-32
Burn centers, 140
Burns, 66-67, 145, 201

C
Calcium, 154, 155, 171
Calorie intake, for weight gain and loss, 151
Cancer. *See also specific types*
　information services on, 21-22

treatment centers for, 17, 65-66, 67
  warning signs of, 17-18, 20-21
CancerFax, 21
Cancer Information Service (CIS), 21
Cancer Rehabilitation Center, 262
Cardiac catheterization specialists, 50
Cardiac/thoracic surgery specialists, 56
Cardiology specialists, 50
Cardiovascular disease, 156, 157
Center for Advancement in Cancer Education, The, 22
Center for Continuing Health, 77
Center for Women's Health, 79
Cerebral Palsy Clinic, 63
Cervical cancer, 20, 169-70
Change of life, 177, 179-85
Charter Fairmount Institute, 225
Checkups, medical, 11, 12, 263
Chester County Hospital, 115
Chestnut Hill Hospital, 97-98
Chestnut Hill Rehabilitation Hospital, 260
Chest pain, as emergency, 144
Childbirth. *See also* Pregnancy
  women's health services for, 192-93
Children. *See also pediatric entries*
  emergency care for, 145-46, 199-202
  as finicky eaters, 152-53
  sick, day care for, 266
Children's Hospital of Philadelphia, 62, 63, 67, 98, 141, 209
Children's Regional Hospital at Cooper, 129
Children's Seashore House, 63, 68, 138-39, 208-9
Cholesterol, 153, 156-57, 182
Chronically ill adults, emergency care for, 146
Colon cancer, 20, 92
Colonoscopy, 92
Colon/rectal surgery specialists, 56
Common Thread, The, 22
Comprehensive Epilepsy Center, 69
Comprehensive Headache Center, 71, 265
Computerized axial tomography, 83-84
Continuing care retirement communities, 241, 243-48
Cooper Health System, 128-29

Cooper Hospital/University Medical Center, 64, 128-29, 141
Cooper Institute for In Vitro Fertilization, 73
Cosmetic medicine, 42, 58, 67
Counseling, as diagnostic tool, 12, 14-15
Craniofacial Clinic, 63
Cravings, for sweets, 152
CRISP (Computer Retrieval of Information on Scientific Projects), 45
Crozer-Chester Medical Center, 66, 77, 117, 140, 141
CT scans, 83-84
Cystic Fibrosis Center, 64

D

Day care, for sick children, 266
Deborah Heart and Lung Center, 139
Delaware County Memorial Hospital, 117-18
Delaware Valley Medical Center, 111
Dental care, at home, 258
Depression, 215, 220-22
Dermatology specialists, 50
Diabetes, 67, 146
  specialists in, 51
Diabetes Center for Children, 67
Diagnostic tests. *See* Medical tests
Diet, questions about, 150-55
Dining out, guidelines for, 156-60
Dining With Heart program, 158-59, 160
Disabilities, pregnant women with, 73-74
Doctors
  board certification of, 42
  choosing, 41-45, 47-48
  firing, 43
  malpractice charges against, 43
  top specialists, 47-59
Doppler echocardiography, 88
Doppler ultrasound, 88
Doylestown Hospital, 112
Drucker Brain Injury Center, 65
Drugs. *See* Medications

E

Eagleville Hospital, 122
Ear infections, 202
Eastern Pennsylvania Psychiatric Institute, 225-26

Eating, questions about, 150-55
Eating disorders, 68, 193-94, 265
Eating out, guidelines for, 156-60
Echocardiography, Doppler, 88
Edwin and Fannie Gray Hall Center for Human Appearance, 67
Elderly adults
 continuing care retirement communities for, 241, 243-48
 emergency care for, 146
 medications contraindicated for, 239-40
 nursing home care evaluations for, 277-78
 resources for, 248-49, 275-76
Elkins Park Hospital. *See* Allegheny University Hospitals, Elkins Park
ELM Lifelines, 22
Emergencies, 142-47, 199-202
Emergency medicine specialists, 50-51
Endocrinology specialists, 51
Endometrial ablation, 174
Endometrial cancer, 180, 182
Endoscopy, 91-92
Energy, foods to increase, 151
Epilepsy, 69
Episcopal Hospital, 99
Equipment, medical, 257
Estrogen replacement therapy, 172, 177, 179-85
Examinations, physical, 11, 12, 263
Exercise, for elderly, 77
Eye care, 53-54, 69, 258, 266
Eyesight, impaired, resources for, 283

F

Family practice specialists, 51
Fat, dietary, 150, 156-57
Fat-free foods, 155
Fever, in children, 145-46, 201
Fibroid tumors, 173, 174
Fitzgerald Mercy Hospital, 118
Fox Chase Cancer Center, 17, 65-67, 139
Frankford Hospital, 99-100, 141
Friends Hospital, 68, 226
Fruit, calories from, 153

G

Gastroenterology, 69-70
 specialists in, 51
Gastrointestinal endoscopy, 92
General practice specialists, 51
General surgery specialists, 56
Geriatrics. *See also* Elderly adults
 facilities for, 70
 top specialists in, 51
Germantown Hospital and Medical Center, 71, 100, 265
Girard Medical Center, 104
Graduate Health System City Avenue Hospital, 100-101
Graduate Health System Parkview Hospital, 101
Graduate Health System Rancocas Hospital, 128
Graduate Hospital, The, 69, 74, 78, 79, 101-2
Grand View Hospital, 112-13
Gynecology, 79
 specialists in, 51-52

H

Hahnemann University Hospital. *See* Allegheny University Hospitals, Center City
Hair transplantation specialists, 50
Hampton Hospital, 227
Hand care, 70-71
Headaches, 71, 265
Head trauma, as emergency, 145
Health care, changes in, 41
HealthSouth Rehabilitation Hospital of New Jersey, 260
Heart, treatment centers for, 71-72, 265
Heart disease, 156, 157, 182
Heart Hospitals, The, 71-72
Hematology-oncology specialists, 52
High-Risk Obstetrics Program, 73
Hip replacements, 75
HIV, women's health services for, 190-92
Hodgkin's disease, signs of, 21
Holy Redeemer Hospital and Medical Center, 122-23
Home-care services, 253-58
Hormone replacement therapy, 172, 177, 179-85

Horsham Clinic, 227-28
Hospice programs, 282
Hospital of the University of Pennsylvania.
   See University of Pennsylvania
   Medical Center
Hospitalizations, home-care services
   after, 253-58
Hospitals. See also individual hospitals
   Atlantic County, N.J., 125-27
   Bucks County, 110-14
   Burlington County, N.J., 127-28
   burn centers, 140
   Camden County, N.J., 128-31
   Cape May County, N.J., 131-32
   Chester County, 114-17
   Cumberland County, N.J., 132-33
   Delaware County, 117-20
   Delaware state, 136-38
   Gloucester County, N.J., 133
   Mercer County, N.J., 133-35
   Montgomery County, 120-25
   Philadelphia, 95-110
   Salem County, N.J., 136
   skilled nursing facilities, 141
   specialty, 138-40
   trauma centers, 141
Hotlines, 278-81
   cancer, 21-22
   suicide, 283
Human papilloma virus (HPV), cervical
   cancer from, 169, 170
Hyperactivity disorder, 203, 205-10, 219
Hyperthermia, as emergency, 145
Hysterectomy, 172-75, 194

I

Imaging techniques, 83-92
Immunizations, recommendations for,
   14
Infant mortality, women's health services
   for, 194
Infections, ear, 202
Infectious disease specialists, 52
Infertility, 72-73
   specialists in, 52
Information services. See Hotlines
Inner-ear disorders, 63
Inoculations, recommendations for, 14
Insect stings, 200

Insomnia, 76
Institute of Pennsylvania Hospital, 228
Insurance coverage, for emergency
   treatment, 143
Internal medicine specialists, 52-53
Interventional radiology, 86-87

J

Jeanes Hospital, 102
Jefferson MS Comprehensive Clinical
   Center, The, 74-75

K

Kennedy Health System, 129-30
Kennedy Memorial Hospital, 141
Kessler Memorial Hospital, 126
Knee replacements, 75

L

Lankenau Hospital, 77, 123-24, 159
Laparoscopic surgery, 45, 175
Laparoscopy/hysteroscopy specialists, 52
Learning problems, 266
Leukemia, signs of, 21
Life-care communities, 241, 243-48
Limbs with Restricted Motion Program,
   75
Liver transplants, 76
Lou Gehrig's disease, 62-63
Lower Bucks Hospital, 77, 113
Low-fat foods, 155
Lung cancer, signs of, 20
Lupus, women's health services for, 194
Lymphoma, non-Hodgkin's, signs of, 21

M

Magee Rehabilitation, 260-61
Magnetic resonance imaging (MRI), 85
Malpractice, 43
Malvern Institute, 228
Mammography, 11-12, 166-67, 182
Managed care, 41, 44, 48-49
Manic depression, drugs for, 219-20
Maternity services, 73-74, 192-93
Meal size, calorie burning and, 151
Medical Center at Princeton, 133-34
Medical College of Pennsylvania. See
   Allegheny University Hospitals,
   East Falls

Medical equipment, 257
Medical imaging techniques, 83-92
Medical research, obtaining information about, 45
Medical specialists, 49-56
Medical tests, 9-15. *See also* Medical imaging techniques
  questions to ask about, 45
  timetable for performing, 13
Medications
  psychotropic, 214-15, 218-23
  questions to ask about, 45
  safety guidelines for, 234-40
  stocking medicine cabinet with, 23-24
Medicine cabinet, recommendations for stocking, 23-24
Melanoma, 12, 18, 19
Memorial Hospital of Burlington County, 127-28, 159
Memorial Hospital of Salem County, 136
Menopause, 172, 177, 179-85
Mental disorders, 214-23
Mental treatment centers, 216-18, 224-30, 266
Mercer Medical Center, 134-35
Mercy Haverford Hospital, 124
Methodist Hospital, 102-3
Miscarriages, 74
Misericordia Hospital, 103
Moles, cancerous, 12, 19
MOM (Making Options for Motherhood), 73-74
Monell/Jefferson Chemosensory Clinical Research Center, 78
Montgomery Hospital Medical Center, 124
MossRehab, 75, 261
Mount Sinai Hospital, 229, 261-62
Movement disorders, 74
MRI, 85, 167
Multiple sclerosis, 74-75
Myomectomy, for fibroid tumors, 174

N
Nathan Speare Regional Burn Treatment Center, 66
Nazareth Hospital, 103-4
Nephrology specialists, 53
Neuro-Implant Center, 75

Neurology specialists, 53
Neurosurgery specialists, 57
Newcomb Medical Center, 132
Non-Hodgkin's lymphoma, signs of, 21
Northeastern Hospital, 105
North Penn Hospital, 118-19
North Philadelphia Health System, 104
Northwestern Institute, 229
Nosebleeds, 201
Nuclear medicine, 88-89
Nursing home care, 277-78
Nutrition, questions about, 150-55

O
Obstetrics. *See also* Maternity services; Pregnancy
  specialists in, 51-52
Older adults. *See* Elderly adults
Oncology, specialists in, 52, 57
Ophthalmology specialists, 53-54
Oral cancer, signs of, 21
Organ transplantation specialists, 57
Orthopedics, 75
  specialists in, 57-58
Osteoporosis, 155, 170-72, 183
Otolaryngology specialists, 54
Our Lady of Lourdes Medical Center, 130
Ovarian cancer, 168

P
Pain, 75, 144, 145, 146
Panic disorders, 214, 215
Paoli Memorial Hospital, 79, 115-16
Pap smear, 169
Parkinson's Disease and Movement Disorders Center, The, 74
Parkview Hospital, 101
Pathology specialists, 54
Patient responsibilities, 44-45
Pediatric Center for Dysphagia and Feeding Management, 68
Pediatric emergency care, 145-46, 199-202
Pediatric issues. *See* Children
Pediatric Transplant Institute, 76
Pediatric transplants, 76
Pelvic pain, as emergency, 145
Pennsylvania College of Optometry, The Eye Institute, 140

Pennsylvania Hospital, 73, 75, 105-6
PET scans, 89-91
Philadelphia Center for Aquatic
   Rehabilitation, 262
Philadelphia Child Guidance Center, 229
Philadelphia Fertility Institute/Pennsylvania Reproductive Associates, 72
Philadelphia Geriatric Center, 70
Philadelphia Hand Center, P.C., 70-71
Phoenixville Hospital, 116
Physical examinations, 11, 12, 263
Physical medicine specialists, 54
Physical rehabilitation, 259-62
Physicians. *See* Doctors
Physicians Data Query (PDQ), 21
Plastic surgery, 42, 58, 67
PMS, 175-76
PMS Access, 176
Poison Control Center, 24
Poisoning, 24, 145, 201-2
Positron emission tomography, 89-91
Pottstown Memorial Medical Center, 124-25
Pregnancy
   emergencies during, 146-47
   health care during, 51-52, 73-74, 192-93
   weight control during, 154
Pregnancy Loss Center, The, 74
Premenstrual syndrome, 175-76
Prenatal care, 51-52, 73-74, 192-93
Presbyterian Medical Center, 70, 106
Prescriptions. *See* Medications
Progesterone, 175, 182-83, 184
Progressions Health Systems Behavioral Health Centers, 230
Prostate cancer, 12, 20
Prozac, for PMS treatment, 175
PSA blood test, 12
Psychiatric disorders, 214-23
Psychiatric specialists, 55
Psychiatric treatment centers, 216-18, 224-30, 266
Psychological problems, 214-23
Psychological treatment centers, 216-18, 224-30, 266
Psychotropic drugs, 214-15, 218-23
Pulmonary medicine specialists, 55

R
Radiology
   interventional, 86-87
   specialists in, 56
Rancocas Hospital, 128
Rape, 188-89
Raynaud's phenomenon, 76
Rectal cancer, signs of, 20
Reduced-fat foods, 155
Referral services, women's, 194
Regional Spinal Cord Injury Center of the Delaware Valley, The, 77
Rehabilitation, physical, 259-62
ReMed Recovery Care Centers, 262
Retinoic acid, for skin cancer reversal, 20
Rheumatology specialists, 56
Riddle Memorial Hospital, 119
Ritalin, 206-7, 219
Rothman Institute, 75
Roxborough Memorial Hospital, 106-7

S
St. Agnes Medical Center, 107, 140
St. Christopher's Hospital for Children, 64, 66-67, 76, 107-8, 140
St. Francis Hospital, 137-38
St. Francis Medical Center, 135
St. Joseph's Hospital, 104-5
St. Luke's Quakertown Hospital, 113-14
St. Mary Medical Center, 114, 141
Scheie Eye Institute, 140
Schizophrenia, drugs for, 222-23
Scleroderma, 76
Second opinions, 43-44, 173
Senior citizens. *See* Elderly adults
Sexual assault, as emergency, 144
Sexually transmitted diseases, 169-70
Shore Memorial Hospital, 126-27
Shots, recommendations for, 14
Sigmoidoscopy, 92
Skilled nursing facilities, 141
Skin cancer, 12, 18, 19, 20
Sleep disorders, 76-77
Smell disorders, 78
Smoking cessation and treatment programs, 267-68
Snacks, healthful, 153
Southern Chester County Medical Center, 116-17

South Jersey Hospital, 132-33
Spastic disorders, 75
Specialists
  choosing, 47-48
  medical, 49-56
  surgical, 56-59
Spinal cord injury, 77
Sports medicine, 77
  specialists in, 58
Sprains, 201
Squamous cell carcinoma, 18, 39
Stings, insect, 201
Stroke, 78, 87, 144
Stuart J. Hulnick Burn Center, 66-67
Suburban General Hospital, 125
Suicide hotlines, 283
Sunburns, 201
Supplements, vitamin, 152
Support groups, 208, 268-74
Surgery
  questions to ask about, 45
  second opinions for, 43
  specialists in, 56
Sweets, cravings for, 152

T
Tamoxifen, 167
Taste and smell disorders, 78
Taylor Hospital, 119-20
Temple University Hospital, 64, 69-70, 72, 77, 108, 141
Tests, medical. See Medical tests
Thomas Jefferson University Hospital, 66, 73-74, 76, 77, 108-9, 141, 158, 159
Ticks, 200
Transplantation
  bone marrow, 64
  hair, 50
  pediatric, 76
  specialists in, 57
Trauma, 144, 145, 147
Trauma centers, 141
Trauma surgery specialists, 58

U
Ultrasonography, 87-88, 92
Underwood-Memorial Hospital, 133
University of Pennsylvania Cancer Center, 17, 65, 67

University of Pennsylvania Medical Center, 63, 64, 68, 69, 72-73, 77, 109-10, 141, 176
Urinary tract infections, emergency care for, 146
Urology, 78
  specialists in, 58-59
Uterine artery embolization, 174
Uterine cancer, signs of, 20

V
Vascular surgery specialists, 59
Vegetarianism, 151-52
Violence
  emergency care after, 144
  workplace, 266-67
Vision care, 53-54, 69, 258, 266
Visual impairment, resources for, 283
Vitamins, 152

W
Weight and Eating Disorders Program, 68
Wellness Community, 22
West Jersey Health System, 131
Wills Eye Hospital, 69, 110
Wills Geriatric Psychiatry Program, 70
Women's health, 165-76. See also Breast cancer; Gynecology; Hormone replacement therapy; Infertility; Osteoporosis; Pregnancy
Women's health services, 79, 187-94, 266
Women's International Pharmacy, 176
Workplace violence, 266-67
Wound Care Center, 79
Wound Healing Clinic, 79
Wounds, 79, 145

X
X-rays, 83

Y
Young Stroke Program, 78